Current Topics in Microbiology and Immunology

132

Editors

Mechanisms in B-Cell Neoplasia

Workshop
at the National Cancer Institute,
National Institutes of Health,
Bethesda, MD, USA, March 24–26, 1986

Organized and Edited by
F. Melchers and M. Potter

With 156 Figures

Springer-Verlag
Berlin Heidelberg New York
London Paris Tokyo

Professor Dr. Fritz Melchers
Basel Institute for Immunology
Grenzacherstr. 487, CH-4005 Basel

Michael Potter, M. D.
Chief, Laboratory of Genetics, National Institutes of Health
National Cancer Institute, Bethesda, MD 20892, USA

ISBN-13:978-3-642-71564-8 e-ISBN-13:978-3-642-71562-4
DOI: 10.1007/978-3-642-71562-4

Softcover reprint of the hardcover 1st edition 1986

Library of Congress Catalog Card Number 15-12910

2123/3130-543210

Preface

The fourth workshop on Mechanisms in B-Cell Neoplasia was held in Bethesda, Maryland, at the National Institutes of Health on March 24, 25 and 26, 1986. The meeting was attended by approximately 150 participants and 58 presentations were given.

The purpose of these workshops and the yearly publications has been to provide a means for exchanging the rapidly developing information in this field and to bring major problems into focus. Edited transcripts of the 1983 and 1985 workshops were published by Editiones Roche Basle, Switzerland. Papers brought to the 1984 workshop were published in Current Topics in Microbiology and Immunology, Vol. 113.

Numerous retroviral recombinant viral constructs are now in general use in a variety of test systems, both *in vivo* and *in vitro*. These are proving to have interesting biological properties.

Recently developed systems for inducing B cell tumors are described: 1) The development of spontaneous B-cell tumors in transgenic mice carrying deregulated *myc* genes and the Ig heavy chain promoter; 2) a method for inducing plasmacytomas in BALB/c mice with short latent periods of *ca* 70 days by infecting pristane treated mice with retroviruses carrying various types of deregulated *myc* genes; 3) induction of pre-B cell tumors with erbB containing recombinant retroviruses; 4) induction of B-cell and other tumors by infection of neonates with recombinant retroviruses. Several retroviral constructs containing *myc* sequences do not induce B-cell tumors in pristane conditioned mice, but rather resemble the experiences in the avian system, where viruses containing v-*myc* induce myelomonocytic tumors. The determinants of tropism in *myc* containing retroviral constructs have not yet been established. It appears the presence of Ig enhancers can insure expression in B-lymphocytes.

There is growing evidence from the following examples that the presence of integrated deregulated c-*myc* genes in B-lymphocytes does not bring about an immediate autonomous state. In transgenic mice carrying c-*myc* genes associated with the Ig heavy chain enhancer, B cell tumor formation is preceded by pre-B cell hyperplasia, suggesting this may be the primary biological action of the *myc* gene expression. Avian lymphotropic v-*myc* viruses induce multiple transformed follicles in the Bursa of Fabricius that are considered to be a stage in the progression to bursal lymphoma development. However, very few of these transformed follicles progress to autonomy. In plasmacytomagenesis induced by pristane and J-3 virus, the latent period is short but not as short as might be expected with a direct one hit transformation.

The myc gene continues to be a major focus of research in B-cell neoplasia. All aspects of myc gene activation, transcription, post-transcription are being intensively investigated. The regulation of c-myc expression by various growth factors and mitogens has been described in several systems providing a more complete understanding of how this gene normally operates. Study of the myc genome and the definition of cis acting regulative elements located at the 5' end of the gene is revealing newer components and the possibility of identifying the important negative controlling element. Transacting factors affecting c-myc transcription are not defined though they are suspected. Several papers discuss aspects of stability of c-myc transcripts from normal and mutant c-myc genes. Some rearrangements of c-myc can produce transcripts with long half-lives. Thus the effect of chromosomal translocations can affect transcription and modify the stability and half life of myc RNA in the nucleus and cytoplasm as well. An exciting development has been the binding activity of the myc protein. Early studies demonstrated myc protein was located in the nucleus and bound weakly to DNA. Newer evidence suggests that the myc protein may bind to RNP particles in the nucleus. This possibility opens up new concepts of myc gene function. Understanding in biochemical terms the function of c-myc presents one of the outstanding challenges in this field.

Normal B-lymphocyte activation requires a series of exogenous factors to drive the cells through the mitotic cycle. Many B-cell lymphocytic tumor cells are factor independent. However, some plasmacytomas and hybridomas do require factors for in vitro growth. Three factors were described that are required by plasmacytomas for growth in vitro: HGF (hybridoma growth factor), PCT-GF that appear to have similar properties, and α-factors, some of which may be related to C3 complement components.

We are very grateful to Professor Dietrich Götze and Springer-Verlag for their willingness to rapidly publish these papers. This is very important to the development of this field. We also express special gratitude to Ms. Victoria Rogers for her help in preparing, collecting and editing the manuscripts for this book.

Fritz Melchers

Michael Potter

Table of Contents

B-Lymphocyte/Plasma Cell Growth Factors, Receptors

Chromosome Translocations, Breaks

Regulation of c-myc Expression

Myc Transcription, Post Transcription

Myc Gene Product

Indexed in Current Contents

List of Contributors

You will find the addresses at the beginning of the respective contribution

c-*Myc*-Induced Lymphomagenesis in Transgenic Mice and the Role of the *Pvt*-1 Locus in Lymphoid Neoplasia

Jerry M. Adams, Alan W. Harris, Wallace Y. Langdon, Carl A. Pinkert*, Ralph L. Brinster*, Richard D. Palmiter**, Lynn Corcoran, Warren S. Alexander, Michael W. Graham and Suzanne Cory.

The Walter and Eliza Hall Institute of Medical Research, P.O. Royal Melbourne Hospital, Melbourne, Victoria 3050, Australia.

*Laboratory of Reproductive Physiology, School of Veterinary Medicine, University of Pennsylvania, Philadelphia, Pennsylvania, U.S.A.

**Howard Hughes Medical Institute, Department of Biochemistry, University of Washington, Seattle, Washington, U.S.A.

Dysregulated expression of the c-myc proto-oncogene has been strongly implicated in lymphoid neoplasia, as reviewed by Leder et al (1984), Klein and Klein (1985), Adams and Cory (1985) and Cory (1986). In plasmacytomas of the mouse and Burkitt lymphomas of man, a predominant form of chromosomal translocation couples the c-myc gene to the IgH constant region locus, presumably bringing c-myc under the control of factors that regulate immunoglobulin expression. In some T lymphomas induced by retroviruses, a provirus has inserted near c-myc (e.g. Corcoran et al 1984). Thus strong circumstantial evidence links altered regulation of myc with lymphomagenesis. Typically, the alterations occur in the immediate vicinity of c-myc, but another class may involve long-range effects within the myc-bearing chromosome, as exemplified by the changes within the pvt-1 locus discussed later.

To seek direct evidence that c-myc can induce lymphomas in vivo, we turned to transgenic mice. It has been reported that characteristic tumors arise in transgenic mice bearing the SV40 T antigen gene (Brinster et al 1984; Hanahan, 1985), and that the c-myc gene coupled to the long terminal repeat of the mouse mammary tumor virus promotes mammary carcinomas in certain lineages (Stewart et al 1984). Our own results, summarized here, have established that the c-myc gene linked to an immunoglobulin enhancer is a potent lymphomagenic agent (Adams et al 1985). Moreover, our findings bear upon the issue of whether c-myc is sufficient for tumorigenesis and whether the normal c-myc gene is subject to autoregulation. The high predisposition of these mice to malignancy offers a new approach to dissecting the earliest stages of lymphomagenesis.

IMMUNOGLOBULIN ENHANCERS MAKE c-MYC TUMORIGENIC

Transgenic mice were produced by injecting various c-myc DNA constructs into the pronuclei of (C57BL/6 x SJL/J)F_2 eggs. The constructs tested included the normal c-myc gene, a truncated form analogous to the segment translocated in most plasmacytomas and two forms with c-myc coupled to immunoglobulin enhancers (Fig. 1). Significantly, both the μ and κ enhancer constructs (Eμ and Eκ) elicited tumors and all were lymphomas. The form bearing Eμ upstream of c-myc exon 1, precisely analogous to that found in the mouse plasmacytoma ABPC17 (Corcoran et al 1985), was particularly potent: nearly all the primary transgenic mice succumbed to lymphomas within a few months of birth (Fig. 1). The construct bearing the κ enhancer (Eκ) was also effective, although the frequency was lower and the latency longer (median 23 weeks vs. 11 weeks).

Current Topics in Microbiology and Immunology, Vol. 132

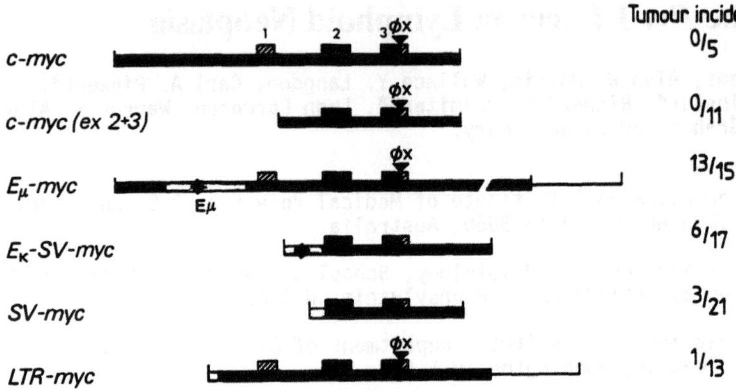

Figure 1. Frequency of tumours in primary transgenic mice bearing the indicated c-myc constructs (from Adams et al. 1985). ØX denotes a phage ØX174 marker. Eκ-SV-myc has an SV40 promoter; SV-myc, the SV40 promoter-enhancer; LTR-myc, an LTR enhancer. Only one tumor induced by SV-myc was a lymphoma.

The efficacy and specificity of these constructs are almost certainly due to the immunoglobulin enhancers, because no tumors have arisen in 12 months of observation in the mice carrying either the normal c-myc gene and its 5' flanking region, or the truncated form lacking the non-coding first exon. These results argue that the major effect of most translocations is not merely to dissociate the myc coding region from a putative negative regulatory element within myc exon 1 or its 5'-flanking region. The immunoglobulin locus must provide a positive regulatory input, and not simply act as a passive bystander, caught up because of its propensity for rearrangement. In the transgenic mice, regulation is presumably mediated through interaction of lymphoid factors with the Ig enhancers. The regulatory element involved in the vast majority of the lymphoma translocations, which do not couple Eμ or Eκ to c-myc, remains obscure, as discussed further elsewhere (Adams 1986).

TUMORS REPRESENT MALIGNANT CLONES OF B-CELL LINEAGE

To evaluate the heritability of the predisposition to malignancy, we established breeding lines of Eμ-myc mice by successive matings of transgenic animals with (C57BL/6 x SJL)F_1 hybrids. In the eight lineages examined, the predisposition was very high. Indeed, in the best studied lineage, involving five generations of descendants, about 94% of transgenic mice have developed lymphomas by six months of age. However, the time of onset, assessed by palpation of the inguinal lymph nodes, ranges from three weeks to as much as six months (Fig. 2). Since the Eμ-myc gene should be activated in concert with lymphoid ontogeny, which commences before birth, the variable latency argues that tumorigenicity requires some additional events (see below).

The pathology elicited by the Eμ-myc construct is most frequently a disseminated lymphoma (Fig. 3). Most lymph nodes become massively enlarged; the spleen is variably enlarged and, in more than half the animals, the thymus is also notably enlarged. The blood almost always contains large numbers of lymphoblast-like cells, so the disease is also a leukemia. Transplantation into syngeneic (C57 x SJL)F_1 mice established that the enlarged lymphoid organs bear bona fide tumors rather than expanded populations of 'normal' cells. Typically, disseminated tumors arise in the recipients within a few weeks.

The IgH enhancer is thought to be active in some T cells and probably in certain myeloid cells (e.g. Kemp et al 1980; Grosschedl et al 1984). Hence tumors of any of these cell types might also have been expected, but in fact all thirty

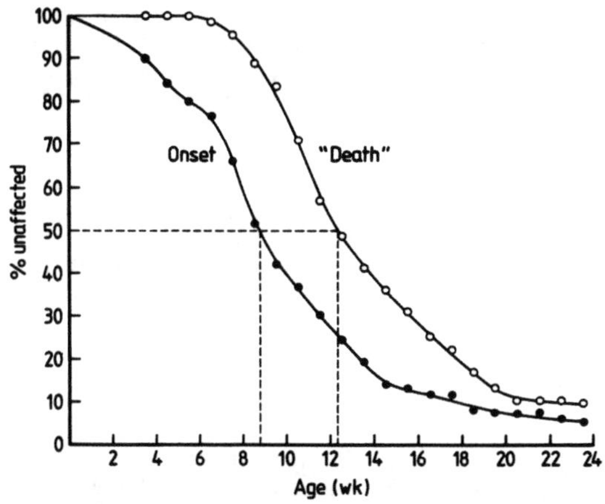

Figure 2. Kinetics of lymphomagenesis in an Eμ-myc lineage, including the appearance of enlarged nodes and the time of sacrifice due to terminal illness.

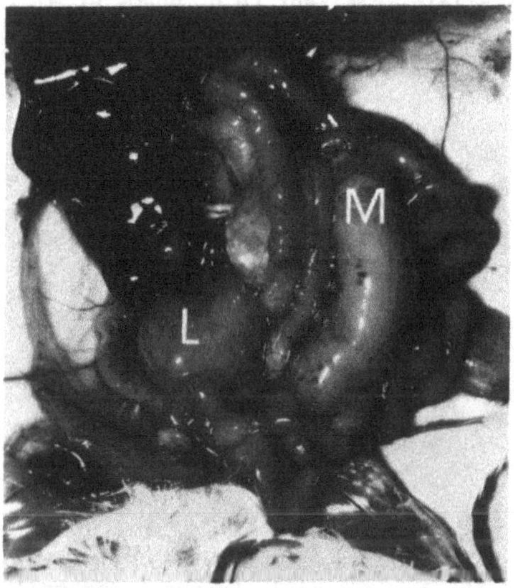

Figure 3. Enlarged mesenteric (M) and lumbar (L) lymph nodes in an Eμ-myc mouse.

tumors that we have so far analysed appear to be of the B-cell lineage. On the basis of the presence or absence of surface immunoglobulin, the types of rearrangement at the J_H and/or Jκ locus in the tumors, and the kinds of Ig mRNA that they make, we conclude that about 60% of the tumors are of the pre-B type, i.e. lacking surface Ig, and the others are B lymphomas. Interestingly, in contrast to nearly all lymphomas induced by Abelson virus, several of the Eμ-myc tumors spontaneously differentiate from a pre-B to a B-cell phenotype on growth in culture. Hence c-myc-induced tumorigenicity is not restricted to a single stage of differentiation and need not freeze the neoplastic cell at one stage. The absence of plasmacytomas among the tumors so far examined might be related to the genetic background of the mice, since plasmacytomas arise only rarely in mouse strains other than BALB/c and NZB.

Since myc expression driven by an immunoglobulin enhancer should be constitutive throughout the B lymphoid compartment, it was conceivable that Eμ-myc mice would bear polyclonal tumors. Our analysis of J_μ and J_κ rearrangement in the tumors indicates, however, that all are monoclonal or oligoclonal (Adams et al 1985).

Thus, in each mouse, one cell within the B-cell lineage has gained a strong growth advantage, presumably as a result of genetic alteration. This evidence that myc alone is not fully tumorigenic is supported also by the variable latency of tumor onset (Fig. 2) and the observation that the lympho-hematopoietic tissue (including bone marrow) of young Eμ-myc mice without overtly swollen nodes does not contain transplantable tumor cells (A.H., unpublished results).

REGULATION of c-MYC EXPRESSION

Abundant c-myc RNA was present in all Eμ-myc tumor cell lines examined. Because the introduced gene contains a 0.6 kb sequence from phage ØX174 within its 3' untranslated region, the transgene generates ~2.9 kb rather than ~2.3 kb transcripts (Fig. 4). Significantly, no normal 2.4 kb myc transcripts are detectable in any tumor cell line, whether of pre-B or B lymphoma type. Hence both normal alleles are silent in the face of the constitutive transgene expression. This result is highly reminiscent of that in tumors bearing myc translocations, where the unaffected myc allele is silent (e.g. Adams et al 1983; Bernard et al 1983).

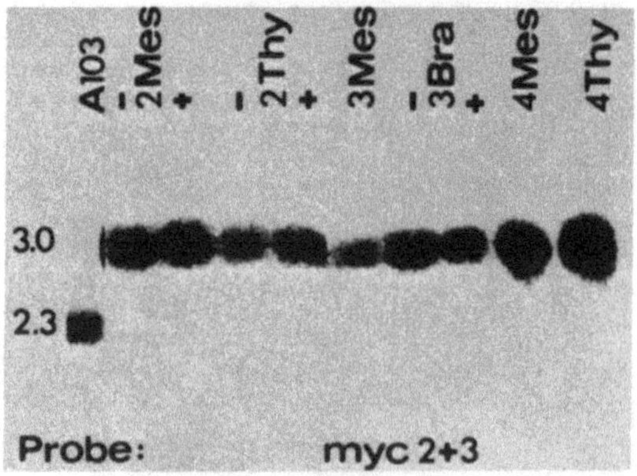

Figure 4. Expression of the c-myc gene in Eμ-myc tumor cell lines. The transgene is expressed (~2.9 kb mRNA) but not the endogeneous myc gene (~2.3 kb mRNA). A103 is a conventional tumor expressing the normal gene.

One model to account for such observations is that the neoplastic transformation occurred in a cell at a stage when c-myc is not normally expressed. On this model, the normal allele simply remains silent after transformation. A corollary would be that c-myc expression should be tumorigenic only at a stage where it is normally silent. This model appeared tenable when c-myc had been associated only with tumors of mature stages of B-cell development, but our findings with the Eμ-myc mice indicate that the earliest stages are also susceptible. We therefore favor the hypothesis advanced by Leder et al (1983) and Rabbitts et al (1984) that c-myc is subject to negative feedback regulation. On this model (Fig. 5), c-myc expression above some threshold level induces a repressor-like activity that restricts further transcription of a normal c-myc allele. The typical translocated myc gene, and the transgene, presumably cannot respond to the repression.

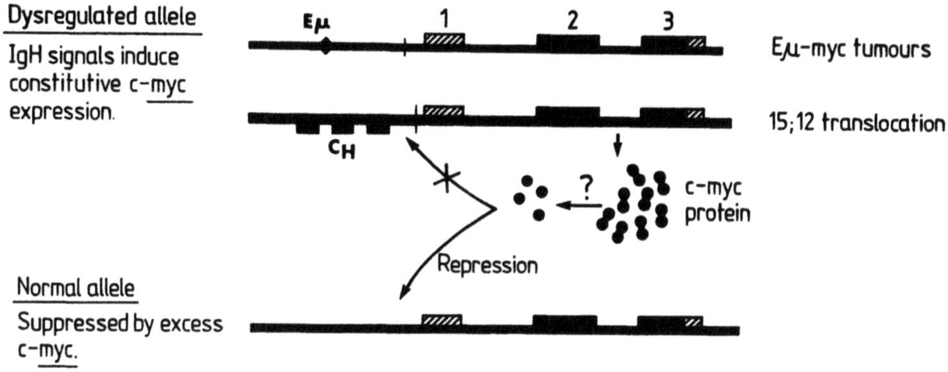

Figure 5. Feedback repression model to account for the absence of expression of the normal c-myc gene in tumors bearing a constitutively activated myc gene.

THE PRE-NEOPLASTIC STATE IN Eμ-MYC MICE

Young, non-lymphomatous Eμ-myc mice provide novel opportunities for learning how constitutive myc expression perturbs hemopoiesis. It is already clear that the bone marrow of young non-tumor-bearing Eμ-myc mice differs dramatically from that of their normal littermates. The cell size profile revealed by analysis with a Coulter counter (Fig. 6) indicates that the bone marrow of Eμ-myc mice lacks the small lymphocyte peak present in the normal mice. This population has been replaced by a large population of blast cells which lack surface immunoglobulin but express the Ly 5 (B220) surface marker characteristic of cells of the B lineage (W.L., unpublished results). These observations suggest that a marked expansion of pre-B cells occurs in Eμ-myc mice well before any neoplastic cells are generated.

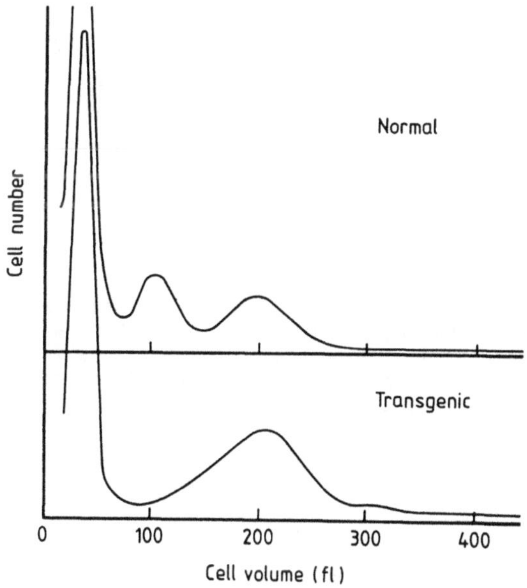

Figure 6. Altered size distribution of bone marrow cells in Eμ-myc mice.

The elevated levels of early cells of the B lineage in Eμ-myc mice encourage us to think that the level of myc expression is a prime determinant of the probability of self-renewal on cell division. In other words, myc expression above a threshold may promote cell division at the expense of differentiation. Hence constitutive myc expression may increase the proportion of immature cycling cells and thereby generate a population vulnerable to further genetic alteration.

Our studies to date with the Eμ-myc mice lead us to think that these mice provide novel opportunities for studying the biological function of the myc gene, the early stages of lymphoma development, and early events in lymphoid ontogeny.

THE ENIGMA OF THE PLASMACYTOMA VARIANT TRANSLOCATIONS

Although the typical 15;12 translocation in plasmacytomas clearly represents an exchange between the c-myc and IgH constant region loci, the nature of the variant (15;6) translocations remains an enigma. It was widely expected that these translocations would represent an exchange between c-myc and the IgK locus and we have indeed shown that C_K is one of the partners (Webb et al, 1984). The chromosome 15 breakpoint region was shown by cloning, however, to lie at least 72 kb from the c-myc gene and was denoted the pvt (plasmacytoma variant translocation) locus (Cory et al 1984). To date, seven 15;6 translocation breakpoints have been mapped within an 18 kb region of the 108 kb pvt locus defined by cloning (Cory et al 1984). Recent cytogenetic analysis of the t(15;6) by Banerjee et al (1985), and the results of Erikson et al (1985), make it clear that pvt lies 3' to c-myc. Our cloning data therefore place pvt at least 85 kb 3' to the c-myc promoters (Fig. 7). Thus the murine 15;6 translocation may be closely analogous to the Burkitt t(8;2), which couples a region that lies more than 20 kb 3' of c-myc to the C_K locus (Taub et al 1984).

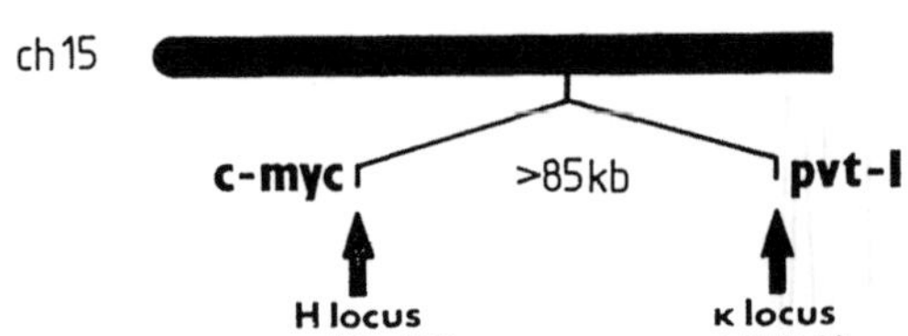

Figure 7. Relation of the typical 15;12 translocation to the variant (15;6) translocation.

Pvt-1 is implicated in T-cell as well as B-cell neoplasia because we have identified several T lymphomas bearing proviral inserts within pvt-1 (Graham et al. 1985). Indeed, our recent results indicate that pvt-1 is the murine equivalent of a common proviral insertion region (mis-1) identified independently in rat T lymphomas (Villeneuve et al 1986).

The c-myc gene is expressed in most of these tumors, but it remains unclear how, or indeed whether, the pvt-1 alterations influence c-myc expression. One model would be that pvt-1 bears an independent oncogene. Another would be that the effect of pvt-1 alterations can be transmitted to c-myc along the chromosome over a remarkable distance.

REFERENCES

Adams JM, Gerondakis S, Webb E, Corcoran LM and Cory S (1983) Cellular myc oncogene is altered by chromosome translocation to an immunoglobulin locus in murine plasmacytomas and is rearranged similarly in human Burkitt lymphomas. Proc Natl Acad Sci USA 80:1982-1986.

Adams JM, Harris A, Pinkert C, Corcoran L, Alexander W, Cory S, Palmiter R and Brinster RL (1985) C-myc oncogene driven by immunoglobulin enhancers induces lymphoid malignancy in transgenic mice. Nature 318:533-538.

Adams JM and Cory S (1985) Myc oncogene activation in B and T lymphoid tumours. Proc R Soc Lond 226:59-72.

Adams JM (1986). The influence of immunoglobulin genes in lymphoid oncogenesis. BioEssays (in press).

Banerjee M, Wiener F, Spira J, Babonits M, Nilsson M-G, Sumegi J and Klein G (1985) Mapping of the c-myc, pvt-1 and immunoglobulin κ genes in relation to the plasmacytoma-associated variant (6;15) translocation breakpoint. EMBO J 4:3183-3188.

Bernard O, Cory S, Gerondakis S, Webb E and Adams JM (1983) Sequence of the murine and human cellular myc oncogenes and two modes of myc transcription resulting from chromosome translocation in B lymphoid tumours. EMBO J 2: 2375-2383.

Brinster RL, Chen HY, Messing A, Van Dyke P, Levine AS and Palmiter RD (1984) Transgenic mice harboring SV40 T-antigen genes develop characteristic brain tumors. Cell 37:367-379.

Corcoran LM, Adams JM, Dunn AR and Cory S (1984) Murine T lymphomas in which the cellular myc oncogene has been activated by retroviral insertion. Cell 37: 113-122.

Corcoran LM, Cory S and Adams JM (1985) Transposition of the immunoglobulin heavy chain enhancer to the myc oncogene in a murine plasmacytoma. Cell 40:71-79.

Cory S, Graham M, Webb E, Corcoran L and Adams JM (1985) Variant (6;15) translocations in marine plasmacytomas involve a chromosome 15 locus at least 72 kb from the c-myc oncogene. EMBO J 4:675-681.

Cory, S (1986) Activation of cellular oncogenes by chromosome translocation in haematological malignancies. Adv Cancer Res (in press).

Erikson J, Miller DA, Miller JO, Abcarian PW, Skurla RM, Mushinski, JF and Croce CM (1985) The c-myc oncogene is translocated to the involved chromosome 12 in mouse plasmacytoma. Proc Natl Acad Sci USA 82:4212-4216.

Graham M, Adams JM and Cory S (1985) Murine T lymphomas with retroviral inserts within the chromosome 15 locus for plasmacytoma variant translocations. Nature (London) 314:740-742.

Grosschedl R, Weaver D, Baltimore D and Costantini F (1984) Introduction of a μ immunoglobulin gene into the mouse germ line: specific expression in lymphoid cells and synthesis of functional antibody. Cell 38:647-658.

Hanahan D (1985) Heritable formation of pancreatic β-cell tumours in transgenic mice expressing recombinant insulin/simian virus 40 oncogenes. Nature 315:115-122.

Kemp D, Harris AW and Adams JM (1980) Transcripts of the immunoglobulin Cμ gene vary in structure and splicing during lymphoid development. Proc Natl Acad Sci USA 77:7400-7404.

Klein G and Klein E (1985) Myc/Ig juxtaposition by chromosome translocations: some new insights, puzzles and paradoxes. Immunology Today 6:208-215.

Leder P, Battey J, Lenoir G, Moulding C, Murphy W, Potter H, Stewart T and Taub R (1983) Translocations among antibody genes in human cancer. Science 222:765-771.

Rabbitts TH, Forster A, Hamlyn P and Baer P (1984) Effect of somatic mutation within the translocated c-myc genes in Burkitt's lymphoma. Nature 309: 592-597.

Stewart T, Pattengale P and Leder P (1984) Spontaneous mammary adenocarcinomas in transgenic mice that carry and express MMTV/myc fusion genes. Cell 38: 628-637.

Taub R, Kelly K, Battey J, Latt S, Lenoir GM, Tantravahi U, Tu Z and Leder P (1984). A novel alteration in the structure of an activated c-myc gene in a variant t(2;8) Burkitt lymphoma. Cell 37:511-520.

Villeneuve L, Rassart E, Jolicoeur P, Graham M and Adams JM (1986). Proviral integration site mis-1 in rat thymomas corresponds to the pvt-1 transloca-tion breakpoint in murine plasmacytoma. Molec Cell Biol (in press).

Webb E, Adams JM and Cory S (1984) Variant (15;6) translocation in a murine plasmacytoma occurs near immunoglobulin C_κ gene but far from the myc oncogene. Nature (London) 312:777-779.

Lymphohematopoietic and Other Malignant Neoplasms Occurring Spontaneously in Transgenic Mice Carrying and Expressing MTV/myc Fusion Genes

P. Pattengale,** A. Leder, A. Kuo, T. Stewart,*** and P. Leder[1]

Department of Genetics, Harvard Medical School, 25 Shattuck Street, Boston, Massachusetts 02115 USA

INTRODUCTION

Transgenic mice carrying and expressing exogenously introduced cellular oncogenes offer the opportunity to study oncogenesis in the context of the living organism (Stewart et al., 1984; Adams et al., 1985). To this end, we have produced various strains of transgenic mice that carry a normal mouse c-myc gene in which increasingly larger portions of the myc promoter region have been replaced by a hormonally inducible mouse mammary tumor virus promoter (Stewart et al., 1984). Two of these transgenic strains were of considerable interest, since virtually all of the available female progeny, which were in their second and third pregnancies, spontaneously developed mammary adenocarcinomas of the breast (Stewart et al., 1984). It was also of interest that the MTV/myc fusion gene was expressed both in non-neoplastic and neoplastic mammary glands, and with the exception of the normal salivary gland, was not significantly expressed in any other tissue (Davis et al., 1986). In contrast, another transgenic strain, hereafter referred to as the "K" strain, expresses MTV/myc fusion gene mRNA in a much wider range of tissues, with the subsequent development of a high spontaneous incidence of malignant neoplasms (Leder et al., 1986). Although the largest portion of malignant neoplasms are lymphoid cell neoplasms of B cell derivation, we also have observed smaller numbers of T and non-B, non-T lymphomas as well as mast cell sarcomas, testicular neoplasms of Sertoli cell type, and mammary adenocarcinomas. We have described our experience with this strain in detail elsewhere (Leder et al., 1986).

EXPRESSION OF THE MTV/myc GENE IN NORMAL TISSUES

The K-strain of transgenic mice is derived from a founder animal, which received into its germline DNA, a gene formed by joining the MTV promoter and glucocorticoid responsive enhancer segments to a SmaI site 5′ to the normal mouse c-myc gene (Figure 1) (Stewart et al., 1984). This particular construct is noteworthy since, in contrast to other tumorigenic constructs, it retains about .7 kb of 5′ c-myc flanking sequences including the two normal c-myc promoter initiation sites (P-1 and P-2).

[1]**Department of Pathology, University of Southern California School of Medicine, Los Angeles, CA 90033 USA and supported in part by a grant from the Margaret Early Medical Research Trust; ***Genentech, 460 Point San Bruno Blvd., South San Francisco CA 94080 USA.

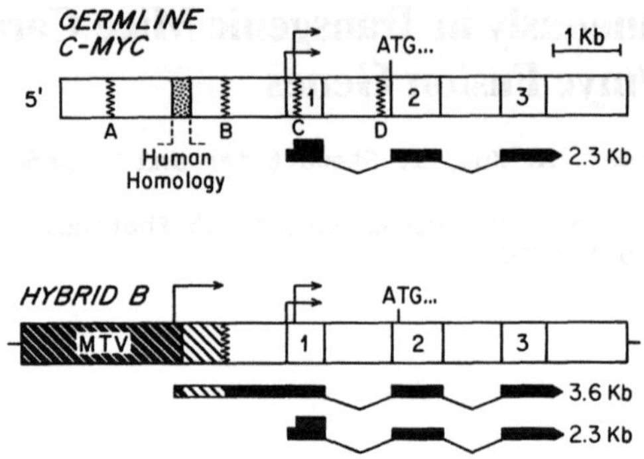

Fig. 1. Diagrammatic representation of murine c-myc gene and the MTV/myc hybrid transgene (hybrid B). The three exons of the gene are indicated as numbered boxes. The two normal promoters of the c-myc gene are indicated as arrows within exon one. The stippled area in the 5′ flanking region of the germline c-myc gene is a region of homology preserved in the human c-myc gene. The letters A,B,C, and D represent sites used in constructing other lines of MTV/c-myc transgenic mice (Stewart et al., 1984). The heavy line beneath each gene map represents the expected mRNA produced from each potentially active promoter. The dark hatched area in the fusion gene is the MTV LTR; the light hatched area is an unrelated DNA fragment carried over from one of the parental constructs (pA-9) (Huang et al., 1981) used in making the fusion gene.

Using a combination of Northern analysis and the more sensitive S-1 nuclease protection assay, it is therefore possible to distinguish among mRNA transcripts arising from either the MTV transgene promoter(s) or the normal myc promoters (transgene or endogenous) (Leder et al., 1986). Using a combination of these techniques, we have been able to detect constitutive production of transgenic message arising from the MTV promoter in breast, testis, lung, brain, salivary gland, spleen, preputial glands, pancreas, and kidney. As expected, transgenic animals injected with 500 micrograms of dexamethasone over a 48 hour time period, quantitatively express more transgenic mRNA arising from the MTV promoter. Interestingly, and in contrast to other tissues, the spleen from transgenic mice constitutively produced significant amounts of normal sized c-myc transcripts, which were also inducible to greater quantities after dexamethasone treatment. Although glucocorticoid (dexamethasone) inducibility is consistent with the normal sized c-myc transcripts arising from normal c-myc promoters on the transgene, it is impossible to exclude the participation of the normal, endogenous c-myc gene in mRNA expression.

Table 1. Histopathology of Spontaneous Neoplasms Occurring in Transgenic K Mice

Type of Neoplasm	Number of Tumors[1]	Comments
1. Adenocarcinoma of breast	4	Moderately well differentiated; locally invasive in breast and surrounding tissues (Stewart *et al.*, 1984)
2. Stromal cell neoplasm of testis, Sertoli cell type	4	Low grade, slow growing *in situ* neoplasms of Sertoli cells
3. Malignant lymphoma	12	See Table 2
4. Malignant mast cell neoplasm	5	High grade malignant neoplasm derived from tissue mast cells
5. Uncharacterized	2	Animals not autopsied

[1]Total of 24 transgenic mice (K) (10 males and 14 females; mean age of 12 months [range of 3-25 months]); with a cumulative total of 27 neoplasms. One animal had both a lymphoblastic lymphoma and an adenocarcinoma of the breast; another animal had both a follicular center cell lymphoma and an adenocarcinoma of the breast; while another had both a lymphoblastic lymphoma and a Sertoli cell neoplasm of the the testis.

OCCURRENCE OF SPONTANEOUS NEOPLASMS IN K MICE

In the most extensively studied pedigree, fourteen (7 males and 7 females) of 35 homozygous and heterozygous transgenic K strain mice (40% incidence) spontaneously developed a wide variety of malignant neoplasms at a mean age of 14 months. We have, to date, observed a total of 27 neoplasms occurring spontaneously in a total of 24 transgenic K mice (11 males and 13 females at mean age of 12 months) (Table 1). Strikingly, three mice each had two separate and distinct histologic malignancies at autopsy (see footnote, Table 1). Of the 27 malignant neoplasms observed to occur in transgenic K mice, four were adenocarcinomas of the breast, four were testicular neoplasms of the Sertoli cell type, 12 were malignant lymphomas, five were malignant mast cell neoplasms, and two were uncharacterized (probable lymphomas) (Table 1). Because of the even sex distribution, and the fact that not all transgenic mice developed malignancies, the transgene in the K strain behaves as an autosomal dominant with variable penetrance. In marked contrast to the transgenic K strain, only two malignancies (lymphomas) spontaneously occurred in approximately 200 age-matched control animals over a 30 month observation period. Both animals were very old at the time of diagnosis (30 months each).

Table 2. Correlation of Lymphoma Morphology with Genotype and Differentiation State

Morphology[1]	No.	Genotype[2]	Diff. State	Comments
Lymphoblastic Lymphoma	3	IgH rearranged; κ deleted or germline; λ germline	Pre-B	Similar to childhood ALL[3]
	3	IgH rearranged; κ deleted or rearranged; λ germline or rearranged	Early B	Similar to Burkitt's lymphoma
	1	IgH, κ, λ germline; T γ gene expressed	T	Probable early T cell
	1	IgH, κ, γ, T γ gene not expressed	Non-B,Non-T	Probable uncommitted lymphoid stem cell
	1	Not Done	?	Morphology unpredictive
Follicular Center Cell (FCC) Lymphoma	1	IgH rearranged; κ rearranged; λ Not Done	Activated B	Derived from germinal center cells
	1	Not Done	Activated B	Morphology predictive
Immunoblastic Lymphoma	1	IgH rearranged; κ rearranged; λ germline	Activated, Late B	Has class-switched; secretes Ig

[1]Classified according to Pattengale and Taylor (1983)

[2]Tumor genomic DNAs were cut with restriction endonucleases (EcoRI for IgH locus, EcoRI and BamHI for κ locus, and EcoRI for the λ locus), size separated on .9% agarose gels, blotted to nitrocellulose, and hybridized to either the 1.5 kb PstI/PstI fragment containing J-H sequences (Early et al., 1980), the 2.4 kb HindIII/BamHI fragment containing C-κ sequences (Seidman et al., 1979), and the .8 kb XbaI/XbaI fragment containing Vλ-2 sequences (Blomberg et al., 1981). Expression of the gene coding for the γ chain of the T cell receptor was performed on Northern analysis using a cDNA probe corresponding to the γ subunit of the T cell receptor (Murre et al., 1985).

[3]Abbreviations used: ALL = acute lymphoblastic leukemia; FCC = follicular center cell; IgH = immunoglobulin heavy chain locus

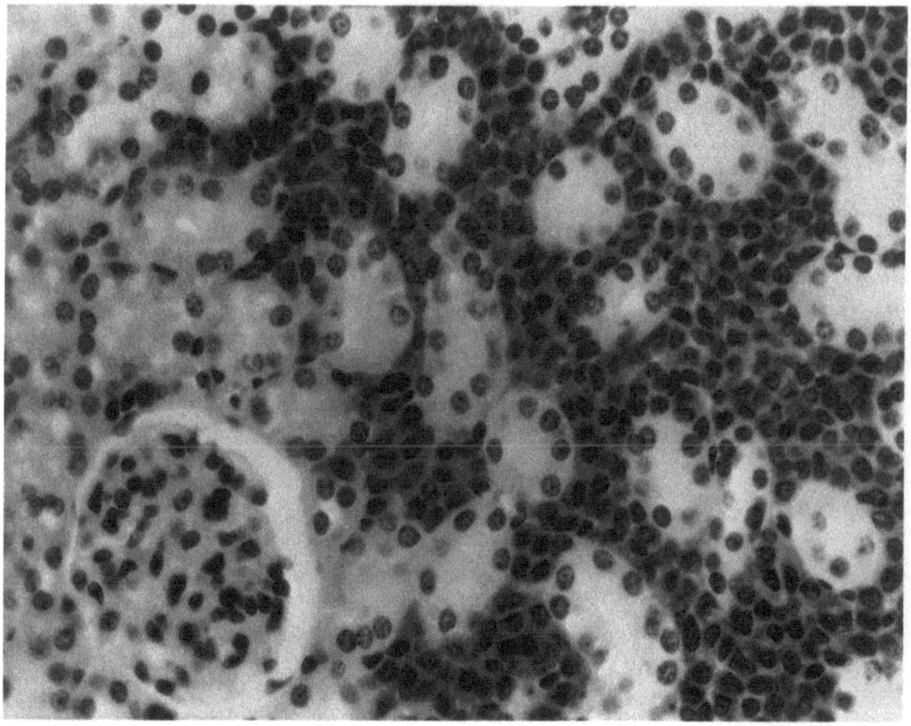

Figure 2. Follicular center cell (FCC) lymphoma. Infiltration of kidney with malignant lymphoid cells. Note the characteristic irregularly-shaped nuclear morphology and conspicuous cytoplasm of malignant follicular (germinal center) B cells. These cells characteristically have both easily detectable surface and cytoplasmic immunoglobulin (Hematoxylin and eosin, kidney, mouse K-331, x 500). DNA from this tumor showed rearrangement of both heavy and light chain loci (see Table 2).

CHARACTERIZATION OF MALIGNANT LYMPHOMAS

Lymphoid cell neoplasms (malignant lymphomas and related leukemias) are considered to be monoclonal proliferations of malignant lymphoid cells, which are arrested at various stages of lymphocyte differentiation. Because lymphomas represent malignant outgrowths of lymphocytes, it is possible to assign a particular lymphoma to a particular stage of differentiation using a combination of morphologic, phenotypic, and genotypic parameters. Using combinations of these techniques, it has been possible to biologically characterize spontaneous non-Hodgkins lymphomas and related leukemias in man and mouse. As in man, it is now clear in the mouse that the majority of spontaneously occurring lymphoid cell neoplasms are B-cell derived (Pattengale and Taylor, 1983). It is therefore, of interest, that the spontaneous malignant lymphomas occurring in K strain transgenic mice are also primarily of B cell derivation (see Table 2, above). As seen in Table 2, which correlates the lymphoma cell morphologic type with the presence or absence of immunoglobulin (Ig) gene rearrangement (heavy and light chain), and further attempts to stage the lymphomas at a particular stage of differentiation, it is clear that the majority are B cell derived and corresponds to various stages of B cell differentiation (pre-B, early B, and activated B [intrafollicular] and activated late B [postfollicular]). While

REFERENCES

Adams JM, Harris AW, Pinkert CA, Corcoran LM, Alexander WS, Cory S, Palmiter RD, Brinster RL (1985) The c-myc oncogene driven by immunoglobulin enhancers induces lymphoid malignancy in transgenic mice. Nature 318:533-538

Blomberg B, Traunecker A, Eisen H, Tonegawa S (1981) Organization of four mouse λ light chain immunoglobulin genes. Proc Natl Acad Sci USA 78:3765-3769

Davis LG, Hennighausen L, Woychik R, Leder A, Tepler I, Kuo A, Stewart T, Leder P. Tumor formation and elevated myc expression co-segregate in a line of transgenic mice. Submitted.

Early P, Rogers J, Davis M, Calame K, Bond M, Wall R, Hood L (1980) Two mRNAs can be produced from a single immunoglobulin mu gene by alternative RNA processing pathways. Cell 20:313-319

Huang AL, Ostrowski MC, Bernard O, Hager GL (1981) Glucocorticoid regulation of the HaMuSv p21 gene conferred by sequences from mouse mammary tumor virus. Cell 27:245-255

Leder A, Pattengale PK, Kuo A, Stewart T, Leder P. Consequences of widespread deregulation of the c-myc gene in transgenic mice: multiple neoplasms and normal development. Cell, in press.

Murre C, Waldmann RC, Morton CC, Bongiovanni KF, Waldmann TA, Shows TB, Seidman JG (1985) The human gamma chain genes rearrange in leukemic T cells and map to the short arm of chromosome 7. Nature 316:529-533

Pattengale PK, Taylor CR (1983) Experimental models of lymphoproliferative disease: the mouse as a model for human non-Hodgkin's lymphomas and related leukemias. Am J Pathol 113:237-265

Seidman JG, Max EE, Leder P (1979) A κ immunoglobulin gene is formed by site-specific recombination without further somatic mutation. Nature 280:370-375

Stewart TA, Pattengale PK, Leder P (1984) Spontaneous mammary adenocarcinomas in transgenic mice that carry and express MTV/myc fusion genes. Cell 38:627-637

Tumors of Newborn NFS/N Mice Infected with Murine Retroviruses Containing Avian v-*Myc*

H.C. Morse, III, J.W. Hartley, T.N. Fredrickson, R.A. Yetter, J.L. Cleveland, C. Majumdar, U.R. Rapp

Laboratory of Immunopathology, National Institute of Allergy and Infectious Diseases and Laboratory of Viral Carcinogenesis, National Cancer Institute, National Institutes of Health, Bethesda, Maryland

INTRODUCTION

Deregulated expression of the c-myc protooncogene appears to contribute to the development of a great variety of neoplasms in different vertebrate species. Perhaps the strongest evidence in support of this view comes from the observations that chickens infected with retroviruses carrying v-myc rapidly develop a spectrum of hematopoietic neoplasms and solid tumors (1). The indications that altered expression of myc is also an important event in the genesis of mammalian tumors are more circumstantial. They center primarily on the observations that aberrant expression of c-myc is associated with the insertion of proviruses in juxtaposition to this gene in T cell lymphomas (2,3) and the regular translocation of c-myc in specific B cell-lineage neoplasms (4,5). Recently, a number of different approaches have been developed to more clearly define the contribution of altered myc expression to neoplasia. These include the development of in vitro transformation assays of nonestablished cell lines (6,7) and studies of transgenic mice bearing myc genes controlled by different regulatory sequences (8,9). Our attempts to understand the role of deregulated myc expression in transformation have focused on a novel system in mice using recombinant murine retroviruses that contain avian v-myc genes. Here we report that newborn NFS/N mice infected with different pseudotypes of these recombinant viruses develop a wide spectrum of hematopoietic and epithelial tumors.

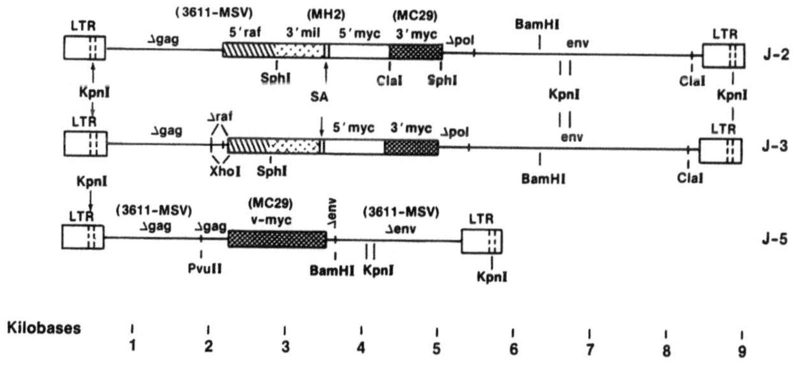

Fig. 1. Genomic structures of recombinant MuLV containing hybrid murine/avian raf/mil and/or avian v-myc genes.

Current Topics in Microbiology and Immunology, Vol. 132

RESULTS AND DISCUSSION

The structures of the recombinant viruses used in these studies are shown in Fig. 1. They include the J-2 virus that contains and expresses v-*raf* and v-*myc*; the J-3 virus, a derivative of J-2 which contains a deletion and frameshift in v-*raf* and expresses v-*myc* from a subgenomic RNA; and the J-5 virus that expresses v-*myc* as a *gag*-*myc* fusion protein (10). These constructs were pseudotyped with a series of replication-competent helper murine leukemia viruses (MuLV) including Moloney, Cas-Br-M, 1504M and C2S ecotropic viruses and 4070A amphotropic MuLV. Newborn NFS/N mice were infected with the pseudotyped viruses and followed for the development of disease in relation to mice infected with the helper viruses alone.

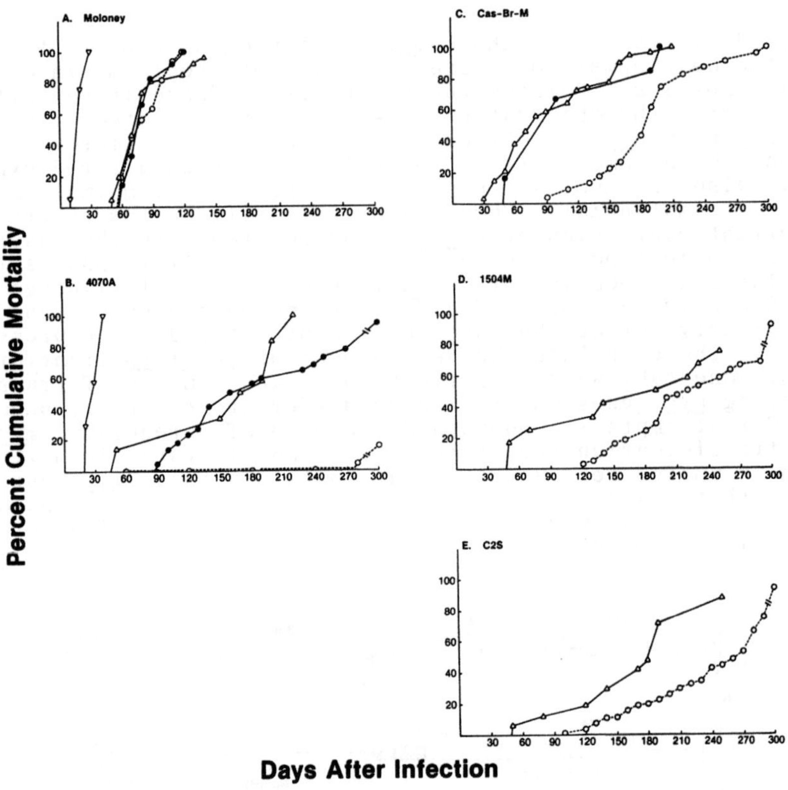

Fig. 2. Cumulative mortalities of mice infected with helper MuLV (o-o), or helper pseudotypes of J-2 (∇-∇), J-3 (●-●) or J-5 (Δ-Δ)MuLV. Helper viruses: Panel A, Moloney; B, 4070A; C, Cas-Br-M; D, 1504M; E, C25.

The results of these studies (Fig. 2, Table I) demonstrated the following points. First, except for mice infected with constructs pseudotyped with Moloney MuLV, the cumulative mortality for mice inoculated with the J-3 and J-5 viruses was variably accelerated over that observed in mice infected with the rescuing viruses alone. This acceleration was most evident for mice infected with 4070A pseudotypes of J-3 and J-5 since the helper virus on its own does not induce disease until more than 9 months after infection (Fig. 2). The data also show that for mice infected with Cas-Br-M pseudotypes of J-3 and J-5, approximately 65% of these animals died before 10% of the mice infected with the helper virus alone had died (Fig. 2). Finally, for mice infected with 1504M or C2S pseudotypes of J-5, the time course of disease was accelerated 50 to 100 days over that induced by the helper viruses alone (Fig. 2).

Table I. Histologic diagnoses of neoplasms induced by pseudotypes of J-3 and J-5

		Percent Histologic Diagnoses*				
Construct	Rescuing Virus	LL	EL	ML	PAC	MAC
None	Moloney	100	0	0	0	0
J-3		100	0	0	0	0
J-5		100	0	0	0	0
None	Cas-Br-M	44	22	30	0	0
J-3		66	17	0	0	0
J-5		69	8	0	23	5
None	C2S	19	0	56	0	0
J-5		47	0	13	13	7
None	1504M	8	55	0	0	0
J-5		44	11	0	11	0
None	4070A	100	0	0	0	0
J-3		45	9	0	32	0
J-5		33	2	16	33	0
Totals-J3 and J-5+		68 (91)	5 (7)	2 (3)	16 (21)	2 (3)

*6-73 mice per group. Diagnoses made on fixed sections of tissues obtained at autopsy of moribund mice. LL = lymphoblastic lymphoma; EL = erythroleukemia; ML = myelogenous leukemia; PAC = pancreatic adenocarcinoma; MAC = mammary adenocarcinoma.

+Numbers in parenthesis indicate the number of mice in each diagnostic category.

Second, many of the neoplasms exhibited at autopsy by mice infected with pseudotypes of J-3 and J-5 differed in several respects from those diagnosed for mice infected with the different helper viruses alone (Table I). Perhaps most striking are the findings that 18% of mice infected with pseudotypes of the J-3 and J-5 constructs died with epithelial tumors including pancreatic and mammary adenocarcinomas. None of the 199 mice infected with the different helper viruses died with a carcinoma of either type. Pancreatic adenocarcinomas are extremely rare spontaneous neoplasms of mice and, in extensive studies of NFS/N mice infected with a variety of viruses, have been observed previously only in mice infected with pseudotypes of J-2 (10). Pancreatic tumors were first observed at 40 days after infection with J-3 or J-5 and developed with a mean latency of 150 days. Only mice infected with Moloney pseudotypes of the v-*myc*-containing constructs did not develop this type of neoplasm.

The three mammary tumors developed at 152, 153 and 241 days after infection with Cas-Br-M and C2S pseudotypes of J-5 (Table I). Remarkably, the first two tumors developed in male mice and the third in a virgin female. This type of neoplasm has not been observed previously in our studies of normal or virus-infected NFS/N mice.

Third, 91% of the J-3 or J-5-infected mice diagnosed with hematologic tumors died with lymphoblastic lymphomas. This result is not unexpected for mice infected with the Moloney helper virus alone as T cell lymphoblastic lymphomas are the only neoplasms induced by this virus in NFS/N mice studied in our laboratories. However, flow cytometry studies of 12 lymphomas induced by Moloney pseudotypes of J-3 and J-5 revealed, unexpectedly, that four of them were of pre-B or B cell origin.

A high proportion of mice infected with Cas-Br-M, C2S and 1504M pseudotypes of J-3 and J-5 also developed lymphoblastic lymphomas, even though the diseases induced by these helper viruses alone were predominantly myelogenous and erythroleukemias (Table I). Flow cytometry studies of 23 of these lymphomas showed that 17 were of T cell origin, 4 were of pre-B or B cell origin and two were mixtures of malignant T and B cells or pre-B and B cells.

The potential for autonomous growth on transplantation or *in vitro* has been documented for a number of the neoplasms induced by pseudotypes of J-3 and J-5. Continuous cell lines of two pre-B cell lymphomas, one B cell lymphoma and three T cell lymphomas were established in vitro in the absence of added growth factors. In addition, two pancreatic adenocarcinomas were successfully passaged *in vivo*.

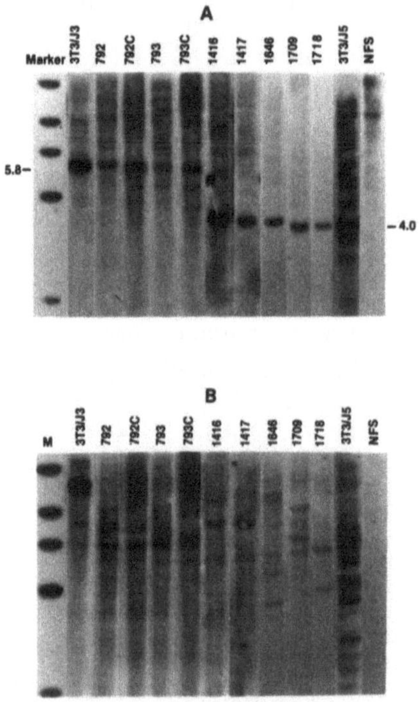

Fig. 3. Southern blot hybridization of cellular DNA digested with KpnI (A) or BamHI (B) with an avian v-*myc* probe. Tumors and continuous *in vitro* cell lines (indicated by "c") derived from them include two pre-B cell lymphomas (792,793) induced by J-3/Moloney, two lymphoblastic lymphomas (1416,1417), a pancreatic adenocarcinoma (1646) and a mammary adenocarcinoma (1718) induced by J-5/Cas-Br-M and a pancreatic adenocarcinoma (1709) induced by J-5/4070A.

A number of tumors induced by different pseudotypes of J-3 and J-5 were analyzed to determine if they contained and expressed v-*myc*.

Southern blot analyses of DNA digested with KpnI and BamHI and probed with v-myc are shown in Fig. 3. Digestion with KpnI produces internal v-myc-containing fragments of 5.8 kb from J-3 and 4.0 kb from J-5. BamHI cuts once within env in both constructs such that v-myc-reactive fragments contain variable amounts of cellular sequences 5' to the virus. The results of these studies showed that each of the primary tumors of hematopoietic or epithelial origin contained v-myc-hybridizing fragments consistent with the size of the viruses used in their induction (Fig. 3A). In addition, all of the primary tumors exhibited one and up to four v-myc integrations (Fig. 3B). It is noteworthy that the integration sites in the two primary tumors (792,793) and their derivative cell lines were identical.

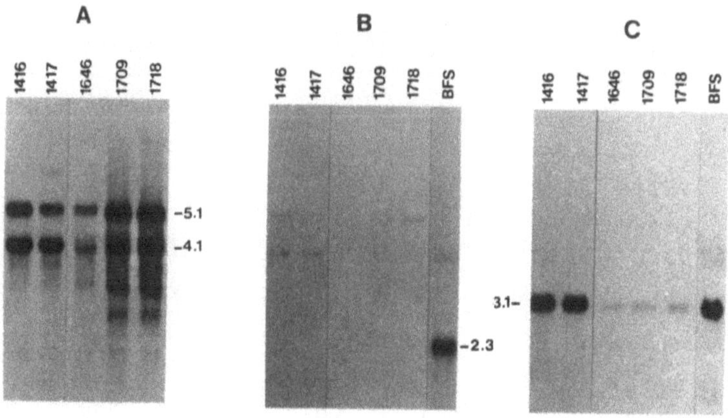

Fig. 4. Northern blot hybridizations of poly-A$^+$ mRNA prepared from some of the primary tumors described in the legend to Fig. 3 and an IL-3-dependent cell line (BFS) with probes specific for avian v-myc (A) murine c-myc (B) and murine c-raf (C).

Poly-A$^+$ RNA prepared from some of the J-5-induced tumors was examined by Northern hybridization with probes specific for v-myc, c-myc and c-raf (Fig. 4). The results show that the lymphoid and epithelial tumors all expressed v-myc-containing messages of 5.1 and 4.1 kpb but that the normal c-myc message of 2.3 was absent. A normal c-raf message of 3.1 kpb was present in all of the tumors although the levels were significantly higher in the lymphoid than in the epithelial tumors.

Taken together, the data presented here indicate that deregulated expression of myc resulting from integration of v-myc-containing viruses in somatic cells is critical to the transformation of T cells, B cells and pre-B cells and the development of pancreatic and mammary adenocarcinomas. The possibility that genetic changes other than deregulated expression of myc may contribute to the development of the fully transformed phenotypes of these cells is suggested by the observations that many of the tumors were mono- or oligoclonal. If genetic changes other than altered expression of myc are required for induction of autonomous growth, it might be expected that these "second signals" would vary for cells belonging to different lineages or for cells at specific states of differentiation within the same lineage. The availability of a variety of tumors expressing myc at high levels may provide an important opportunity to evaluate this question. If a second onc gene were involved in the induction of these tumors, it might be expected that they would have properties similar to those that complement myc for transformation in vitro (6,7).

The wide range of murine cells targeted for transformation by v-myc contrasts with the more limited spectrum of cells affected by other onc genes transduced by MuLV, most of which induce fibrosarcomas or a limited variety of hematopoietic tumors. The basis for these differences in target cell range are not known, but may be related to the position of a particular onc gene in the signal transduction pathway of growth/differentiation factors. Thus, an oncogene that is derived from a ligand gene may be restricted to transformation of cells expressing the corresponding receptor. By comparison, a gene such as myc which can substitute for a variety of growth factors (11,12), presumably due to its role as a central information relay, would supply many cell types with a growth stimulus. Indeed, from earlier studies of chickens infected with myc-containing viruses, the range of cell types susceptible to transformation by these genes (1) may be considerably greater than that revealed by our results. The possibility that other susceptible cell types might be revealed by procedures that alter the normal biology of the mouse is supported by data presented elsewhere in this volume (Potter et al.).

REFERENCES

1. Beard JW (1980) Biology of avian oncornaviruses. In: Klein G (ed) Viral oncology, Raven Press, New York, pp 55-87.
2. Li Y, Holland CA, Hartley JW, Hopkins, N (1984) Viral integrations near c-myc in 10-20% of MCF-247-induced AKR lymphomas. Proc Natl Acad Sci USA 81: 6808-6811.
3. Corcoran LM, Adams JM, Dunn AR, Corey S (1984) Murine T cell lymphomas in which the cellular myc oncogene has been activated by retroviral insertion. Cell 37: 113-122.
4. Shen-Ong GLC, Keath EJ, Piccoli SP, Cole MD (1982) Novel myc oncogene RNA from abortive immunoglobulin gene recombination in mouse plasmacytomas. Cell 31: 443-452.
5. Taub R, Kirsch I, Morton C, Lenoir G, Swan D, Tronick I, Aaronson S, Leder P (1982) Translocation of the c-myc gene into the immunoglobulin heavy chain locus in human Burkitt lymphoma and murine plasmacytoma cells. Proc Natl Acad Sci USA 79: 7837-7841.
6. Land H, Parada LF, Weinberg RL (1983) Tumorigenic conversion of primary embryo fibroblasts requires at least two cooperating oncogenes. Nature 304: 596-602.
7. Ruley HE (1983) Adenovirus early region 1A enables viral and cellular transforming genes to transform primary cells in culture. Nature 304: 602-606.
8. Stewart TA, Pattengale PK, Leder P (1984) Spontaneous mammary adenocarcinomas in transgenic mice that carry and express MTV/myc fusion genes. Cell 38: 627-637.
9. Adams JM, Harris AW, Pinkert CA, Corcoran LM, Alexander WS, Corey S, Palmiter RD, Brinster RL (1985) The c-myc oncogene driven by immunoglobulin enhancers induces lymphoid malignancy in transgenic mice. Nature 318: 533-538.
10. Rapp UR, Cleveland JL, Fredrickson TN, Holmes KL, Morse HC III, Patschinsky T, Bister K.(1985) Rapid induction of hematopoietic neoplasms in newborn mice by a raf(mil)/myc recombinant murine retrovirus. J Virol 55: 23-33.
11. Armelin HA, Armelin MCS, Kelly K, Stewart T, Leder P, Cochran BH, Stiles CD (1984) Functional role for c-myc in mitogenic responses to platelet-derived growth factor. Nature 310: 655-660.
12. Rapp UR, Cleveland JL, Brightman K, Scott A, Ihle JN (1985) Abrogation of IL-3 and IL-2 dependence by recombinant retroviruses expressing v-myc oncogenes. Nature 317: 434-438.

Induction of Clonal Monocyte/Macrophage Tumors *in vivo* by a Mouse c-*myc* Retrovirus: Evidence for Secondary Transforming Events

William R. Baumbach, E. Richard Stanley,* and Michael D. Cole

Department of Molecular Biology, Princeton University, Princeton, NJ and *Department of Microbiology and Immunology, and Department of Cell Biology, Albert Einstein College of Medicine, Bronx, New York

INTRODUCTION

Activation of the c-myc proto-oncogene, in the form of DNA rearrangements that lead to constitutive expression, has been implicated in the genesis of a wide range of tumors. It is therefore of great interest to determine the influence of c-myc oncogene activation on cellular growth control, especially in primary cells. To facilitate the efficient transfer of an activated c-myc oncogene, we have developed a mouse retrovirus that contains the c-myc protein coding sequences and which can be transmitted in the presence of a Mo-MuLV helper virus or established as a helper-free stock using a retroviral packaging cell line. Infection of bone marrow cells gave rise to partially transformed mononuclear phagocytes which were entirely dependent on an exogenous supply of the monocyte specific-growth factor CSF-1 for proliferation. Infection in vivo induced monocyte/macrophage tumors with a latency period of 8-10 wks.

RESULTS AND DISCUSSION

Transformation of bone marrow cells. The majority of the tumors in which activated c-myc genes have been implicated are of the hemopoietic lineage. We therefore assayed the c-myc retrovirus for the ability to induce partial or complete transformation of bone marrow cells from 4 wk old mice. The infected cells were cultured in medium containing 10% fetal calf serum or this same medium supplemented with the growth factor CSF-1 (from L cell conditioned medium). CSF-1 is a principal mitogen for the monocytic lineage in the mouse (Guilbert and Stanley, 1980; Tushinski et al., 1982) and this lineage is the primary target cell type for avian retroviruses (Graf and Beug, 1978).

Bone marrow cells were analysed for both colony formation in soft agar and extended proliferation in culture. In the soft agar colony assay, the c-myc virus induced numerous, tightly packed anchorage-independent colonies, but only in the presence of CSF-1-supplemented medium (not shown). There were no soft agar colonies in the absence of added CSF-1 or with c-myc virus infection alone. A small number of colonies with a more diffuse morphology were found with growth factor supplemented medium. In culture, the c-myc virus induced extensive long term proliferation of mononuclear phagocytic cells, but only in the presence of CSF-1-containing medium. With CSF-1-supplemented medium alone, there was an initial, proliferation of macrophage-like cells, but these cells senesced rapidly. There was no cell growth with the c-myc virus alone, beyond that observed with uninfected primary bone marrow cultures. The bone marrow cells partially transformed in vitro could be propagated in the presence of CSF-1 and had a somewhat rounded morphology, although they were quite adherent and phagocytic (not shown). The myc-trans-

Current Topics in Microbiology and Immunology, Vol. 132

formed bone marrow cells can be assigned to the the mononuclear phagocyte lineage because only cells of this stage express receptors for the growth factor CSF-1 (Guilbert and Stanley, 1980).

The growth of the MRV-transformed macrophages was dependent on a continuous supply of exogenous CSF-1. When cells partially transformed by c-myc in the presence of exogenous CSF-1 are transferred to unsupplemented medium, they stop proliferating and begin to die immediately, while cells cultured with CSF-1 grow vigorously (Baumbach et al., 1986). Thus, the c-myc retrovirus can partially transform macrophage-like cells in culture, but the cells are absolutely dependent on an exogenously supplied hemopoietic growth factor.

Induction of monocytic tumors. We also investigated the in vivo oncogenic potential of the c-myc retrovirus. Filtered supernatants from MRV-infected cells and from control cells producing only the MuLV helper virus were injected intraperitoneally into 8-10 wk old BALB/c mice. Approximately 10(3)-10(4) cfu of c-myc retrovirus was injected per animal. Some animals were also injected with the mineral oil pristane prior to virus infection. As shown in Table 1, pristane-treated mice preferentially showed rapid signs of neoplastic disease, usually from 8 to 10 weeks after infection. Abdominal swelling was followed by rapid loss of vitality (anemia) and death after about two weeks. Ascites fluid, thickening of the peritoneal wall and tumor masses within the abdominal cavity characterized these neoplasia. The ascites fluid was found to contain a high density of transformed cells with monocytic morphology (not shown) and characteristics (see below). No spleen, thymus or lymph node enlargement was observed in MRV-infected mice, which clearly distinguished them from the control mice infected only with Mo-MuLV. The latter displayed the gross enlargement of these organs characteristic of Mo-MuLV induced thymic lymphomas, usually at much later times (3-6 mo.).

Cells derived from the ascites fluid of MRV-infected mice could be passaged intraperitoneally through non-pristane treated mice, causing death within 2 wks. Induction of myeloid tumors was not specific to BALB/c mice because identical results were obtained with MRV infection of pristane-primed DBA mice (Table 1). Tumors were also

TABLE 1: Incidence of neoplastic disease in mice infected with a c-myc retrovirus (MRV), in the presence or absence of helper virus.

Mouse Strain	Virus	Pristane [a]	Tumors	Time (weeks) [b]
BALB/c	MRV	+	11/14	6-12
BALB/c	MRV	-	2/5	12-20
BALB/c	MuLV	+	1/5	13*
BALB/c	MuLV	-	1/3	17*
DBA/2	MRV	+	10/14	12-20
DBA/2	MuLV	+	0/5	20
BALB/c	MRV**	+	10/12	8-13

a : The influence of pristane on tumor incidence was analysed by injection of 0.5 ml intraperitoneally 28 days prior to virus infection.
b : Number of animals with evidence of neoplastic disease/number infected with the virus.
* T cell lymphoma; ** helper-free retrovirus

induced by helper-free c-myc retrovirus infection of bone marrow or spleen cells that were subsequently injected into the peritoneal cavity of pristane treated mice.

Stage-specificity of the transformed cells. The c-myc retrovirus-induced tumor lines were tested cytologically to define the specificity of their hemopoietic lineage and stage. Wright's staining revealed morphologies generally characteristic of more differentiated mononuclear phagocytes (not shown). Some lines contained substantial numbers of cells which appeared to be morphologically similar to terminally differentiated macrophages, while others contained more rounded cells that appear to be less mature, although all were quite adherent. The tumor cells were analysed for several markers of myeloid cell differentiation. The Mac-1 cell surface antigen is diagnostic of cells of the myeloid series (Ho and Springer, 1982). Lysozyme activity, nonspecific esterase staining and phagocytosis are specific markers for mononuclear phagocytes (Osserman and Lawler, 1966; Rashke et al., 1978; Yam et al., 1971). Analysis of each of these markers place the MRV-induced tumor cells in the monocytic or macrophage differentiation pathway (Baumbach et al., 1986). For comparison, control cell lines were included which represent known differentiative stages of murine hemopoiesis. The myelomonocytic leukemia WEHI-3 represents a stage prior to commitment to either granulocytic or mononuclear phagocytic pathways (Metcalf et al, 1969) and P388D1 is a murine macrophage cell line (Koren et al., 1975).

Clonality of the monocyte/macrophage tumors. Analysis of c-myc proviral sequences in DNA from the ascites cells confirmed the involvement of the virus in the neoplastic transformation and indicated that nearly all of the tumors were clonal. DNA was extracted directly from ascites cells and subjected to Southern analysis to determine the frequency of proviral integration within the tumor cell populations. Using a c-myc exon 2 probe, one novel myc-containing restriction fragment was found in 12/14 tumors, with a unique junction fragment in each tumor (Figure 1). These unique proviral junction fragments were found even when DNA was isolated from primary ascites cells. Conversely, digestion with Xba I gave an identical myc fragment of 1.9 kb for each tumor (Figure 1), which was consistent with the provirus structure (Keath et al., 1984; Baumbach et al., 1986). Only one of the tumors gave submolar or no myc proviral bands with single cleavage enzymes, but gave the expected proviral fragment with Xba I (not shown), indicating a possible multiclonal origin. In addition, at least one cell line derived from a single soft agar colony (3.1.1) displayed two exogenous c myc proviruses (Figure 1). Thus, the MRV-induced tumor populations were monoclonal, with one exception. The cell lines analyzed below were derived either from tumor cell populations displaying a single exogenous c-myc band (e.g. 1.1 and 2.3) or from single soft agar colonies (e.g. 3.1.1, 7.1.3).

RNA expression in the mononuclear phagocytic tumor cells. RNAs from the MRV-induced tumor lines were analyzed using several oncogene probes to examine the expression of cellular genes that are associated with the control of cell proliferation. In order to distinguish between mRNA levels of the endogenous and exogenous c-myc genes, identical filters were probed with nick-translated fragments corresponding to c-myc exons 1 or 2. Both the viral and cellular myc RNAs contain the 2nd exon while only the endogenous transcripts contain the noncoding exon 1. Figure 2a shows that all cell lines express high levels of c-myc, but the levels are less than or, at

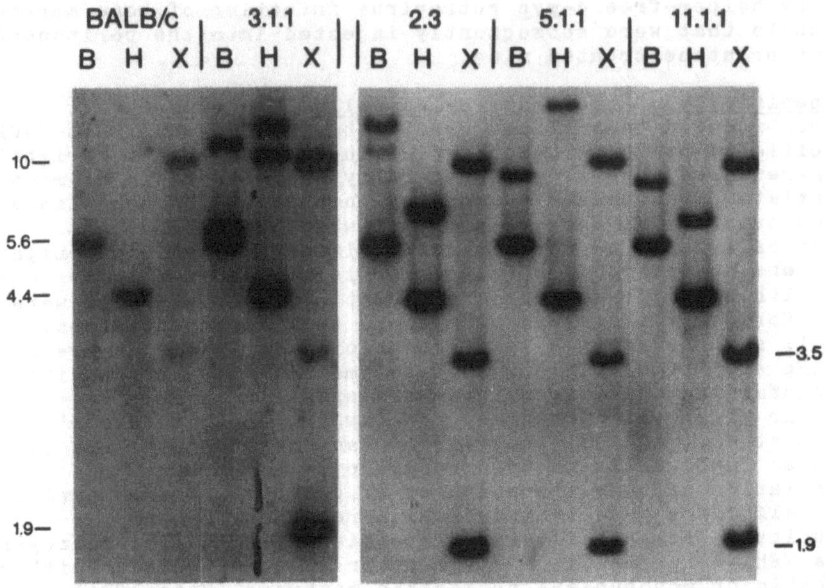

Figure 1: Southern blots of DNA from monocyte/macrophage tumors showing a single c-*myc* provirus in each line. The DNAs were digested with either Bam HI (B), Hind III (H) or Xba I (X), electrophoresed on 0.7% agarose gels and hybridized to a probe from the c-*myc* second exon (1.4 kb Sac I-Sac I). The endogenous c-*myc* bands at 10.0 kb (Xba I), 5.6 kb (Bam HI) and 4.4 kb (Hind III) are indicated. The 1.9 kb Xba I band in each tumor line derives from the identical proviruses.

most, equal to those found in plasmacytomas or *myc*-transformed fibroblasts. The MRV-induced tumor lines express the 2.5 and 3.0 kb RNAs that are consistently found with the c-*myc* retrovirus construct (Baumbach et al., 1986). WEHI-3 and P388D1 express the normal 2.4 kb c-*myc* transcript. *myc*XH2-T is a tumor derived from an NIH/3T3 line stably transformed by the pEVX-XH construct and it expresses the same two *myc* RNAs as the MRV infected lines. In contrast, none of the MRV-induced tumor lines express detectable endogenous c-*myc* transcripts, with the exception of 9.1.1 which has a low but significant level (Figure 2b). The latter line consistently exhibited lower levels of mature macrophage-specific markers, indicating a slighly early stage of differentiation. The endogenous c-*myc* gene is also inactive or expressed at a low level in MOPC 315 and *myc*XH2-T, as described previously (Keath et al., 1984).

We also examined the expression of three other cellular proto-oncogenes, c-*myb*, c-*fos* and c-*fms*, which have been linked to different stages of myeloid cell differentiation. For c-*myb*, only WEHI-3, which is at the earliest stage of differentiation of the lines tested here, displays evidence of transcriptional activity (Figure 2c). On the other hand, high constitutive levels of c-*fos* mRNA were uniformly observed in all of the MRV-induced tumors,

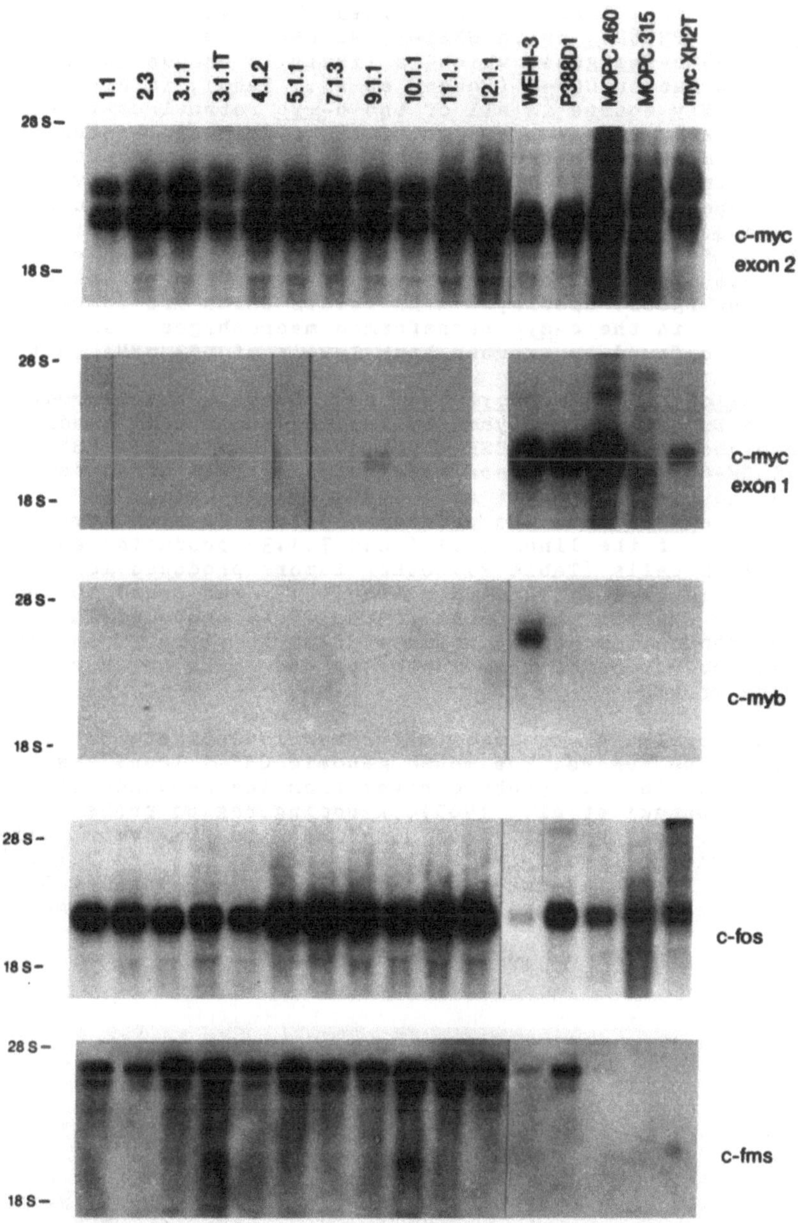

Figure 2: Northern blots of monocyte/macrophage tumor RNAs with cellular oncogene probes. A) c-*myc* second exon (0.98 kb Xba I-Sac I); B) c-*myc* first exon (0.45 kb Bam HI-Bgl II); C) v-*myb* (1.3 kb Kpn I-Sac I, Klempnauer et al., 1982); D) v-*fos* (1.0 kb Pst I, Curran et al., 1982); E) v-*fms* (1.6 kb PstI from pSM3, Hampe et al., 1984). For comparison, RNA is also included from WEHI-3, a monomyelocytic cell line; P388D1, a macrophage tumor line; MOPC 315, a plasmacytoma with a c-*myc* translocation (Shen-Ong et al., 1982) and *myc*XH2-T, a nude mouse tumor induced by transfection of the pEVX-XH *myc* construct into NIH/3T3 cells (Keath et al., 1984).

(Figure 2d), in some lines at many times the level found in the macrophage line P388D1, or in WEHI-3, where virtually no c-fos RNA was found. The c-fms gene, which is likely to encode the receptor for the growth factor CSF-1 (Scherr et al., 1985), is also transcriptionally active in all of the c-myc retrovirus-induced tumor lines (Figure 2e). The expression of the c-fms gene by the tumor cells is consistent with their characterization as mononuclear phagocytes, since the CSF-1 receptor and/or c-fms mRNA have been shown to be specifically expressed at high levels in mononuclear phagocytes and at substantially lower levels in more primitive cells (Guilbert and Stanley, 1980; Byrne et al., 1981; Sariban et al., 1985). Correspondingly, a lower level of c-fms expression was found in WEHI-3, but P388D1 displayed mRNA levels which are comparable to the levels seen in the c-myc transformed macrophages. All of the lines were also found to express high levels of p53 mRNA (not shown).

CSF-1 expression in the monocyte tumors. Growth factor production by the monocyte tumors was analysed by testing tumor cell conditioned medium or by Northern blot. CSF-1 was determined by RIA (Stanley, 1979), and GM-CSF and IL-3 were assayed using cell lines dependent the growth factors (Dexter et al., 1980; Ihle et al., 1982). Four of the tumor lines were found to produce moderate to high levels of CSF-1, with two of the lines (9.1.1 and 7.1.3) producing as much of the factor as L cells (Table 2). Other tumors produced lower but still detectable levels. One tumor line (2.3) was found to produce both CSF-1 and GM-CSF, while none of the lines produced IL-3. As mononuclear phagocytes do not produce CSF-1 in vitro (Tushinski et al., 1982), production of this factor by the tumor cells could lead to autocrine growth.

Northern blot analysis was used to further investigate CSF-1 production in the tumors. The mouse genomic CSF-1 locus was cloned using an oligonucleotide probe derived from the sequence of a human CSF-1 cDNA (Kawasaki et al., 1985). A coding region probe was then used to examine the production of CSF-1 mRNA in the tumor cells. L cells were found to transcribe two CSF-1 mRNAs (4.3 and 2.3 kb), with the 4.3 kb species being more abundant (Figure 3). The level of CSF-1 mRNA in the tumors was found to correspond well with the amount of

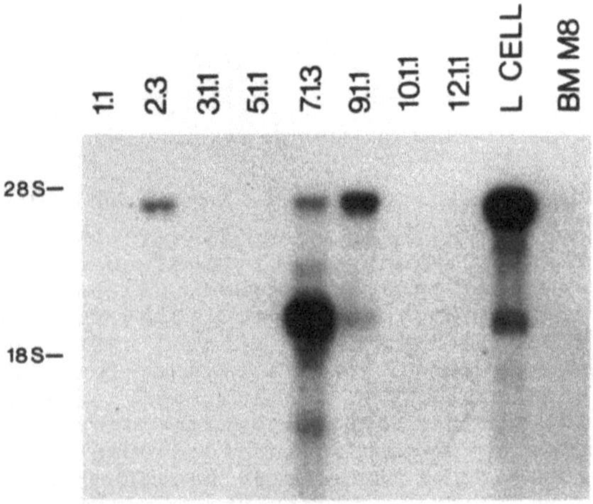

Figure 3: Northern blot of monocyte/macrophage tumor RNA hybridized with an oligonucleotide probe corresponding to the mouse colony stimulating factor-1 gene. BM-M8 is a cell line derived from bone marrow cells infected in vitro with a helper-free c-myc retrovirus and grwon in the presence of CSF-1.

TABLE 2: Hemopoietic growth factor production by c-myc retrovirus-induced monocyte/macrophage tumors.

Tumor Line	CSF-1 (u/ml) [a]	GM-CSF [b]	IL-3 [b]
2.3	257	+	-
3.1.1	221	-	-
4.1.2	70	-	-
5.1.1	137	-	-
7.1.3	1496	-	-
9.1.1	2391	-	-
10.1.1	18	-	-

a : CSF-1 production was assayed from medium conditioned by confluent tumor cells in RPMI 1640 for two days. CSF-1 concentrations were determined on triplicate sets of CM by RIA (Stanley, 1979). 1 unit = 0.44 fmoles CSF-1 protein.
b : Production of the hemopoietic growth factors GM-CSF and IL-3 was assayed as described in the text.

factor secreted into the medium, with the exception of tumor line 9.1.1. This tumor line produced the highest levels of the factor, yet had only a moderate level of CSF-1 mRNA. Notably, tumor line 7.1.3 had an altered pattern of CSF-1 RNA, with extremely abundant 2. kb RNA and a lower level of 4. kb RNA. The production of high levels of CSF-1 RNA and protein is not a consequence of c-myc retrovirus infection or culturing the tumor cells because in vitro transformed macrophages grown for a similar length of time in culture (in the presence of CSF-1) do not express CSF-1 RNA (Figure 3).

Anti-CSF-1 serum blocks the growth of 7.1.3. We next wished to test if the production of CSF-1 contributed to tumor cell growth. To this end, we analysed the anchorage-independent growth of several tumor lines in response to conditioned medium (CM) and purified CSF-1. Table 3 shows that the growth of 7.1.3 is stimulated dramatically by self-conditioned medium (8.0% versus 0.8%) and to a lesser extent by purified CSF-1 (2.5%). Greater than 80% of the response to CM (both number and size of colonies) was blocked by anti-CSF-1 serum. The

TABLE 3: Anchorage-independent growth response of monocyte tumor lines to conditioned medium and blocking by anti-serum to CSF-1.

Additions [a]	Tumor Line 7.1.3	2.3	9.1.1	3.1.1
none	0.8	0.3	1.1	7.5
CM (20% v/v)	8.0	2.5	16.0	12.6
CM + pre-immune serum	5.9	2.0	13.5	11.7
CM + anti-CSF-1 antiserum	1.6	2.5	9.1	9.7
CSF-1 (2000 u/ml)	2.5	13.0	0.6	3.8
CSF-1 + anti-CSF-1 antiserum	<0.01	1.4	0.4	4.6

a : Tumor cells were plated in 0.26% agar with DMEM and 10% fetal calf serum plus the indicated additional reagents. Values represent the percentage of the cells plated which formed colonies of >30 cells.

anti-serum also completely blocked the response to purified CSF-1 to yield an anchorage-independent cloning efficiency lower than with medium alone (<0.01%). Thus, tumor line 7.1.3 exhibits a substantial autocrine growth response.

Other tumor lines exhibited a different response to CSF-1 and CM (Table 3). Tumor line 2.3, which produces both CSF-1 and GM-CSF, was dramatically stimulated by both CM and by purified CSF-1, but the response to CM was not blocked by anti-CSF-1 serum, suggesting that the cells may possess receptors, and respond to, both GM-CSF and CSF-1. On the other hand, 9.1.1 failed to respond to purified CSF-1 and growth was not blocked by anti-CSF-1 serum, even though this line produced the highest level of CSF-1 in the medium and growth was stimulated dramatically by CM. Tumor lines which produced only low levels of CSF-1, such as 3.1.1, did not respond to purified CSF-1 and exhibited only a limited growth stimulation in response to CM.

Numerous studies, largely from Graf, Beug and coworkers, have investigated the transforming activity of the avian myc-containing retroviruses both in vivo and in vitro (reviewed in Graf and Beug, 1978). The principal disease induced by the prototype myc virus, MC29, is myelocytomatosis, with which the neoplasm described in this study shares many features. One of the most striking aspects is the uniformity of the specific maturational stage and lineage of the transformed cells, in particular the mononuclear phagocytic target cells. In each case, the transformed cells resemble fully differentiated macrophages for the majority of the myeloid cell stage-specific markers. However, chicken myelocytomatosis is a somewhat more rapid disease, killing the animals in 4-5 weeks as compared to visible ascites formation usually in 8-10 weeks in BALB/c mice or 12-20 wks in DBA/2, and death 2-3 weeks later. It is possible that transformation by MC29 may result from a higher level of expression in virus-infected cells, and/or mutations within the v-myc protein, as compared to the cellular myc protein (Watson et al., 1983; Hayflick et al., 1985). In contrast, the murine virus used in this study expressed c-myc at a level at most 4-fold higher than that of the endogenous gene in proliferating cells lacking activated c-myc genes (Figure 2). The distinct lag time associated with the induction of myeloid tumors by the murine c-myc retrovirus most likely reflects the acquisition of additional genetic changes that contribute to full malignant transformation. The production of high levels of hemopoietic growth factors by some tumor lines suggests that the secondary changes may involve an autocrine growth response.

ACKNOWLEDGEMENTS

We would like to thank Tom Curran, Charles Scherr and Jacalyn Pierce for oncogene probes and cell lines, and Claudia Saez for technical assistance. MDC is the recipient of a Faculty Research Award from the American Cancer Society and is a Pew Scholar in the Biomedical Sciences. WRB is supported by a training grant from the National Institutes of Health and ERS is a recipient of an Irma T. Hirschl Career Scientist Award. This work was supported by grants from the American Cancer Society (CD-236) and the National Institutes of Health (CA39550) to MDC, and the National Institutes of Health (CA26504) to ERS and by an AECOM Cancer Center Core grant (Albert Einstein College of Medicine, ERS).

References

Baumbach, W. R., Keath, E. J., Cole, M. D. (1986) A mouse c-myc retrovirus transforms established fibroblast lines in vitro and induces monocyte/macrophage tumors in vivo. J. Virol., in press.
Byrne, P. V., Guilbert, L. J., Stanley, E. R. (1981) Distribution of cells carrying receptors for colony-stimulating factor (CSF-1) in murine tissues. J. Cell Biol. 91: 848-853.
Curran, T., Peters, G., Van Beveren, C., Teich, N. M., Verma, I. M. (1982) FBJ murine osteosarcoma virus: identification and molecular cloning of biologically active proviral DNA. J. Virol. 44: 674-682.
Dexter, T. M., Garland, J., Scott, D., Scolnick, E., Metcalf, D. (1980) Growth on factor-dependent hemopoietic precursor cell lines. J. Exp. Med. 152: 1036.
Graf, T., Beug, H. (1978) Avian leukemia viruses: interaction with their target cells in vivo and in vitro. Biochim. Biophys. Acta 516: 269-299.
Guilbert, L. J., Stanley, E. R. (1980) Specific interaction of murine colony-stimulating factor with mononuclear phagocytic cells. J. Cell Biol. 85: 153-159.
Hampe, A., Gobet, M., Scherr, C. J., Galibert, F. (1984) Nucleotide sequence of the feline retroviral oncogene v-fms shows unexpected homology with oncogenes encoding tyrosine-specific protein kinases. Proc. Natl. Acad. Sci. USA 81: 85-89.
Hayflick, J., Seeburg, P. H., Ohlsson, R., Pfeifer-Ohlsson, S., Watson, D., Papas, T., Duesberg, P. H. (1985) Nucleotide sequence of two overlapping myc-related genes in avian carcinoma virus OK10 and their relation to the myc genes of other viruses and the cell. Proc. Natl. Acad. Sci. USA 82: 2718-2722.
Ho, M.-K., T. A. Springer. (1982) Mac-1 antigen: quantitative expression in macrophage populations and tissues, and immunofluorescent localization in spleen. J. Immunol. 128: 2281-2286.
Ihle, J. N., Keller, J., Greenberger, J. S., Henderson, L., Yetter, R. A., Morse III, H. C. (1982) Phenotypic characterization of cell lines requiring Il-3 for growth. J. Immunol. 129: 1377.
Kawasaki, E. S., Ladner, M. B., Wang, A. M., Van Arsdell, J., Warren, M. K., Coyne, M. Y., Schweickart, V. L., Lee, M.-T., Wilson, K. J., Boosman, A., Stanley, E. R., Ralph, P., Mark, D. F. (1985) Molecular cloning of a complemantary DNA encoding human macrophage-specific colony stimulating factor (CSF-1). Science 230: 291-296.
Keath, E. J., Caimi, P. G., Cole, M. D. (1984) Fibroblast lines expressing activated c-myc oncogenes are tumorigenic in nude mice and syngeneic animals. Cell 39: 339-348.
Klempnauer, K. H., Gonda, T. J., Bishop, J. M. (1982) Nucleotide sequence of the retroviral leukemia gene v-myb and its cellular progenitor c-myb: the architecture of a transduced oncogene. Cell 31: 453-463.
Koren, H. S., Handwerger, B. S., Wunderlich, J. R. (1975) Identification of macrophage-like characteristics in a cultured murine tumor line. J. Immunol. 114: 894-897.
Metcalf, D., Moore, M. A. S., Warne, N. L. (1969) Colony formation in vitro by myelomonocytic leukemia cells. J. Natl. Can. Inst. 43: 983-988.
Osserman, E. F., D. F. Lawlor. (1966) Serum and urinary lysozyme (muramidase) in monocytic and monomyelocytic leukemia. J. Exp. Med. 124: 921-952.
Raschke, W. G., S. Baird, P. Ralph, I. Nakoinz. (1978) Functional macrophage cell lines transformed by Abelson leukemia virus. Cell 15: 261-267.

Sariban, E., Mitchell, T., Kufe, D. (1985) Expression of the c-fms proto-oncogene during human monocytic differentiation. Nature 316: 64-66.
Shen-Ong, G. L. C., Keath, E. J., Piccoli, S. P., Cole, M. D. (1982) Novel myc oncogene RNA from abortive immunoglobulin-gene recombination in mouse plasacytomas. Cell 31: 443-452.
Sherr, C. J., Rettenmier, C. W., Sacca, R., Roussel, M. F., Look, A. T., Stanley, E. R. (1985) The c-fms proto-oncogene product is related to the receptor for the mononuclear phagocyte growth factor, CSF-1. Cell 41: 665-676.
Stanley, E. R. (1979) Colony-stimulating factor (CSF) radioimmunoassay: Determination of a CSF subclass stimulating macrophage production. Proc Natl. Acad. Sci. USA 76: 2969-2993.
Stanley, E. R. (1985) The macrophage colony stimulating factor, CSF-1. In Methods in Engymology-Immunochemical Techniques, Vol. 116 (Colwick and Kappler, eds.) Harcourt, Brace Janovich, New York. pp. 564-587.
Tushinski, R. L., Oliver, I. T., Guilbert, L. J., Tynan, P. W., Warner, J. R., Stanley, E. R. (1982) Survival of mononuclear phagocytes depends on a lineage-specific growth factor that the differentiated cells selectively destroy. Cell 28: 71-81.
Vennstrom, B., Kahn, P., Adkins, B., Enrietto, P., Hayman, M. J., Graf, T., Luciw, P. (1984) Transformation of mammalian fibroblasts and macrophages in vitro by a murine retrovirus encoding an avian v-myc oncogene. EMBO J. 3: 3223-3229.
Watson, D. K., Reddy, E. P., Duesberg, P. H., Papas, T. S. (1983) Nucleotide sequence analysis of the chicken c-myc gene reveals homologous and unique coding regions by comparison with the transfroming gene of avian myelocytomatosis virus MC29. Proc. Natl. Acad. Sci. USA 80: 2146-2150.
Yam, L. T., C. Y. Li, W. H. Crosby. (1971) Cytochemical identification of monocytes and granulocytes. Am. J. Clin. Pathol. 55:283-297.

Addendum

The c-myc retrovirus (MRV) used in this study is derived from the pEVX-mycXH construct described previously (Keath et al., 1984). This plasmid contains the translocated c-myc gene from plasmacytoma line MOPC 104E (Shen-Ong et al., 1982), cloned into the pEVX vector (Kriegler et al., 1984) as shown below. Proviral forms of MRV lack the c-myc second intron, and the provirus produces two RNAs of 3.0 and 2.5 kb, the latter due to splicing of the MuLV/c-myc intron (Baumbach et al., 1986). No mutations have been found in the MOPC 104E c-myc gene (S. Piccoli, pers. comm.). Splice donor and acceptor sites are indicated by open and filled triangles; restriction enzyme sites are indicated: B, BamHI, Bg, BglII; H, HindIII; R, RsaI; S, SstI; X, XbaI.

Kriegler, M., Perez, C. F., Hardy, C. and Botchan, M. (1984) Transformation mediated by SV40 T antigens: Separation of overlapping SV40 early genes with a retroviral vector. Cell 38, 483-491.

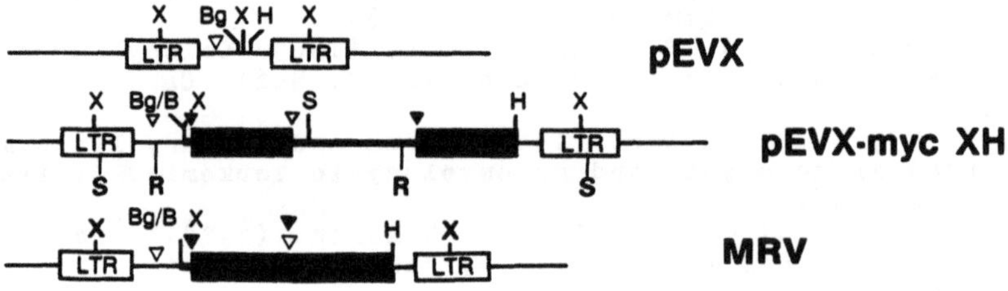

Induction of Hematopoietic Tumors Using a Viral Construct Containing c-*myc* cDNA from Normal Mouse Spleen

Linda Wolff[1], J. Frederic Mushinski[1], Eli Gilboa[2] and Herbert C. Morse, III[3]

[1]Laboratory of Genetics, National Cancer Institute, National Institutes of Health, Bethesda, MD 20892 USA; [2]Department of Molecular Biology, Princeton University, Princeton, NJ 08544 USA; [3]Laboratory of Immunopathology, National Institute of Allergy and Infectious Diseases, National Institutes of Health, Bethesda, MD 20892 USA

INTRODUCTION

Deregulated expression of the c-myc protooncogene is assumed to be a major contributing factor to the development of plasmacytomas in pristane-primed BALB/c mice (reviewed in Potter, 1986) and murine T cell lymphomas induced by AKR and Moloney murine leukemia viruses (MuLV) (Steffen 1984, Selden et al. 1984, Li et al. 1984, Corcoran et al. 1984). Studies on the c-myc expression in plasmacytomas suggest that myc can be deregulated by a variety of mechanisms. These include stabilization of the myc message due to an altered transcriptional unit (Piechaczyk et al. 1985), removal of cis-acting regulatory sequences (Yang et al. 1985) and augmentation of transcriptional activity resulting from apposed IgH enhancer sequences (Corcoran, 1985). These studies provide substantial inferential support for the view that aberrant expression of myc is central to the transformation of murine plasma cells and T cells but direct evidence to buttress this argument has been lacking. Efforts to develop this evidence have taken several complementary directions, all resulting in abnormally high levels of myc expression in somatic cells. These include the development of transgenic mice with murine or human c-myc genes driven by selected promoter/enhancer sequences (Stewart et al. 1984; Adams et al. 1986) or infection of mice with recombinant murine retroviruses containing avian v-myc genes (Morse et al. 1986; Potter et al. 1986). The avian v-myc genes are known to contain numerous coding region mutations in comparison to normal avian c-myc sequences and also differ from normal murine c-myc genes (Papas and Lautenberger, 1985). Since sequence differences among avian v-myc genes appear to contribute to variations in their oncogenic potentials (Enrietto et al. 1984), we wished to determine if overexpression of a normal murine c-myc gene in mice would result in the development of tumors. This report describes the features of two new recombinant murine retroviruses containing normal mouse c-myc coding sequences and the results obtained when pseudotypes of these viruses were used to infect adult, pristane-primed BALB/c mice.

VIRUS CONSTRUCTION

Two retroviral vectors were constructed as shown in Fig. 1. In both cases the myc sequences were placed in a Moloney MuLV-based

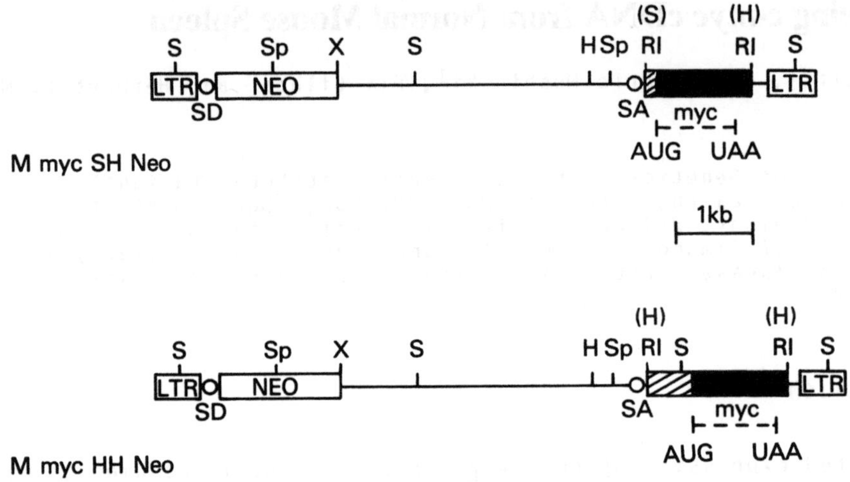

Figure 1. Retrovirus vectors containing c-myc cDNA. The Moloney leukemia based virus contain neomycin resistance gene sequences downstream from the 5' LTR and splice donor site (SD) and c-myc cDNA downstream from the slice acceptor site (SA). c-myc coding sequences and 3' untranslated regions are indicated by a shaded box. c-myc 5' nontranslated sequences are indicated by a box containing cross-hatches. The c-myc coding sequences are designated by a dotted line. H, Hind III; RI, EcoRI; S, SacI; Sp, Sphl; X, Xhol.

vector which was modified from a double expression vector previously reported by Gilboa et al. (1982). In these retroviruses, the neomycin resistence gene (Beck et al. 1982) was positioned in the gag region of the MuLV where it could be translated directly from the major viral genomic transcript. This gene was included for subsequent selection of cells containing the virus and for the determination of viral titers (see below). Both the Mmyc SH Neo virus and the Mmyc HH Neo virus had at their 3' ends c-myc cDNA isolated from a normal BALB/c spleen (Stanton et al. 1983). These sequences replace retroviral env sequences which are expressed on a spliced, subgenomic transcript. Both of these vectors include the c-myc coding regions of Exons 2 and 3 but differ in that the Mmyc SH Neo virus is missing almost all of Exon 1 (except for 50 bp), whereas the Mmyc HH Neo virus contains most of Exon 1. We were interested in comparing constructs with and without the 5' noncoding sequences in Exon 1 since it has been proposed that these sequences may be involved in post-transcriptional regulation of the gene (Piechaczyk et al. 1985). The viral DNAs were transfected, by calcium phosphate precipitation, into NIH 3T3 cells productively infected with Moloney MuLV and cells containing the DNAs were selected for one week using the neomycin analogue, G418. Titers of viruses harvested from 24 hr confluent cultures were determined by the ability of the viruses to confer G418 resistance to other cultures of NIH 3T3 cells. The titer of the Mmyc SH Neo virus in culture medium was 1.5 x 10^5/ml, whereas that of the Mmyc HH Neo virus was 7.2 x 10^4/ml.

TUMOR INDUCTION IN PRISTANE-PRIMED BALB/c MICE

To determine if the c-myc viruses could contribute to neoplastic disease in vivo, we used Moloney helper MuLV pseudotypes of the viruses to infect adult BALB/c mice. These mice had been primed i.p. with 0.5 ml of pristane for one month at the time of infection. Fifty two days after infection with the Mmyc SH Neo virus (minus Exon 1) eight mice with distended abdomens were shown to have rapidly proliferating neoplasms. Their Wrights-Giemsa stained ascites cells appeared morphologically to be a mixture of myeloid cells at various stages of differentiation. Large cells with a more mature phenotype had monocyte/macrophage characteristics with large vacuoles and a granulated cytoplasm. Additional mice subsequently developed the same type of tumor and as shown in Table 1, the overall frequency for this type of tumor was 64% (16 out of 25 mice injected with an average latency of 68 days). Some mice injected with the other c-myc vector, which contained most of Exon 1 (Mmyc HH Neo), developed myelogenous leukemias also. However the disease incidence was significantly lower (26%) and tumors did not appear until day 102 (Table 1). Mice with primary neoplasms and tumors that were transplanted in pristane-primed mice showed extensive growth of solid tumor tissue throughout the whole peritoneal cavity including the mesenteric connective tissue, the peritoneal wall and the diaphragm. It appears that the pristane-induced inflammatory response and the formation of an extensive oil granuloma, throughout the peritoneal cavity (Potter, 1986), is required for rapid development of this myeloid disease, since injection of virus in the absence of pristane did not result in myeloid tumor induction.

Two mice in this study developed T cell lymphomas with latencies of 115 and 150 days. It is probable that these were induced by the Moloney MuLV helper virus which is known to cause T-cell lymphomas. To test this possibility a control group of pristane-primed mice were injected i.p. with helper virus alone; these experiments are presently two months in progress, with no evidence of tumors.

CHARACTERIZATION OF TUMOR CELLS

Cells from six first generation transplants, were analysed for expression of cell surface antigen markers by flow microfluorometry using a large panel of monoclonal, allo- and xenoantibodies (Davidson et al. 1984, Holmes et al. 1986). The spectrum of reactivity with these antibodies was the same for all of the neoplasms. Although all were negative for B and/or T specific cell surface antigens such as Thy-1, Ly-1, kappa, IgM, Ly-5(B220) and ThB, they were all reactive with monoclonal antibodies to Mac-1, Fc receptor (Ly-17) and Ia. This confirmed the morphological characterization indicating that the tumors were composed of monocyte/macrophage cells. Subpopulations of

Table 1. Tumor induction by *myc* viruses in pristane-primed BALB/c mice

Virus[a]	Pristane (1 mo)	No. of mice	Tumor Type Myeloid	Tumor Type Lymphoid	Latency[b] in days Aver. (range)
M*myc* SH Neo (- Exon 1)	+	25	16	0	68 (52-107)
M*myc* SH Neo (- Exon 1)	-	10	0	0	-
M*myc* HH Neo (+ Exon 1)	+	15	4	1	110 (102-115)
M*myc* HH Neo (+ Exon 1)	-	13	0	1	150
None	+	5	0	0	-

[a]Route of injection was i.p. Moloney MuLV was employed as a helper virus. Mice received 0.5 ml of undiluted virus from 24 hr culture supernatant.
[b]Post virus infection.

cells in two of the tumor samples were negative for Mac-1 and Ia but positive for Ly-17, suggesting that the neoplasm contained a population of immature myeloid cells as well as the more mature Mac-1 and Ia positive cells. Cell lines from 8 tumors were established in liquid culture and have continued to grow under conditions of minimal growth requirements (Dulbecco's minimal essential medium with 10% fetal calf serum) for greater than 2 months. These semi-adherent cells have the Mac-1, Ly-17 and Ia markers that were demonstrated to be present on the *in vivo*-derived tumor cells and in addition, have been shown to be positive for Mac-2. The monocyte/macrophage nature of these cells was further supported by a lyso-plate assay (Osserman and Lawlor 1966) which demonstrated the production of lysozyme and by the staining of the cells for nonspecific esterase (α-naphthylacetate esterase) (Yam et al. 1971).

MOLECULAR STUDIES

Monocyte-macrophage tumors do not occur normally as a consequence of pristane treatment, and the pristane controls in this experiment did not develop neoplasms by day 150. This implies that the recombinant virus used to infect the mice is the causative agent of the disease. To provide support for this conclusion, we have performed Southern blot analyses to look for integrated viral DNA in the tumors and have analyzed them for the expression of viral *myc* messenger RNA. Southern blots of three primary tumor DNAs contained virus-specific SacI and EcoRI bands that hybridized with a c-*myc* probe. The c-*myc* sequences that were inserted into the vector appeared to be unaltered in every case, but the integrated virus in one of the tumors was deleted in the intronic region upstream from the splice acceptor site. Expression of viral c-myc was demonstrated on a Northern blot of total RNA where a 2.4 kb message that hybridizes with both a c-myc probe and a Moloney MuLV probe was evident.

CONCLUSION

The data presented here demonstrate that infection of adult pristane-primed BALB/c mice with recombinant murine retroviruses containing normal murine c-myc coding sequences results in the development of myelomonocytic leukemias (Table I). Baumbach, Stanley and Cole (1986) obtained similar tumors in both BALB/c and DBA/2 mice using a retrovirus construct containing a mouse plasmacytoma derived c-myc gene. These results differ in part, however, from those obtained by infecting pristane-primed mice with retroviruses containing avian v-myc genes which showed that they develop predominantly plasmacytomas and a lower frequency of myelomonocytic tumors (Potter et al. 1986). The basis for the differences between these results is not known but may be related to coding or noncoding region sequence differences in the constructs, or their relative levels of myc expression.

The possibility that non-coding region sequences may affect the oncogenic potential of recombinant myc retroviruses is indicated by our observation that mice infected with pseudotypes of Mmyc HH Neo developed a significantly lower frequency of disease than mice infected with Mmyc SH Neo (Table I). The lower frequency of disease in mice infected with Mmyc HH Neo, which contained the most Exon 1 sequences could be explained by the possibilities that (1) these 5' noncoding sequences made the transcript more unstable, as it may in the case of normal myc message from the endogenous gene (Piechaczyk et al. 1985) or (2) that translation of the c-myc protein was less efficient due to the increased distance between the splice-acceptor site and the ATG initiation codon.

Although further work is required to resolve these issues, this study provides direct evidence that a homologous, nonmutated myc gene, devoid of its own regulatory sequences and expressed in abundance, can induce neoplastic disease in mice. The possibility that aberrant expression of myc may be insufficient to induce these neoplasms without alterations of other onc genes is also being studied.

ACKNOWLEDGEMENTS

We would like to thank Dr. Michael Potter for support and helpful discussions regarding this work and Judith Wax for assistance in organizing and carrying out the animal experiments.

REFERENCES

Adams JM, Gerondakis S, Webb E, Corcoran LM, Cory S (1983) Cellular myc oncogene is altered by chromosomal translocation to an immunoglobulin locus in murine plasmacytomas and is rearranged similarly in human Burkitt's lymphomas. Proc Natl Acad Sci USA 80:1982-1986

Adams JM, Harris AW, Pinkert CA, Corcoran LM, Alexander WS, Cory S, Palmiter RD, Brinster RL (1985) The c-myc oncogene driven by immunoglobulin enhancers induces lymphoid malignancy in transgenic mice. Nature 318:533-538
Baumbach WR, Stanley ER, Cole MD (1986) Induction of clonal monocyte macrophage tumors in vivo by a mouse c-myc retrovirus: evidence for secondary transforming events. Current Topics in Microbiology and Immunology (this volume)
Beck E, Ludwig G, Auerswald EA, Reiss B, Schaller H (1982) Nucleotide sequence and exact location of the neomycin phosphotransferase gene from transposon Tn5. Gene 19:327-336
Corcoran LM, Adams JM, Dunn AR, Cory S (1984) Murine T lymphomas in which the cellular myc oncogene has been activated by retroviral insertion. Cell 37:113-122
Corcoran LM, Cory S, Adams JM (1985) Transposition of the immunoglobulin heavy chain enhancer to the myc oncogene in a murine plasmacytoma. Cell 40:71-79
Davidson WF, Frederickson TN, Rudikoff EK, Coffman RL, Hartley JW, Morse HC, III (1984) A unique series of lymphomas related to the Ly-1^{+} lineage of B lymphocyte differentiation. J Immunol 133:744-753
Enrietto PJ, Payne LN, Hayman MJ (1983) Recovered avian myelocytomatosis virus that induces lymphomas in chickens: pathogenic properties and their molecular basis. Cell 35:369-379
Gilboa E, Park J, Kolbe M, Hwang S, Kucherlapati R, Noonan K, Freeman H (1982) Transduction and expression of nonselectable genes using retrovirus-derived vectors. In: Gluzman Y (ed) Eukaryotic viral vectors. Cold Spring Harbor Laboratory, Cold Spring Harbor, NY, p 145-151
Holmes KL, Pierce JH, Davidson WS, Morse HC, III (1986) Murine hematopoietic cells with Pre B or Pre B/myeloid characteristics are generated by in vitro transformation with retroviruses containing Fes, Ras, Abl and Src oncogenes. J Exp Med (in press)
Li Y, Holland CA, Hartley JW, Hopkins N (1984) Viral integration near c-myc in 10-20% of MCF 247-induced AKR lymphomas. Proc Natl Acad Sci USA 81:6808-6811
Morse HC, III, Hartley JW, Frederickson TN, Yetter RA, Cleveland JL, Majumdar C, Rapp UR (1986) Tumors of newborn NFS/N mice infected with murine retroviruses containing avian v-myc. Current Topics in Microbiology and Immunology (this volume)
Osserman EF, Lawlor DF (1966) Serums and urinary lysozyme (muramidase) in monocytic and monomyelocytic leukemia. J Exp Med 124:921-952
Papas TS, Lautenberger JA (1985) Sequence curiosity in v-myc oncogene. Nature 318:237
Piechaczyk M, Yang J-Q, Banchard J-M, Jeanteur P, Marcu KB (1985) Post-transcriptional mechanisms are responsible for accumulation of truncated c-myc RNAs in murine plasma cell tumors. Cell 42:589-597
Potter M (1986) Progression in plasmacytoma development. Adv in Viral Onc, Vol 6 (in press)
Potter M, Wax J, Mushinski E, Brust S, Babonits M, Wiener F, Mushinski JF, Mezebish D, Skurla R, Rapp U, Morse HC, III (1986) Rapid induction of plasmacytomas in mice by pristane and a murine recombinant retrovirus containing an avian v-myc and a defective raf raf oncogene. Current Topics in Microbiology and Immunology (this volume)
Selten G, Cuypers HT, Zijlstra M, Melief C, Berns A (1984) Involvement of c-myc in MuLV-induced T cell lymphomas in mice: frequency and mechanisms of activation. EMBO J 3:3215-3222

Stanton LW, Watt R, Marcu KB (1983) Translocation, breakage and truncated transcripts of c-myc oncogene in murine plasmacytomas. Nature 303:401-406
Steffen D (1984) Proviruses are adjacent to c-myc in some murine leukemia virus induced lymphomas. Proc Natl Acad Sci USA 81:2097-2101
Stewart TA, Pattengale PK, Leder P (1984) Spontaneous mammary adenocarcinomas in transgenic mice that carry and express MTV/myc fusion genes. Cell 38:627-637
Yam LT, Li CY, Crosby WH (1971) Cytochemical identification of monocytes and granulocytes. Am J Clin Pathol 55:283-297
Yang J-Q, Bauer SR, Mushinski JF, Marcu KB (1985) Chromosomal translocations clustered 5' of the murine c-myc gene qualitatively affect promotor usage: implications for the site of normal c-myc regulation. EMBO J 4:1441-1447

Rapid Induction of Plasmacytomas in Mice by Pristane and a Murine Recombinant Retrovirus Containing an Avian v-*myc* and a Defective *raf* Oncogene

M. Potter, J. Wax[1], E. Mushinski, S. Brust, M. Babonits[2], F. Wiener[2], J. F. Mushinski, D. Mezebish, R. Skurla, U. Rapp[3], and H. C. Morse, III[4]

Laboratory of Genetics, National Cancer Institute, National Institutes of Health, Bethesda, MD USA*

Plasma cell tumors can be induced in genetically susceptible BALB/cAn mice by the intraperitoneal injection of various kinds of mineral (paraffin) oils or available components of these oils. Currently, the most widely used agent is pristane 2,6,10,14 tetramethylpentadecane. The incidence of plasma cell tumors obtained in BALB/cAn mice varies according to the dose of pristane. The highest incidence of plasmacytomas occurs when mice are given three 0.5 ml i.p. injections of pristane, spaced 2 months apart (Potter and Wax 1983). Approximately 60% of the mice treated with this regimen develop plasmacytomas with a minimal latent period of 120 days and a mean latent period of 210-220 days. In contrast, when mice are given a single injection of 0.5 ml pristane i.p., only 25-30% develop plasmacytomas. The minimal latent period is 140 days and the mean latent period ca. 215 days.

A low yield of plasmacytomas with shorter latent periods have been induced in BALB/cAn by infecting the mice with Abelson virus 20 to 40 days after pristane injection (Potter et al. 1973; Ohno et al. 1984). When mice that had been given 0.5 ml pristane and infected with Abelson virus 39 to 58 days post pristane the mean latent period of plasmacytoma development was 52 post virus, and 93 days post pristane. Over 95% of plasmacytomas induced by pristane and Abelson virus have non-random chromosomal translocations rcpt(12;15) and rcpt(6;15), that are associated with deregulation of c-myc gene transcription (Ohno et al. 1984).

The availability of recombinant retroviruses carrying functional myc gene sequences provides an opportunity to determine if these sequences, under the control of viral promoters, could induce plasmacytomas in BALB/c mice. In the present experiments we have used the J-3 recombinant virus, a variant of J-2 that was constructed by one of us (Rapp et al. 1985a; Rapp et al. 1985b). J-2 virus was derived from the murine 3611 (which contains a v-raf oncogene) and the avian viruses MH2 and MC29 (which contain v-myc) (Fig. 1). MH2 carries two

*[1]Hazleton Laboratories, Rockville, MD USA; [2]Karolinska Institute, Stockholm, Sweden; [3]Frederick Cancer Research Center, Frederick, MD USA; [4]National Institute of Allergy and Infectious Diseases, National Institutes of Health, Bethesda, MD USA

Current Topics in Microbiology and Immunology, Vol. 132

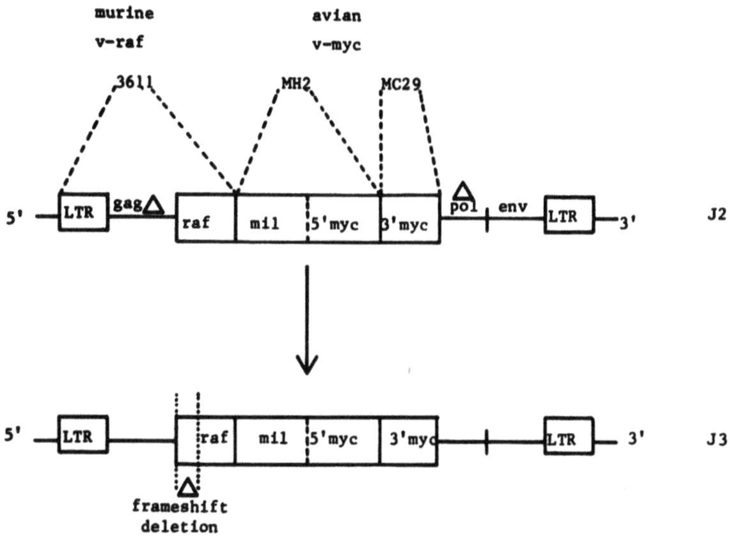

oncogenes, v-mil (the avian homologue of raf) and v-myc, while MC29 contains only v-myc. J-3 virus was modified from J-2 by deleting 200 bp from the 5' end of the raf element. This deletion disrupted the reading frame of the raf/mil hybrid gene (Fig. 1).

Plasmacytomas were induced in 20.5% of 114 BALB/cAn mice by a single 0.5 ml i.p. injection of pristane and infection with J-3 virus 7 to 33 days later. The plasmacytomas developed 42 to 117 days after virus infection (mean 71 days) or 54 to 150 days after pristane. The plasmacytoma cells contained less cytoplasm than the pristane induced plasmacytomas and the cytoplasm stained a very intensive dark blue with Wright's-Giemsa stain suggesting a plasmablast like morphology. All of the tumors have grown rapidly in pristane conditioned syngeneic transplant recipients. J-3 virus alone did not induce tumors in 45 non-pristane treated mice.

Six percent of the BALB/c mice also developed myeloid tumors during the same time periods. Myeloid tumors were diagnosed on the basis of characteristic monocyte/macrophage-like cells in ascites and tissue sections. Some of these tumors were also examined by flow cytometry for expression of cell surface antigens and were shown to be Mac-1$^+$, Fc receptor$^+$ and Ia$^+$.

Twelve plasmacytomas were transplanted and characterized for the presence of immunoglobulin (Ig) heavy and light chains by immunoperoxidase staining of fixed tissue sections. Cytoplasmic Ig was demonstrated in ten of the tumors by immunoperoxidase staining in fixed tissue sections. Eight tumors produced only IgA, three IgM and 2 produced more than two Ig classes; two tumors were non-producers. J3PC2095 was biclonal and contained two separate populations, one an IgA, the other IgM. The J3PC2094 contained a mixture of cells that contained IgG1 or IgM. It was not determined if the 2094 tumor cells produced both IgG1 and IgM.

Cytogenetic analysis of 9 of the plasmacytomas revealed eight of them did not have reciprocal translocations rcpt(12;15) or rcpt(6;15). The J3PC2095 did have rcpt(12;15) and a rearranged c-myc gene and did not produce avian myc mRNA. The other plasmacytomas (Table 2) transcribed abundant avian myc mRNAs and the c-myc loci were not rearranged.

Avian v-myc insertions were found in all of the tumors, usually revealed by a distinctive restriction fragment. This suggested the tumors were clonal and contained relatively few inserts.

The findings strongly suggest that avian c-myc sequences transduced into appropriate target B-cells by the Moloney retroviral helper played a role in plasmacytoma devlopment. The introduction and integration of J-3 virus into the genome of the B-cell target may not, however, have resulted in the development of an autonomous tumor in a single step. The relatively long mean latent period for most of the tumors suggests that other changes were required to convert the cell to a fully malignant status. The J-3 infected B-cell target cells may, however, express the changes that are related to the "immortalization-establishment phenomenon" described by others in transformation of rat embryo fibroblasts (Land et al. 1983), i.e., they may maintain B-cells in continuous cell cycle, thereby making these cells candidates for further mutations. Not all retroviruses that contain myc sequences are able to induce plasmacytomas (see Wolff 1986 and Baumbach et al. 1986, this book). This suggests that the hybrid MH2/MC29 v-myc gene in the absence of a function raf gene has special plasmacytomagenic properties.

This method for inducing plasmacytomas, i.e., injecting retroviruses 7 days post pristane provides several experimental advantages. First, plasmacytomas can be induced rapidly. Secondly, the requirement for chromosome 15 translocations is circumvented. Third, these tumors can be useful for defining second biochemical changes that are critical for plasmacytoma development and, finally, the role of other oncogenes and deregulated genes in plasma cell development can be explored.

REFERENCES

Land H, Parada LF, Weinberg RA (1983) Tumorigenic conversion of primary embryo fibroblasts requires at least two cooperating oncogenes. Nature (London) 304:596-602

Ohno S, Migita S, Wiener F, Babonits M, Klein G, Mushinski JF, Potter M (1984) Chromosomal translocations activating c-myc sequences and transduction of v-abl are critical events in the rapid

Potter M, Wax JS (1983) Peritoneal plasmacytomagenesis in mice. A comparison of three pristance dose regimens. J Natl Cancer Inst 71:391-395

Potter M, Sklar MD, Rowe WP (1973) Rapid viral induction of plasmacytomas in pristane primed BALB/c mice. Science 182:592-594 induction of plasmacytomas by pristane and Abelson virus. J Exp Med 159:

Rapp UR, Cleveland JL, Frederickson TN, Holmes KL, Morse HC III, Patschinsky T, Bister K (1985a) Rapid induction of hematopoietic

neoplasms in newborn mice by a raf(mil)/myc recombinant murine retrovirus. J Virol 55:23-33
Rapp UR, Cleveland JL, Brightman K, Scott A, Ihle JN (1985b) Abrogation of IL-3 and IL-2 dependence by recombinant murine retroviruses expressing v-myc oncogenes. Nature 317:434-438

Transformation and Insertional Mutagenesis In Vitro of Primary Hematopoietic Stem Cell Cultures

J.L. Cleveland*, Y. Weinstein**†, J.N. Ihle**, D.S. Askew**, and U.R. Rapp*

*Laboratory of Viral Carcinogenesis, National Cancer Institute, Frederick, Maryland 21701, USA.

INTRODUCTION

Deregulated expression of proto-oncogenes alone or in concert appears to be causally related to the development of many neoplasias in vertebrates. We have previously shown that the combination of two oncogenes, v-*raf* and v-*myc*, in an infectious murine retrovirus (the J-2 virus) is cumulative in terms of the types of tumors that are induced and synergistic in terms of the latencies with which the tumors develop relative to those induced by retroviruses carrying only v-*raf* and v-*myc* (Rapp et al., 1985b; Cleveland et al., 1986). Specifically, the v-*raf* carrying viruses, 3611 and J-1, induce fibrosarcomas and erythroid hyperplasia (Rapp et al., 1983a, 1983b, 1985b), whereas v-*myc* expressing viruses (J-3 and J-5) induce T and B cell lineage lymphomas, and more rarely, pancreatic and mammary carcinomas (Morse et al., submitted). The dual oncogene retrovirus, J-2, induced all of these neoplasms with a greatly reduced latency. Moreover, mice inoculated with J-2 virus generally die of multiple neoplasias. However, all neoplasms induced by this recombinant virus were clonal or oligoclonal in nature, suggesting that even the deregulated expression of two oncogenes was perhaps insufficient to maintain the transformed state and that unidentified additional events were also necessary.

The lymphomas of pre-B, B and T cell lineage caused by the J-2, J-3 and J-5 viruses were able to be established in culture without the addition of specific growth factors required by normal lymphocytes for viability. In experiments which utilized IL-3 and IL-2 dependent hematopoietic and lymphoid cells, we demonstrated that high levels of expression of v-myc can abrogate the requirements for these growth factors (Rapp et al., 1985c). In conjunction with the complementation between raf and myc in J-2 disease induction *in vivo*, these data were interpreted to indicate that v-*myc* and v-*raf* provided constitutive competence and progression signals, respectively, in driving transformed cells through the G_1 phase of the cell cycle (Rapp et al., 1985a).

Because of the preponderance of hematopoietic/lymphoid neoplasms induced by these viruses *in vivo*, we wished to test their transforming properties *in vitro* by infecting primary hematopoietic

**LBI-Basic Research Program, NCI-Frederick Cancer Research Facility, P.O. Box B, Frederick, Maryland 21701 USA.
†Faculty of Health Sciences, Unit of Microbiology and Immunology, Ben Gurion University of the Negev, Beer Sheva, Israel.

Current Topics in Microbiology and Immunology, Vol. 132

stem cell cultures. Two regimens were examined; the first involved infection of primary bone marrow from weanling C3H mice in the absence of exogenous growth factors and the second involved infection of murine fetal liver cultures in the presence of the growth factor interleukin-3 (IL-3) (Fig. 1).

TRANSFORMATION OF PRIMARY BONE MARROW CULTURES

Primary bone marrow (BM) cultures were infected overnight in the absence of exogenous growth factors with retroviruses carrying v-*raf* and/or v-*myc* or with helper virus alone and then were cultured in standard medium lacking exogenous growth factors. Under these conditions no growth was observed with untreated BM cells or with cells infected with helper virus, or with retroviruses carrying only v-*raf* (3611, J-1) or v-*myc* (J-3, J-5). In contrast, J-2 BM cells proliferated rapidly reaching a peak in cell number and rate of proliferation 14 days after infection and then decreased in their rate of proliferation. This decrease in proliferation was not due to changes in viral replication as assessed by infectious cell center assays. Following the proliferative phase of growth, during which there were free floating clusters of cells, the J-2 BM cells formed an adherent monolayer. These cultures then either became spontaneously proliferative or could be induced to proliferate by adding dextran based (cytodex) culture beads. Morphologically, J-2 BM cells were mature macrophages. Comparable results have been obtained in 10 independent experiments. By immunoflouresence and Northern blot hybridization the cells were found to express J-2 v-*raf* and v-*myc* RNA and protein (Blasi et al., 1985). Interestingly, neither J-2 infected BM cells nor J-2 infected mouse fibroblast cells expressed detectable levels of the endogenous c-*myc*. The observation that high levels of v-*myc* expression is associated with c-*myc* suppression has been shown in three different lineages of cells (Rapp et al., 1985c). Nuclear run on experiments indicate that the suppression of c-*myc* expression is at the level of transcription (unpublished results). Taken together, these data support a potential autoregulatory mechanism in the regulation of c-*myc* expression.

Several conclusions can be drawn from the above studies. First, there is an absolute requirement for expression of both v-*raf* and v-*myc* in the transformation of primary bone marrow cultures in the absence of specific growth factors. Second, these immortalized macrophages do not require specific growth factor supplements nor do they produce factors which are mitogenic for infected or uninfected cultures. Third, the lineage or target stem cell which the J-2 virus can infect and transform under the culture conditions used appears to be restricted to macrophages. Finally, when tested for clonality by Southern blot analysis of virus integrations, we have observed that one line is clonal and two others are pauciclonal. This indicates that either one or a few infected cells had a selective growth advantage and outgrew other infected cohorts or that an additional event(s), such as the activation of another proto-oncogene, could have allowed selective outgrowth of infected cells.

TRANSFORMATION OF PRIMARY FETAL LIVER CULTURES

In a second series of experiments, fetal liver cultures were infected with various transforming viruses in the presence of the stem cell growth factor interleukin-3 (IL-3). In these studies the viruses used have included helper virus alone or viruses carrying v-raf (3611 MSV and J-1), v-myc (J-3 and J-5), v-raf and v-myc (J-2), v-mos (Mo-MSV), v-Ha-ras (Ha-MSV), and v-abl (Ab-MuLV). The cultures were maintained in the presence of IL-3 for periods ranging from 2 weeks to 3 months and then characterized. To date, four lineages of cells have been isolated from these experiments, the more common ones being immortalized mast cells and macrophages and the rare ones being of myeloid and B cell lineage (Fig. 1).

The predominant cell types arising during the first 1-3 weeks in IL-3 supported fetal liver cultures are granulocytes and macrophages (Ihle et al., 1984, 1985). These cells lose their proliferative ability with terminal differentiation and become replaced by cells committed to the mast cell lineage which after 4 weeks become the exclusive cell type (Ihle, 1985). These mast cells persist in culture for up to 2-5 months then senesce and die out. Infection of fetal liver cultures with MuLV helper virus alone, or with Moloney pseudotypes of the v-myc J-3 and J-5 viruses failed to overtly transform fetal liver cultures. In contrast, when fetal liver cultures were infected with viruses carrying v-raf, v-Ha-ras, v-mos, and v-abl oncogenes, immortalized mast cell lines were consistently obtained (Rapp et al., 1985a; Ihle et al., 1985; Rein et al., 1985; Pierce et al., 1985). The mast cell lines immortalized by infection with v-raf, v-mos, and v-Ha-ras containing viruses required IL-3 for viability whereas the v-abl immortalized mast cells had lost their requirements for IL-3 for growth (Pierce et al., 1985). In contrast, when fetal liver cultures were infected with the J-2 virus factor independent macrophage-like cell lines were obtained which were morphologically similar to those obtained from the transformation of primary bone marrow cultures. Therefore, the specific transformation of macrophages in a second in vitro culture system also required expression of both raf and myc. J-2 transformed macrophages from fetal liver cultures were not growth factor independent due to an autocrine type of mechanism as conditioned medium from these cultures is not mitogenic when placed back upon these cultures.

INSERTIONAL MUTAGENESIS IN VITRO OF THE C-MYB PROTO-ONCOGENE

In the course of culturing J-2 infected fetal liver cultures, we obtained three unusual factor independent variant cell lines which appeared clonal according to the kinetics of their emergence. The properties of these cells are shown in Table 1. The IFLJ-2 cell line was clearly lymphoblastic and expressed markers such as Igμ, Ly-5 B220, and 6C3 which identified it as an early B cell. The IIFLJ-2 and IIIFLJ-2 cell lines, however, were clearly myeloblastic in morphology and expressed markers characteristic of IL-3 lineage related myeloid leukemia cells including RB6-8C5 and IL-3 receptors. However, neither the IIFLJ-2 nor the IIIFLJ-2 cell line requires exogenous IL-3 for growth in vitro. In addition, neither of the cell lines produced growth factors which were mitogenic for themselves or for factor dependent myeloid cell lines.

Since myeloid tumors have been shown to have rearrangements in the 5' (ABPL lymphosarcomas, Mushinski et al., 1984; Sheng-Ong et al., 1986; Reddy et al., 1986) and 3' regions of the c-myb proto-oncogene (Weinstein et al., 1986; Sheng-Ong et al., 1986; Reddy et al., 1986), we examined the c-myb gene in IFLJ-2, IIFLJ-2 and IIIFLJ-2 (Fig. 2) for possible rearrangements. Using a 5' 4.2 EcoRI c-myb gene probe no rearrangements were detected in any of the cell lines. However, when a 3' 1.5 kb EcoRI probe was used we observed rearrangements in IIFLJ-2 in EcoRI digests (a 9.2 kb fragment) and rearrangements in both IIFLJ-2 and IIIFLJ-2 in BamHI digests. As the IIIFLJ-2 c-myb rearrangement was only detected in BamHI but not in EcoRI digests this places this rearrangement 3' of the 1.5 kb c-myb EcoRI fragment. This rearrangement is currently being cloned and characterized. The rearrangement occurring in one allele of the 1.5 kb EcoRI c-myb fragment in IIFLJ-2 was very similar to that previously observed in another myeloid leukemia cell line, NFS-60 (Weinstein et al., 1986). This line had been shown to have a rearranged 10 kb EcoRI fragment. In the case of NFS-60 cell line it was demonstrated that the alteration was due to the insertion of a Cas-Br-M-MuLV type provirus in a 5' to 3' orientation within one allele of the 1.5 kb EcoRI fragment in the sixth exon of c-myb. Associated with proviral integration into this allele was the production of a truncated c-myb RNA containing LTR sequences (Weinstein et al., 1986) and protein (W. Boyle, Y. Weinstein, J. Ihle, unpublished data).

To assess the effects of the rearrangements in the IIFLJ-2 and IIIFLJ-2 cell lines on the transcription of c-myb, poly(A)$^+$ mRNAs was analyzed by Northern blot hybridization (Figure 3). The IFLJ-2 lymphoid cell line, as well as the myeloid leukemia cell lines FDC-P1 and NFS-58 expressed a normal sized c-myb mRNA of 3.6 kb. In contrast, the IIFLJ-2 cell line expressed high levels of a 2.0 kb transcript and lower levels of an RNA of 9.0 kb. Interestingly, no 3.6 kb c-myb mRNA was detectable, even though one allele is unaltered in this cell line (Figure 2). The IIIFLJ-2 cell line expressed appreciable levels of a slightly smaller c-myb mRNA of about 3.5 kb (Fig. 3).

The finding that the IIFLJ-2 cell line made a truncated mRNA of 2.0 kb similar to that previously observed with NFS-60 (Weinstein et al., 1986; Shen-Ong et al., 1986), was confirmed by a direct comparison of c-myb RNA from the two cell lines (Fig. 4). Both cell lines had high levels of transcript of 2.0 kb and undetectable levels of normal c-myb mRNA.

To further characterize the rearrangement in IIFLJ-2 cells, we cloned the rearranged 9.2 kbp c-myb fragment. Southern blot analysis of this fragment demonstrated that it contained LTR and env sequences detectable with MoLV specific probes. As shown in Figure 5, restriction enzyme mapping demonstrated that a 7.6 kbp MuLV provirus containing a 1.0 kb deletion in the pol gene, integrated in a 5' to 3' orientation within the 1.5 kb EcoRI c-myb fragment, approximately 500 bp from the 5' end. This insertion was indistinguishable from that of Cas-Br-M-MuLV occurring in the in vivo transformed NFS-60 myeloid cell (Fig. 6). Preliminary evidence indicates that the insertion occurred at the same nucleotide (unpublished results). This deleted provirus, as well as the defective J-2 and undeleted helper virus were expressed in IIFLJ-2 cells as assessed by Northern blot hybridization with LTR-specific probes (Fig. 3).

CONCLUSIONS

Our results suggest that the *in vitro* transformation of hematopoietic cells may require the alteration of several cellular functions. Similar to the adaptation of fibroblasts for long-term growth *in vitro*, an immortalizing event is required for establishing long-term cell lines. Immortalized hematopoietic cells generally retain an absolute dependence for growth factors and the abrogation of this factor dependence requires an additional change. Finally, specific events may also be associated with altering the hematopoietic stem cell intermediates ability to continue to terminally differeniate.

In primary hematopoietic stem cell cultures containing IL-3, a variety of lineages are observed including macrophages, granulocytes, megakaryocytes, eosinophils and mast cells. Among these only mast cells normally retain the ability to proliferate for a limited time *in vitro* as fully differentiated cells. In previous studies we have demonstrated that a variety of oncogenes can immortalize mast cells and allow the establishment of cell lines. These oncogenes include Ha-*ras*, v-*mos*, v-*abl* and v-*raf*. None of these oncogenes has been shown to affect the differentiation of normal hematopoietic cells and, with the exception of v-*abl*, the immortalized mast cell lines still require IL-3 for growth. In these cultures, v-*myc* only viruses have not yielded continuous cell lines. However, the combination of v-*myc* and v-*raf* in primary cultures in the presence or absence of IL-3 have consistently yielded continuous macrophage cell lines. The predominance of J-2 macrophage cell lines is possibly due to several factors. First, the proliferation and differentiation of hematopoietic stem cell progenitors is absolutely dependent on growth factors. Thus, in the absence of IL-3, the target cell populations available for transformation may be limited to cells such as macrophages which can survive in tissue culture long enough to be infected. In the presence of IL-3, we had expected that continuous mast cell lines would be obtained with the v-*raf*/v-*myc* virus. Since macrophage differentiation occurs early in IL-3 driven cultures prior to the emergence of mast cells it is possible that the outgrowth of J-2 transformed macrophages may either inhibit the growth of mast cell progenitors or, alternatively, that J-2 transformed macrophages simply outgrow mast cell components.

The precise contributions of v-*raf* and v-*myc* in the transformation of primary macrophages is not known. The cell lines differ from normal macrophages in at least two regards. First, the cells are "immortalized" for growth *in vitro*. As noted above, this property has been ascribed to v-*raf* in the establishment of mast cell lines and has not been shown to be a property of v-*myc*. Consistent with this, Vennstrom et al., (1985) demonstrated that while v-*myc* constructs altered the growth of primary macrophages no cell lines were obtained. Second, the macrophage lines we obtain do not require exogenous growth factors. The ability to abrogate the requirement for growth factors of established hematopoietic/lymphoid cell lines has been shown to be a property of the v-*myc* only viruses (Rapp et al., 1985). In the studies of Vennstrom et al., (1985) it was demonstrated that in primary cultures growth factors increased the frequency of macrophage colonies after infection with v-*myc* constructs; however, whether these infected macrophages continued to require growth factors was not addressed. From our results we speculate that the v-*raf* contributed an immortalizing "progression type" function whereas v-*myc* provides a "competence type" growth factor signal for these cells.

In addition to the macrophage cell lines, 3 cell lines were obtained which arose in a manner consistent with a clonal outgrowth. Initially the lines were striking in that they were either early B cells or early myeloid cells and were not differentiated macrophages or mast cells. In hematopoietic stem cell cultures, IL-3 supports the growth and continued differentiation of early myeloid cells and has been speculated to support the early differentiation of pre-B cells (Palacios and Steinmetz, 1985). Normally such cells continue to terminally differentiate thus suggesting that in the 3 lines the ability of the cells to continue differentiation had been altered. The clonal nature of the lines as well as the frequency with which they arose, suggests that activation of additional oncogenes may have occurred in these lines.

In previous studies, rearrangements of the c-*myb* gene by retroviral insertions have been implicated in the transformation of myeloid progenitor cells. For this reason the 3 lines were examined for potential rearrangements of the c-*myb* gene. Strikingly the two myeloid lines had rearrangements and one that was characterized (IIFLJ-2) had a retroviral insertion which resulted in a truncation of the c-*myb* gene product. Thus, in this line, there are three activated transforming genes each of which can be speculated to have contributed to the transformed phenotype in different ways. Specifically, v-*raf* immortalized the cells for growth *in vitro*, v-*myc* abrogated the requirement for growth factors and the rearranged c-*myb* altered the ability of the cells to terminally differentiate.

These results represent the first demonstration that one can activate protooncogenes by retroviral insertions in *in vitro* cultures of hematopoietic cells. We have also demonstrated the effectiveness of this approach in MuLV-mediated transformation of epitheleal rodent MMCE cells, but have as yet not identified the targets of insertional mutagenesis (Rapp and Keski-Oja, 1982). In the latter experiments, MuLV was used in conjunction with the tumor promoter 12-0-tetradecanoylphorbol 13-acetate (TPA) for the transformation of MMCE cells in culture and yielded cells containing activated oncogene(s) as determined by DNA transfection into NIH 3T3 cells. Therefore, this type of *in vitro* approach, i.e., the use of MuLV together with growth promoting agents for insertional mutagenesis, represents a potentially powerful tool by which one can identify cellular genes which have a selectable function in *in vitro* culture. The IL-3 culture system described here provides a potent mitogen for early stem cells and the growth conditions that are likely required for the occurrence and detection of rare events. In this mileau it appears that the activation of c-*myb* is a highly selectable event. By manipulating the culture conditions it is conceivable that the molecular events in leukemogenesis occurring *in vivo* can be duplicated *in vitro*. For example, the *in vitro* activation of the c-*myb* gene in the IIFLJ-2 myeloid cell line is identical to that observed in an *in vivo* myeloid leukemia (NFS-60). This could indicate that either there is sequence specificity for sites of integration that have not been identified and/or there is a limited number of integrations that are compatible with the activation of c-*myb*.

ACKNOWLEDGEMENTS

The authors gratefully acknowledge Ms. Patricia Borchert for her expert technical assistance, Kevin Holmes and H.C. Morse for flow microfluoremetry determination of Ly5B220 and $6^{C}3$ markers, and and Ms. Pamela Wahl-Lambert for her expert typing of this manuscript. Research sponsored by the National Cancer Institute, DHHS, under contract NO. NO1-CO-23909 with Litton Bionetics, Inc. The contents of this publication do not necessarily reflect the views or policies of the Department of Health and Human Services, nor does mention of trade names, commercial products, or organizations imply endorsement by the U.S. Government.

REFERENCES

Blasi E, Mathieson BJ, Varesio L, Cleveland JL, Borchart PA, Rapp UR (1985) Selective immortalization of murine macrophages from fresh bone marrow by a raf/myc recombinant murine retrovirus. Nature 318:667-670

Cleveland JL, Jansen HW, Bister K, Morse HC III, Ihle JN, Rapp UR (1986) Interaction between raf and myc oncogenes in transformation in vivo and in vitro. J Cell Biochem 30:195-218.

Ihle JN, Morse HC III, Keller J, Holmes K (1984) Interleukin-3 dependent retrovirus induced lymphomas: loss of the ability to terminally differentiate in response to differentiation factors. In: Gillis S, Inman FD (ed) Current Topics in Microbiology and Immunology Plenum Publishing Corporation, New York, vol 113, pp 86-91.

Ihle JN, (1985) Biochemical and biological properties of interleukin-3: A lymphokine mediating the differentiation of a lineage of cells that includes prothymocytes and mastlike cells. In: Gillis S and Inman FP (ed) Contemporary topics in molecular immunology, Plenum Publishing Corporation, New York, vol 10, p 93-119

Ihle JN, Keller J, Rein A, Cleveland J, Rapp U (1985) Interleukin-3 regulation of the growth of normal and transformed hematopoietic cells. In: Feramisco J, Ozanne B, Stiles C (ed) Cancer Cells 3: growth factors and transformation, Cold Spring Harbor Laboratory Publications, Cold Spring Harbor, New York, pp 211-219

Morse HC III, Hartley JW, Fredrickson TN, Yetter RA, Majumdar C, Cleveland JL, Rapp UR (1986) Recombinant murine retroviruses containing avian v-myc induce a wide spectrum of neoplasms in newborn mice. Proc Natl Acad Sci USA Submitted.

Mushinski JF, Potter M, Bauer SR, Reddy EP (1983) DNA rearrangement and altered RNA expression of the c-myb oncogene in mouse plasmacytoid lymphosarcomas. Science 220:795-798.

Palacios R, Steinmetz M (1985) IL-3 dependent mouse clones that express B-220 surface antigen, contain Ig genes in germ-line configuration, and generate B lymphocytes in vivo. Cell 41: 727-734.

Pierce JH, DiFiore PP, Aaronson SA, Potter M, Pumphrey J, Scott A, Ihle JN (1985) Neoplastic transformation of mast cells by Abelson-MuLV: abrogation of IL-3 dependence by a nonautocrine mechanism. Cell 41:685-693.

Rapp UR, Keski-Oja J (1982) Murine leukemia virus-mediated transformation of a mouse epitheleal cell line MMCE. Cancer Res 42:2407-2411.

Rapp UR, Reynolds FH Jr, Stephenson J (1983a) New mammalian transforming retrovirus: Demonstration of a polyprotein gene product. J Virol 45:914-924.

Rapp UR, Goldsborough MD, Mark GE, Bonner TI, Groffen J, Reynolds FH Jr, Stephenson J (1983b) Structure and biological activity of v-*raf*, a unique oncogene transduced by a retrovirus. Proc Natl Acad Sci USA 80:4218-4222.

Rapp UR, Bonner TI, Moelling K, Jansen HW, Bister K, Ihle JN (1985a) Genes and gene products involved in growth regulation of tumor cells. In: Recent Results in Cancer Research, Havemann K,

Rapp UR, Cleveland JL, Fredrickson TN, Holmes KL, Morse HC III, Jansen HW, Patschinsky T, Bister K (1985b) Rapid induction of hemopoietic neoplasms in newborn mice by a *raf*(*mil*)/*myc* recombinant murine retrovirus. J Virol 55:23-33

Sorenson G, Gropp C (eds) Springer-Verlag, Berlin p 221

Rapp UR, Cleveland JL, Brightman K, Scott A, Ihle JN (1985c) Abrogation of IL-3 and IL-2 dependence by recombinant murine retroviruses expressing v-*myc* oncogenes. Nature 317:434-438.

Reddy EP, Lavu S (1986) Structural organization and nucleotide sequence of mouse c-*myb* oncogene: Activation in ABPL tumors is due to viral integration in an intron which results in the deletion of the five prime coding sequence. Nucleic Acids Res, in press

Rein A, Keller J, Schultz AM, Holmes KL, Medicus R, Ihle JN (1985) Infection of immune mast cells by Harvey sarcoma virus: immortalization without loss of requirement for interleukin-3. Mol Cell Biol 5:2257-2264.

Shen-Ong GL, Potter M, Mushinski JF, Lavu S, Reddy EP (1984) Activation of the c-*myb* locus by viral insertional mutagenesis in plasmacytoid lymphosarcomas. Science 226:1077-1080.

Vennstrom B, Kahn P, Adkins B, Enrietto P, Hayman MJ, Graf T, Luciw P (1984) Transformation of mammalian fibroblasts and macrophages *in vitro* by a murine retrovirus encoding an avian v-*myc* oncogene. The EMBO J 3:3223-3229

Weinstein Y, Ihle JN, Lavu S, Reddy EP (1986) Truncation of the c-myb gene by a retroviral integration in an interleukin-3 dependent myeloid leukemia cell line. Proc Natl Acad Sci USA, in press.

Table 1. Properties of transformed fetal liver cell lines

Cell Line	Morphology	Ig	Thy-1	Ly-5 B220	6C3	RB6-8C5	IL 3 Receptors	Factor Dependence
IFLJ-2	Lymphoid	+	-	+	+++	-	-	-
IIFLJ-2	Myeloblast	-	-	-	-	20%	+	-
IIIFLJ-2	Myeloblast	-	-	-	-	20%	+	-
NFS-60	Myeloblast	-	+	-	NT	-	+	+
ABPL-2	Myeloblast	-	-	NT	NT	18%	+	-

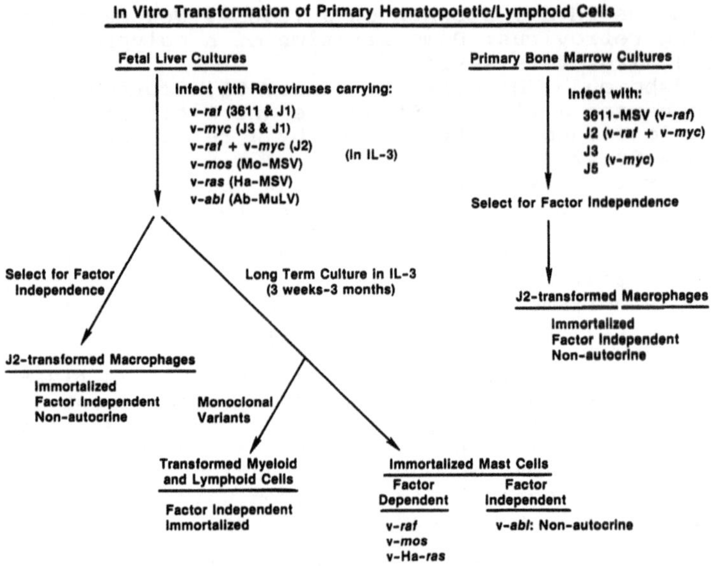

Fig. 1. Derivation of transformed cell lines from murine primary bone marrow or fetal liver cultures by infection with various retroviruses.

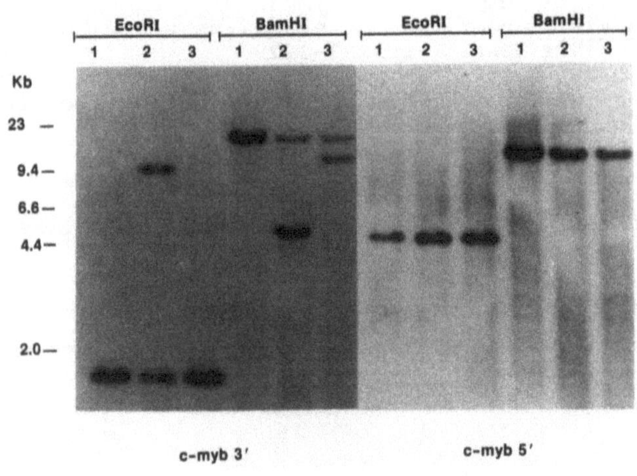

Fig. 2. Rearrangements of the c-myb locus in Southern blots of DNA from transformed myeloid cell lines. DNA was purified from IFLJ-2 (lanes 1), IIFLJ-2 (lanes 2), and IIIFLJ-2 (lanes 3) restricted with EcoRII and BamHI, electrophoresed on agrose gels and transformed to nitrocellulose. The filters were then hybridized with the indicated nick translated ^{32}P probe.

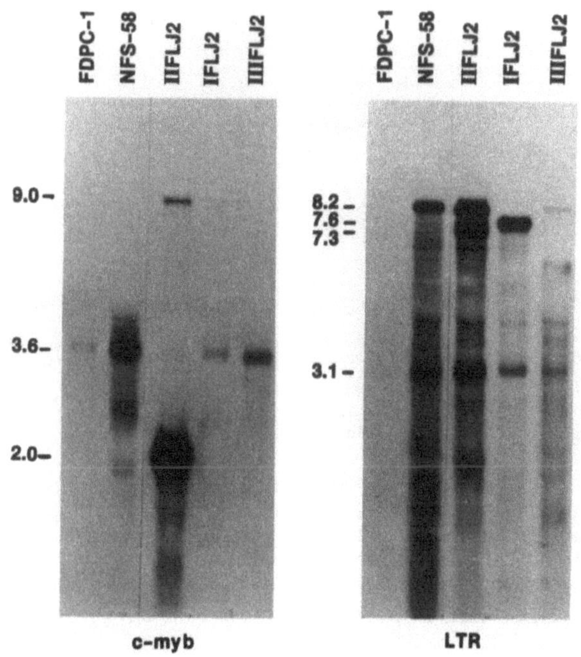

Fig. 3. Expression of c-*myb* and retroviruses in *in vitro* derived transformed pre-B (IFLJ-2) and myeloid (II and IIIFLJ-2) cell lines. PolyA+ RNA (5 mg) was denatured with formamide/formaldehyde, electrophoresed, and blotted into nitrocellulose. Blots were hybridized with ^{32}P-labelled 0.5 kb c-*myb* and Mo-MuLV LTR probes. For comparison, RNAs from myeloid leukemia cell lines FDC-P1 and NFS-58 were also analyzed.

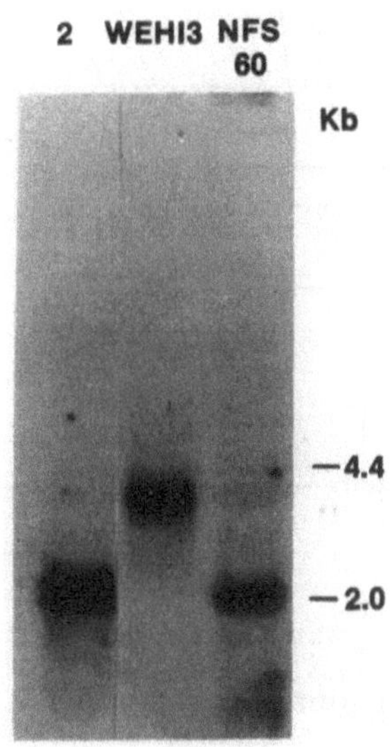

Fig. 4. Comparison of truncated c-*myb* RNAs from IIFLJ-2 and NFS-60 and the normal c-*myb* RNA from the WEHI myelomonocytic leukemia cell line.

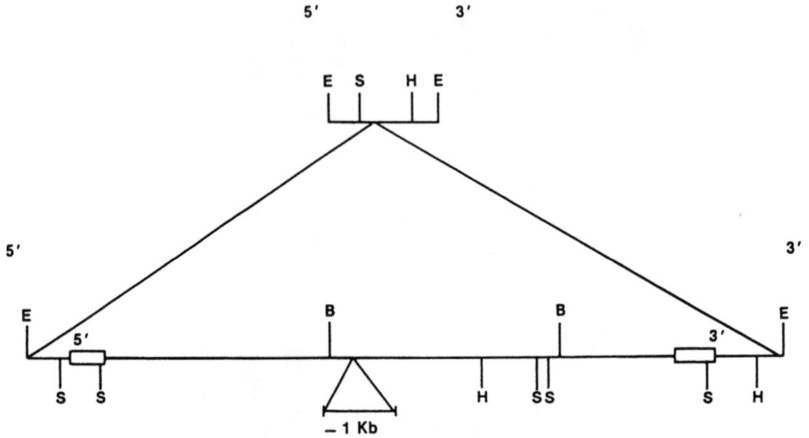

Fig. 5. Restriction enzyme map of the normal and rearranged c-*myb* *EcoRI* fragments from IIFLJ-2 cell line. The restriction maps for the normal 1.5 kbp fragment (top) and the rearranged 9.2 kbp fragment were determined by standard double digests with the indicated enzymes. E, *EcoRI*; H, *HindII*; B, *BglII*; S, *SacI*; X, *XbaI*; P, *PstI*; *Pvu*, *PvuII*.

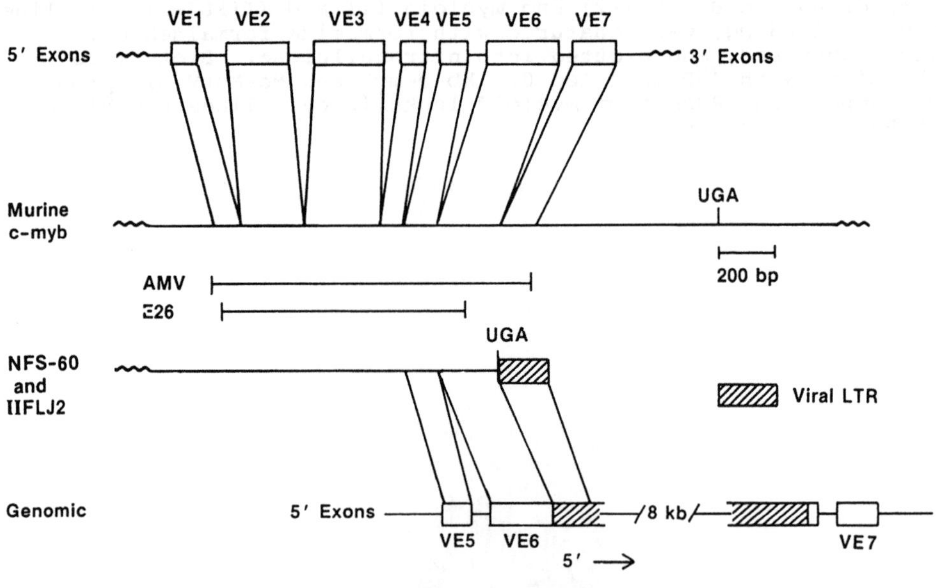

Fig. 6. Comparison of the structure of the normal c-*myb* gene with the rearranged c-*myb* genes in IIFLJ-2 and NFS-60. The structure of the transduced avian v-*myb* genes are also shown for comparison.

Mammalian Cell Transformation by a Recombinant Murine Retrovirus Containing the Avian Erythroblastosis Virus *erb*B Gene

J. H. Pierce, A. Gazit, P. P. Di Fiore, M. Kraus, C. Y. Pennington, K. L. Holmes*, W. F. Davidson*, H. C. Morse III*, and S. A. Aaronson

Laboratory of Cellular and Molecular Biology and *Laboratory of Immunopathology, National Cancer Institute, Bethesda, MD 20892

INTRODUCTION

Avian erythroblastosis virus (AEV) is a replication-defective retrovirus which induces erythroblastosis, sarcomas and carcinomas in chickens and transforms immature avian erythroid and fibroblastic cells in vitro (Graf and Beug, 1978). The genome of AEV contains two distinct oncogenes, v-erbA and v-erbB (Vennström and Bishop, 1982). V-erbB is a member of the src family of retroviral oncogenes (Yamamoto et al., 1983). The products of these src-related oncogenes as well as the receptors for several growth factors have been shown to exhibit tyrosine-specific kinase activity (Hunter and Cooper, 1985). Recently, it has been found that the v-erbB gene sequence possesses extensive homology with the mammalian epidermal growth factor (EGF) receptor gene (Downward et al., 1984). Analysis of the range of mammalian target cells susceptible to transformation by v-erbB has been impaired by difficulties in introducing this avian virus into mammalian cells. Therefore, we constructed a recombinant v-erbB-containing murine retrovirus which has allowed for more extensive investigation of the function of this EGF receptor-related gene as a transforming or growth-promoting gene in well defined mammalian systems.

Construction and Characterization of a Murine Retrovirus Vector Containing the AEV erbB Gene

The strategy employed for construction of a murine retrovirus vector containing the entire v-erbB gene is summarized in Fig. 1. Briefly, a restriction fragment containing the v-erbB gene derived from a molecular clone of AEV (Vennstrom et al., 1980) was inserted into a modified molecular clone of Moloney murine leukemia virus (Mo-MuLV) (Bachelor and Fan, 1981) and designated MuLV/erbB. No v-erbA sequences were present in this construct. MuLV/erbB DNA had a transforming efficiency of 4-15 x 10^3 foci per μg DNA insert in the NIH/3T3 transfection assay (Table 1). Cells from the MuLV/erbB-induced foci exhibited a dense fusiform morphology similar to AEV-transformed chicken embryo fibroblasts and possessed known properties of malignant cells, including their ability to grow in soft agar and form tumors in nude mice (Table 1). Transfectant foci induced by MuLV/erbB vector DNA were nonproductive due to the defective nature of the viral construct. In order to generate infectious transforming virus, nonproducer foci were infected with amphotrophic murine leukemia virus (Amph-MuLV). The presence of rescued murine erbB-containing virus, designated murine-erbB (M-erbB) virus, was detected by the induction of transformed foci on NIH/3T3 cells from culture supernatants of Amph-MuLV-infected transfectants. The transmission of the MuLV/erbB genome into NIH/3T3 cells infected with the rescued M-erbB virus was confirmed by DNA (Fig. 2, lane 7) and protein analysis (Fig. 3, lane 3A).

Current Topics in Microbiology and Immunology, Vol. 132

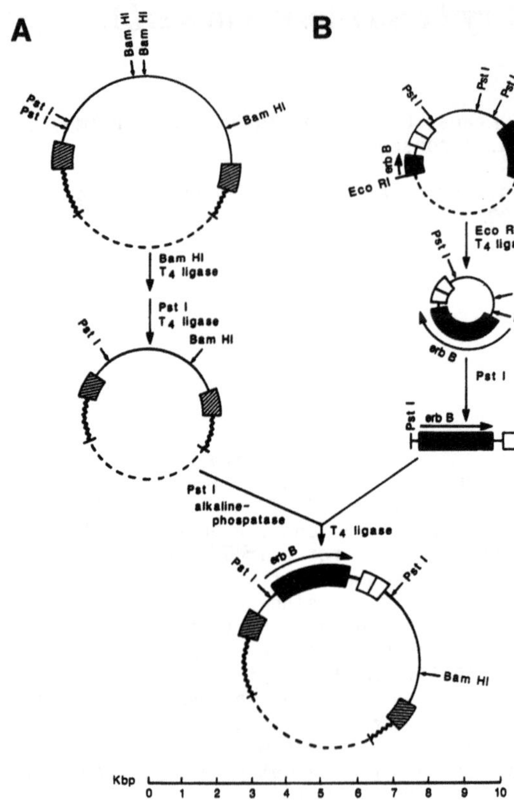

Fig. 1. Construction of MuLV/erbB plasmid. (A) Construction of MuLV vector. Moloney-MuLV integrated DNA subcloned in pBR322 (devoid in Bam HI and Pst I sites) was digested with Bam HI enzyme. Following purification of the 12.4-kbp Bam HI fragment and religation, the DNA was digested with Pst I and the purified 12.2-kbp Pst I fragment was religated. The resulting MuLV vector contained a unique Pst I site. (B) Insertion of v-erbB coding sequence into the MuLV vector. The permuted AEV provirus (Vennström et al., 1980) was purified from pBR313 sequences by Eco RI digestion and religation of the 5.3-kbp Eco RI AEV fragment. The circular AEV provirus molecule was then digested with Pst I, and the 3.5-kbp Pst I fragment encompassing the colinear v-erbB region was purified and inserted into the Pst I site of the MuLV vector DNA. Hatched boxes represent Mo-MuLV LTRs; open boxes are avian LTRs; and black box is the v-erbB gene.

Table 1. Transfection Analysis of MuLV/erbB DNA Constructs

Donor DNA	No. foci per µg DNA	Focus designation	Properties of MuLV/erbB DNA transformed cells: Saturation density (cells x 10^{-5} per cm^2)	% Colony formation in soft agar	Tumor incidence
MuLV/erbB No. 399/2	4 x 10^3	422.12.3	1.5	5-10	10/10
		422.13.1	2.5	5-10	10/10
		422.14.1	2.5	5-10	10/10
		422.15.1	2.0	2-5	10/10
MuLV/erbB No. 399/5	5 x 10^4	NT	NT	NT	NT
Calf thymus	<0.1	NIH/3T3	1.0	<0.01	0/10

Hematopoietic Cell Transformation by M-erbB Virus

To investigate the transforming potential of M-erbB virus for hematopoietic cells, normal NFS/N mouse bone marrow or fetal liver cell suspensions were infected with M-erb virus (Amph-MuLV) and suspended in soft agar medium containing 50 μM 2-mercaptoethanol. By 8 to 12 days, growing colonies were observed in M-erbB virus-infected but not in control cultures (Table 2). Cells from these colonies possessed a blast cell morphology and could be established as continuous cell lines without the use of adherent feeder layers. The hematopoietic cell transformants contained v-erbB DNA sequences (Fig. 2, lanes 2-4) and synthesized v-erbB-related proteins with molecular sizes of 58 and 66 kilodaltons (Fig. 3, lanes 4A-6A). Cells from these lines formed colonies in soft agar at a very high efficiency and large hematopoietic tumors when inoculated subcutaneously into syngeneic mice (data not shown).

Table 2. In Vitro Hematopoietic Colony Formation Induced by M-erbB Virus

Focus-forming units added per plate	Colony formation* (CFU per plate) induced by: M-erbB (Amph-MuLV)		Abelson-MuLV (Amph-MuLV)	
	Bone Marrow	Fetal Liver	Bone Marrow	Fetal Liver
10^5	TMC	TMC	TMC	TMC
10^4	8, 5	8, 6	TMC	TMC
10^3	1, 0	1, 1	9, 18	16, 8
10^2	0, 0	0, 0	1, 2	2, 0
FFU/CFU	2×10^3	10^3	6.7×10^1	10^2

*Bone marrow on fetal liver cell suspensions from NFS/N mice were infected with varying virus dilutions and plated at a concentration of 2×10^6 nucleated cells per plate into soft agar medium containing RPMI-1640 with 20% fetal calf serum and 50 μM 2-mercaptoethanol. Hematopoietic colony formation was scored at day 14.

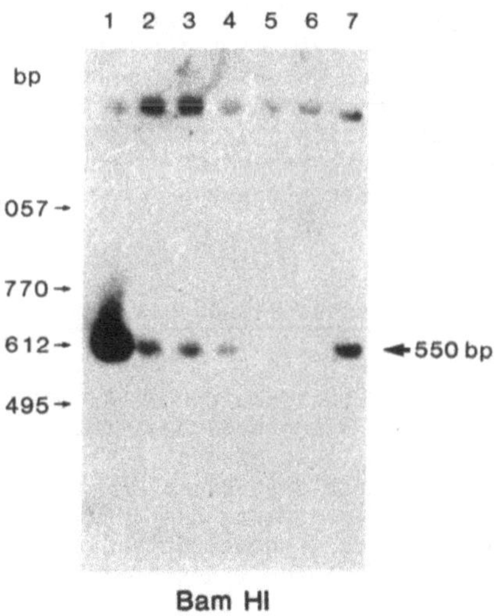

Fig. 2. Detection of v-erbB DNA sequences in individual M-erbB virus-transformed hematopoietic cell lines. High molecular weight DNAs were digested with Bam HI, which generates a 0.55-kbp v-erbB-specific fragment and hybridized to a ^{32}P-labeled nick-translated v-erbB-specific probe. DNAs are from MuLV/erbB-induced transfectant 422.14.1 (lane 1); individual M-erbB-virus-transformed hematopoietic cell lines (lanes 2-4); uninfected NIH/3T3 cells (lane 5); Abelson-MuLV-transformed hematopoietic cell line (lane 6); and M-erbB virus-transformed NIH/3T3 cells (lane 7).

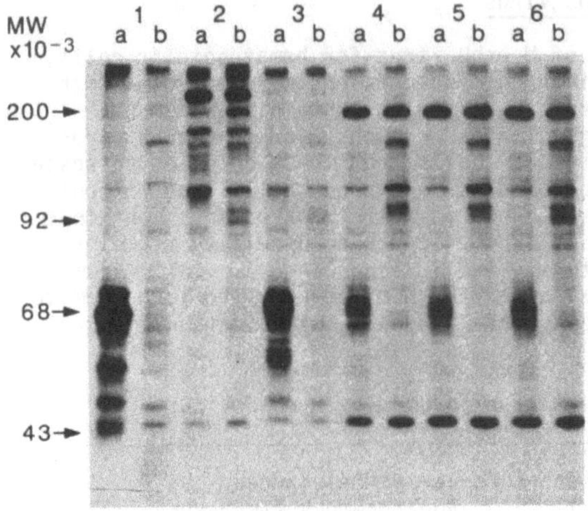

Fig. 3. Immunoprecipitation and electrophoretic analysis of v-erbB-specific translational products in M-erbB virus-transformed hematopoietic cell lines. Cell extracts from [^{35}S]-methionine-labeled AEV-transformed avian erythroblasts (lane 1); Abelson-MuLV-transformed hematopoietic cells (lane 2); M-erbB virus-transformed NIH/3T3 cells (lane 3); M-erbB virus-transformed hematopoietic cell lines (lanes 4-6) were treated with rabbit anti-v-erbB serum (a lanes), or normal rabbit serum (b lanes).

Phenotypic characterization of M-erbB virus induced hematopoietic cell lines revealed that they lacked markers of mature cells within the erythroid and myeloid lineages (Table 3). By contrast, all cell lines analyzed possessed cell surface antigens thought to be specific to early B lymphoid cells, including Lyb2, B220, and 6C3 (Coffman, 1982) (Table 3). In addition, several transformants synthesized high levels of terminal deoxynucleotidyl transferase, a marker associated with immature lymphoid cells (Bollum, 1979). Moreover, all lines analyzed were rearranged for the D-J immunoglobulin heavy chain gene region, and 3/10 lines synthesized cytoplasmic μ chain as determined by radioimmunoassay (Table 3). These results indicate that the M-erbB virus is capable of transforming murine pre-B cells similar to those that are preferentially obtained after Abelson-MuLV infection of normal hematopoietic cells (Siden *et al*., 1979).

Our studies also revealed that M-erbB virus was capable of inducing pre-B cell neoplasia in vivo. Intraperitoneal inoculation of newborn NIH/Swiss mice induced nonthymic lymphomas within 6 to 8 weeks. The pathology of the M-erbB virus-induced disease was remarkably similar to that observed after Abelson-MuLV infection (Abelson and Rabstein, 1970). The majority of M-erbB-infected mice developed swollen heads with lymphomatous infiltrates and some developed subcutaneous masses which were comprised of malignant lymphoid cells. Cells from the bone marrow of these mice also formed colonies in the soft agar assay at a high efficiency and cell lines could easily be established from these tumors. Phenotypic characterization revealed that the in vivo-derived M-erbB virus-induced lines also possessed pre-B cell characteristics (Table 3).

M-erbB Virus-Transformed Hematopoietic Cell Lines do not Possess Detectable Levels of EGF Receptors

In order to determine whether the presence of EGF receptors was required on target cells for transformation by M-erbB virus, we analyzed NIH/3T3 and hematopoietic cell transformants for the presence of such receptors. As illustrated in Table 4, M-erbB virus-infected NIH/3T3 cells possessed readily detectable levels of EGF receptors based on their ability to bind iodinated EGF. By contrast, M-erbB virus-transformed hematopoietic cell lines lacked binding activity, suggesting that the presence of EGF receptors on target cell is not a prerequisite for transformation

Table 3. Phenotypic Characterization of M-*erbB* Virus-Transformed Hematopoietic Cell Lines

Lineage	Marker	No. positive/ No. tested
Erythroid	Hemoglobin	0/10
	+ DMSO	0/10
	+ erythropoietin	0/10
	Spectrin	0/10
Myeloid	Lysozyme	0/10
	Nonspecific esterase	0/10
	Nonspecific phagocytosis	0/10
	Mac-1	0/10
Lymphoid	Thy-1	0/5
	Ly-1	2/5
	Ly-2	0/5
	Lyb-2	5/5
	B220	5/5
	6C3	5/5
	Fc receptor	5/5
	TdT	8/10
	IgJ_H rearrangement	10/10
	$IgJ\kappa$ rearrangement	1/10
	Cytoplasmic μ	3/10
	Cytoplasmic κ	0/10

by this virus. It should be noted that an Abelson-MuLV-induced pre-B cell line also lacked binding activity, indicating that EGF receptors are absent on all pre-B cell transformants. Therefore, the lack of detectable receptors on M-*erbB*-virus-transformed pre-B lines is probably not due to specific down regulation of such receptors.

SUMMARY

AEV is known to transform both avian fibroblasts and erythroblasts in vitro (Graf and Beug, 1978). Although studies employing deletion mutants in v-*erbA* or v-*erbB* have indicated that v-*erbB* is the principal transforming gene of AEV and is sufficient for inducing fibroblast transformation (Frykberg *et al*., 1983; Sealy *et al*., 1983), v-*erbA* is thought to cooperate with v-*erbB* to enhance transformation and block differentiation of avian erythroblasts (Kahn *et al*., 1984). Therefore, we were interested in investigating whether the murine recombinant v-*erbB*-containing retrovirus generated in our laboratory, which does not contain any v-*erbA* sequences, was capable of transforming murine hematopoietic cells. We demonstrated that M-*erbB* virus transformed immature hematopoietic cells both in vitro and in vivo. M-*erbB* virus-induced hematopoietic colonies could be established in culture as continuous clonal lines with high proliferative capacity. Their ability to form rapidly growing tumors of donor origin confirmed their malignant potential.

Table 4. Expression of EGF Receptors on M-*erbB* Virus-Transformed Fibroblast and Hematopoietic Cell Lines

Cell type	Transformant	% EGF binding (relative to uninfected NIH/3T3 cells)
Fibroblasts	M-*erbB* virus	
	1	29.7
	2	48.6
	3	45.9
	4	54.0
Hematopoietic	M-*erbB* virus	
	1	<0.1
	2	<0.1
	3	<0.1
	4	<0.1
	Abelson-MuLV	
	1	<0.1

The hematopoietic blast cell transformants induced by M-*erbB* virus did not express phenotypic markers associated with cells within the erythroid lineage. However, all in vitro and in vivo derived lines analyzed possessed several characteristics of early cells within the B lymphoid lineage. They expressed several pre-B cell-specific antigens (Coffman, 1982), possessed Fc receptors (Kerbel and Davis, 1974), and had detectable levels of TdT (Bollum, 1979). All transformants analyzed were rearranged for the D-J region of the immunoglobulin heavy chain and several synthesized immunoglobulin μ chain in the absence of light chains. Thus, the hematopoietic cells transformed by M-*erbB* virus appeared to be at an early stage of B cell differentiation similar to the pre-B cell phenotype of Abelson-MuLV hematopoietic cell transformants (Siden *et al.*, 1979). Moreover, the pathology of the M-*erbB* virus-induced disease in mice was strikingly similar to that observed after Abelson-MuLV infection (Abelson and Rabstein, 1970).

Although we did not observe any transformation of erythroid cells, it is possible that the culture conditions employed in our assay system lacked specific components required for detection of erythroid colonies (Hankins and Scolnick, 1981). Alternatively, the difference in hematopoietic target cell susceptibility may be due to the absence of v-*erbA* sequences in the murine construct. Finally, recent studies have indicated that the retroviral long terminal repeat may influence the expression of the viral genome in different tissues and play a role in the disease spectrum observed (Chatis *et al.*, 1983; Desgroseiller *et al.*, 1983). We are currently investigating the effects of M-*erbB* virus in an assay developed to detect erythroid burst formation in response to murine retroviruses (Hankins and Scolnick, 1981) in an attempt to resolve this question.

We previously determined that M-*erbB* virus was capable of transforming cells of both fibroblastic and epithelial origin. Since these cell types are known to possess EGF receptors, it was possible that the transforming potential of an oncogene coding for an activated form of a growth factor receptor would be restricted to cells bearing such receptors. However, analysis of M-*erbB* virus-transformed hematopoietic cells revealed that they did not express detectable levels of EGF receptors.

These findings support the concept that the range of target cells whose growth can be altered by an oncogene that possesses homology with growth factor receptor is not limited to cells that utilized that particular growth factor regulatory pathway for proliferation. Therefore, transformation by a growth factor receptor-related oncogene does not necessarily occur by substituting for that particular growth factor receptor function and may act at a point distal to receptor activation.

REFERENCES

Abelson HT, Rabstein LS (1970) Lymphosarcoma: virus-induced thymic-independent disease in mice. Cancer Res 30:2213-2222

Bacheler L, Fan H (1981) Isolation of recombinant DNA clones carrying complete integrated proviruses of Moloney murine leukemia virus. J Virol 37:181-190

Bollum FT (1979) Terminal deoxynucleotidyl transferase as a hematopoietic cell marker. Blood 54:1203-1215

Chatis PA, Holland CA, Hartley JW, Rowe WP, Hopkins N (1983) Role for the 3' end of the genome in determining disease specificity of Friend and Moloney murine leukemia viruses. Proc Natl Acad Sci 80:4408-4411

Coffman RL (1982) Surface antigen expression and immunoglobulin gene rearrangement during mouse pre-B cell development. Immunol Rev 69:5

DesGroseillers L, Rassart E, Jolicoeur P (1983) Thymotropism of murine leukemia virus is conferred by its long terminal repeat. Proc Natl Acad Sci 80:4203-4207

Downward J, Yarden Y, Mayes E, Scrace G, Totty N, Stockwell P, Schlessinger J, Waterfield MD (1984) Close similarity of epidermal growth factor receptor and v-erbB oncogene protein sequences. Nature 307:521:527

Frykberg L, Palmieri S, Beug H, Graf T, Hayman MJ, Vennstrom B (1983) Transforming capacities of avian erythroblastosis virus mutants deleted in the erbA or erbB oncogenes. Cell 32:227-238

Graf T, Beug H (1978) Avian leukemia viruses: interaction with their target cells in vivo and in vitro. Biochim Biophys Acta 516:269-299

Hankins DW, Scolnick EM (1981) Harvey and Kirsten sarcoma viruses promote the growth and differentiation of erythroid precursor cells in vitro. Cell 26:91-97

Hunter T, Cooper JA (1985) Protein-tyrosine kinases. Annu Rev Biochem 54:897-930

Kahn P, Adkins B, Beug H, Graf T (1984) Src- and fps-containing avian sarcoma viruses transform chicken erythroid cells. Proc Natl Acad Sci 81:7122-7126

Kerbel RS, Pross HF, Elliot EV (1975) Origin and partial characterization of Fc receptor-bearing cells found within experimental carcinomas and sarcomas. Int J Cancer 15:918-932

Sealy L, Privalsky ML, Moscovici G, Moscovici C, Bishop JM (1983) Site-specific mutagenesis of avian erythroblastosis virus: erbB is required for oncogenicity. Virology 130:155-178

Siden E, Baltimore D, Clark P, Rosenberg N (1979) Immunoglobulin synthesis by lymphoid cells transformed in vitro by Abelson murine leukemia virus. Cell 16:389-396

Vennström B, Bishop JM (1982) Isolation and characterization of chicken DNA homologous to the two putative oncogenes of avian erythroblastosis virus. Cell 28:135-143

Vennström B, Fanshier L, Moscovici C, Bishop JM (1980) Molecular cloning of the avian erythroblastosis virus genome and recovery of oncogenic virus by transfection of chicken cells. J Virol 36:575-585

Yamamoto T, Nishida T, Miyajima N, Kawai S, Oi T, Toyoshima K (1983) The erbB gene of avian erythroblastosis virus is a member of the src gene family. Cell 35:71-78

Determinants of Abelson Murine Leukemia Virus Pathogenesis

Patrick L. Green, Gina D. Holland, Donal Kaehler, John McKearn*, James McCubrey*, and Rex Risser

McArdle Laboratory for Cancer Research, University of Wisconsin, Madison, WI and *E.I.duPont deNemours & Co., Glenolden Laboratory, Glenolden, PA.

INTRODUCTION

The Abelson murine leukemia virus (A-MuLV) is a rapidly transforming, defective retrovirus that induces pre-B cell tumors in susceptible mice (Abelson and Rabstein 1970, Scher and Siegler 1974, Rosenberg and Baltimore 1976, Risser et al 1978). It encodes the v-abl p160 transforming protein, a tyrosine-kinase viral oncogene product. The v-abl oncogene was formed by the fusion of the Moloney MuLV (M-MuLV) gag gene with cellular c-abl sequences (Reynolds et al 1978, Witte et al 1978). The A-MuLV genome is a genetic recombinant of M-MuLV with the c-abl proto-oncogene (Wang et al 1984), and thus expression of the v-abl gene is controlled by the LTR derived from M-MuLV. Although M-MuLV induces predominantly T-cell tumors, A-MuLV induces pre-B cell tumors. The tissue tropism of M-MuLV is controlled by the LTR (Chatis et al 1983).

Experiments with mutants of A-MuLV have demonstrated that the v-abl protein is required for transformation (Witte et al 1980). Other experiments indicate that initial infection of mouse bone marrow cells is not sufficient for complete in vitro cell transformation (Whitlock et al 1983). Using the NIH3T3 assay for detection of dominant transforming genes Lane et al detected a non-abl transforming gene in A-MuLV tumor DNA (1982). Among other activities A-MuLV has been shown to render IL-3-dependent mast cells and myeloid lines independent of growth factor following infection and subsequent subculture (Cook et al 1985, Pierce et al 1985). In this paper we report our findings on the pathogenesis of A-MuLV tumors as they relate to questions of tumor progression, activation of non-abl transforming genes, the tissue specificity of A-MuLV, the activity of helper-free A-MuLV, and the activity of A-MuLV in IL-3-dependent pre-B cell lines.

RESULTS

Clonal Dominance in A-MuLV Tumors

Most A-MuLV virus pools contain helper virus, frequently M-MuLV. Virus is capable of growth in vivo, and high titers of A-MuLV and M-MuLV are recovered from susceptible infected mice (Risser et al 1978). Thus, one could anticipate that many potential target cells would be transformed in vivo and the resulting tumors would be polyclonal. To test this hypothesis mice were infected with A-MuLV and followed for tumor formation which generally occurred about 30 days post-infection. Primary tumors were excised along with involved peripheral lymphoid organs, and DNAs extracted. DNA was digested with

Current Topics in Microbiology and Immunology, Vol. 132

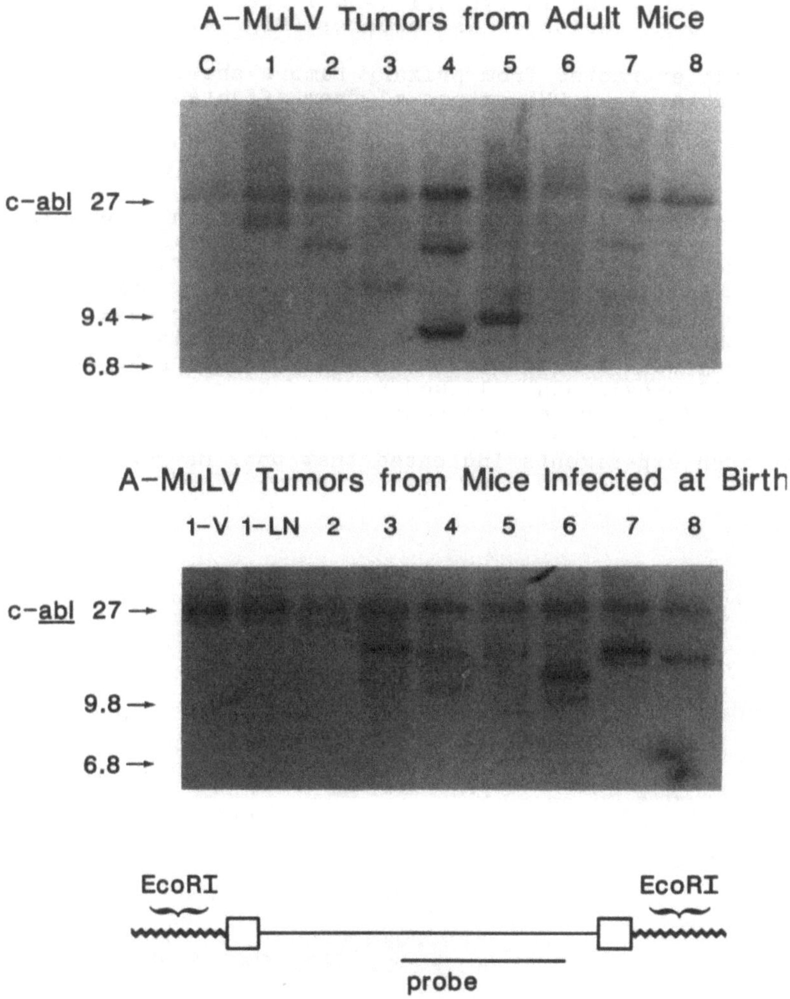

Fig. 1. A-MuLV Proviruses in Primary A-MuLV Tumors

EcoRI, which does not cleave within the A-MuLV provirus, and analyzed by Southern blotting with an A-MuLV-specific probe. The results of such analysis, indicated that each tumor showed 1-3 major hybridizing bands in addition to the 27 kilobase (kb) band expected for c-abl (Fig. 1). These results indicated that A-MuLV tumors were not polyclonal but rather mono- or oligoclonal. The predominance of a few major sites of integration was seen in A-MuLV induced thymomas

(Risser et al 1985), and in typical A-MuLV pre-B cell tumors arising in mice infected as adults or as newborns (Fig. 1, bottom panel).

Analysis of DNA extracted from primary tumors showed the same A-MuLV integration patterns as DNA extracted from affected peripheral tissues of the same mouse (Fig. 1, lower panel 1-V and 1-LN). Thus clones of cells derived from very few (1-3) infected cells dominate the tumor population by the time that tumors are detected by gross pathology.

One possible explanation for clonal dominance is that few cells are infected in vivo. To determine if that were the case we infected mice with A-MuLV and removed bone marrow 14 days after infection, approximately half-way through the latency period. DNA was prepared from total bone marrow, digested with XbaI, which cleaves once in the LTR of A-MuLV, and analyzed by Southern analysis. This experiment done along with a reconstruction analysis using known equivalents of A-MuLV proviruses allowed us to determine the approximate number of A-MuLV proviruses per bone marrow cell. In reconstruction experiments we could detect 0.01 to 0.02 proviruses per cell. The results of such experiments indicated that bone marrow cells from

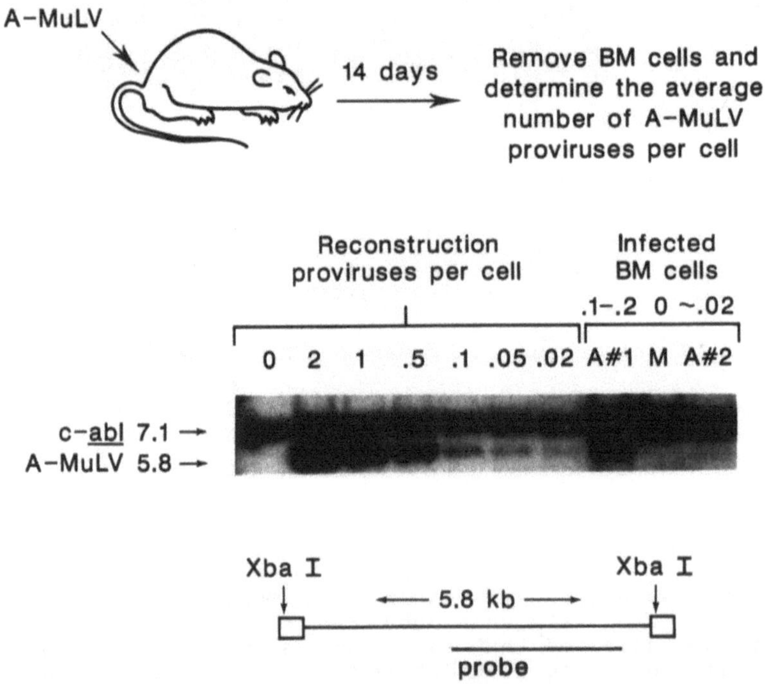

Fig. 2. Quantitation of A-MuLV Proviruses in Preleukemic Bone Marrow of A-MuLV Infected Mice

14-day A-MuLV infected mice carry the equivalent of 0.01 to 0.2 A-MuLV proviruses per cell, or 1-20 % of bone marrow cells are infected (Fig. 2). To determine if particular clones dominate this infected cell population, the DNA of infected bone marrow was cleaved with EcoRI and analyzed as in Fig. 1 along with DNA in a reconstruction experiment. This experiment demonstrated that although we could detect the equivalent of 0.05 proviruses per cell, no distinct integration bands were detected in DNA from infected bone marrow (data not shown). Therefore we conclude that within the limits of resolution of these methods infection of mice *in vivo* by A-MuLV is polyclonal but tumor formation is mono- or oligoclonal.

It is possible that transformation, unlike infection, is a rare event *in vivo*. In that case transformed cells would only predominate shortly before overt tumor formation. To test that hypothesis we have used the *in vitro* transformation assay of Rosenberg and Baltimore (1978) to study the time course of appearance of transformed cells in bone marrow of A-MuLV-infected mice. Bone marrow was removed from mice at 7 and 14 days post-infection and from lymphomatous mice. Bone marrow cells were plated in 0.35% agarose and the number of colonies scored two weeks later. The results of that experiment, presented below in Table 1, indicate that transformed cells are detectable at 7 and at 14 days post-infection and would number 2000 in total mouse bone marrow at 14 days post-infection. Thus transformation *in vivo*, as measured by this assay, is not a rare event. The simplest explanation for the emergence of mono- or oligoclonal A-MuLV tumors is that tumor cells arise by selective outgrowth of a few infected cells. The basis of the selective advantage of particular clones remains to be determined.

Table 1 Transformed Cell Colonies in A-MuLV Infected Mice

Day Post-Infection	Colonies/106 BM Cells	No. Mice
7	0.02	5
14	20	8
25-30 (lymphoma)	510	6
40 (M-MuLV-infected control)	0.0	5

Non-*abl* Transforming Gene in A-MuLV Tumors

One possible explanation for the emergence of clonally dominant A-MuLV tumors is that tumor formation requires more than one oncogenic signal. The activation of a second oncogene could provide such a signal. To determine if activation of a second oncogene could be detected in A-MuLV tumors, we tested DNAs from established and from primary A-MuLV tumors for transforming activity in the NIH3T3 cell assay. The results of that experiment, detailed in Table 2, indicate that most of the A-MuLV cell lines and primary tumors we tested had transforming activity in the NIH3T3 cell assay. The transforming activity was low, usually about 0.01-0.03 foci/ug genomic DNA compared to that observed with the EJ tumor which contains an activated *ras* gene. Foci induced by A-MuLV tumor DNA were slower to appear than those induced by activated *ras* genes, and transformed cells were not as spindle shaped as typical *ras*-transformed cells. The transforming activity was tranferable in secondary rounds of transfection, although at no higher frequencies than with primary tumor DNA.

Table 2 Transforming Activity of A-MuLV Tumor DNA

DNA Source	Total Foci	Total DNA(ug)	Foci/ug
Control	2	1660	0.001
EJ 6-2	46	380	0.12
pUCEJ6.6	217	0.18	1200
pAB4 (A-MuLV provirus)	50	1	50
A-MuLV Cell lines			
E2 and subclone	0	440	.001
4E4 and subclone	60	900	0.07
A-MuLV primary tumors			
2052C	6	120	0.05
2052D	5	120	0.04
2023C	2	60	0.03
2023D	2	60	0.03
Primary foci from A-MuLV tumor DNA			
4E4-11/1	9	170	0.05
4E4-11/2	9	150	0.06
4E4-11/3	18	180	0.1
2052D/1	4	120	0.03

To determine if foci induced by A-MuLV tumor DNAs were tumorigenic we injected 10^6 cells into nude mice and scored the mice for tumor formation at weekly intervals. The results of that experiment indicated that primary foci and secondary foci induced by A-MuLV tumor DNA were tumorigenic in nude mice. The latent period for appearance of tumors was significantly longer than that seen with foci induced with EJ DNA (Table 3). From these results we conclude that DNA of A-MuLV primary tumors and tumor cell lines contain an activated oncogene(s) capable of inducing focus formation and tumorigenicity in NIH3T3 cells.

Table 3 Tumorigenicity of Foci induced by A-MuLV Tumor DNA

Cell Clone	Tumors/Total	Latent Period (days)
4E4-11/1,2	6/7	7-14
2023C/1,2	6/6	4-7
4E4-11/3.1,.2	5/5	10-28

To determine if the gene being transferred was the A-MuLV genome present in the primary tumor DNA, we prepared DNA from several primary transfectants and tested them for the presence of A-MuLV proviral genomes in Southern blots. DNA was digested with EcoRI, fractionated on agarose gels, transferred to nitrocellulose and hybridized with an abl-specific probe. The results of that experiment, presented in Fig. 3, indicate that A-MuLV proviruses are readily detected in the A-MuLV tumor cell line, however they are not detected in transfectants

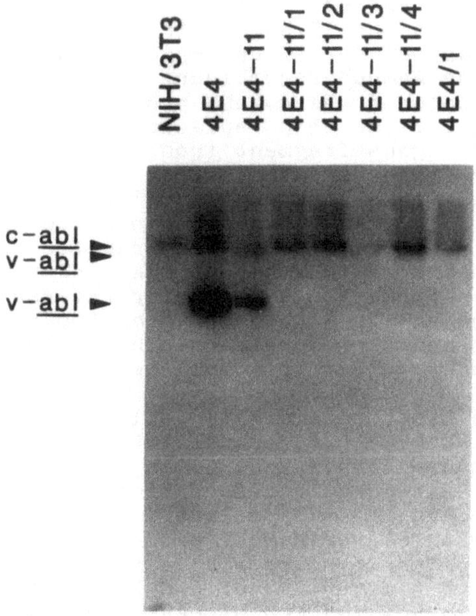

Fig. 3. A-MuLV Proviruses in DNA of NIH3T3 Cells Transfected with A-MuLV Tumor DNA. Genomic DNA was cleaved with EcoRI which does not cleave in the A-MuLV provirus and analyzed in Southern blots with an abl specific probe.

induced by DNA from that tumor line. From these results we conclude that the transforming gene transferred is not v-abl. To determine if the transferred gene was a member of the ras gene family, we metabolically labeled transfectants and immunoprecipitated cell lysates with a monoclonal antibody which reacts with each of the ras proteins. For comparison we also tested foci induced by transfection with EJ DNA. Expression of ras p21 was readily detected in lysates of the ras transfectant however expression of ras p21 was not detected in lysates of foci induced with A-MuLV tumor DNA. Although not definitive these results suggest that the transferred gene is not an activated ras gene.

Tissue Tropism of A-MuLV

Tumors induced by A-MuLV are predominantly of pre-B cell phenotype. The LTR that drives expression of the v-abl gene in these tumors is derived from M-MuLV. M-MuLV induces predominantly T-cell tumors, or other types of lymphoid tumors in some strains of mice. To examine the basis for the tissue tropism of A-MuLV we have constructed molecular recombinants between A-MuLV and Friend MuLV, a replication competent MuLV that induces erythroleukemia in BALB/c mice or occasional myeloid leukemia in C57BL/6 mice.

A biologically active molecular clone of an A-MuLV provirus was recovered from a tumor cell line. We sequenced the LTR of that clone and observed that it differed from the published sequence of M-MuLV in two ways: first it contained 3 point mutations compared to M-MuLV located immediately 5' to the 75 base pair repeat in M-MuLV, second it carried a single copy of the 75 bp repeat found duplicated in M-MuLV. To construct the A-MuLV recombinant carrying F-MuLV U3 sequences we first subcloned the A-MuLV provirus into 5' and 3' halves at the unique Sal I site. We then replaced a Cla I to Kpn I fragment of A-MuLV with the analogous fragment from F-MuLV (kindly provided by N. Hopkins). This fragment extends from sequences immediately 5' to the 3' LTR through U3 and into R. The 3' recombinant was then ligated with the 5' half of A-MuLV and recloned to give an intact A-MuLV-F-MuLV provirus pFARF. This DNA was transfected into NIH3T3 cells along with F-MuLV or M-MuLV helper DNA, and virus pools were prepared from the transformed cells. (During reverse transcription the U3 sequences found at the 3' LTR serve as the source of sequences for the progeny virus and therefore recombinant FARF viruses carry U3 sequences from F-MuLV joined to A-MuLV sequences).

FARF virus pools were titered on NIH3T3 cells and found to have titers somewhat lower than A-MuLV pools. Equal titers of infectious viruses were used to infect mouse bone marrow cells, the cells were plated in the Rosenberg and Baltimore transformation assay (1976), and the number of colonies scored 12-14 days later. We found that FARF genomes pseudotyped with either M-MuLV or F-MuLV were very inefficient in inducing colonies in mouse bone marrow cultures. Bone marrow cells infected with 5 X 10^4 FFU of A-MuLV yielded 150 compact large colonies, whereas 5 X 10^4 FFU of FARF yielded only 1-5 diffuse colonies consisting of several hundred cells. The few macroscopic colonies that developed following FARF infection of bone marrow cells consisted of enucleate cells and large granular cells morphologically distinct from typical A-MuLV-infected lymphocytes.

To determine the activity of FARF virus in mice newborn or adult BALB/c and C57BL/6 mice were injected with virus. The results of that experiment indicated that FARF (F-MuLV) or FARF (M-MuLV) was very effective at tumor induction in vivo. The gross pathological appearance and latency of tumor development were identical to that seen with A-MuLV (Table 4). Eight tumors induced with FARF (M-MuLV) or FARF (F-MuLV) were placed into culture and the cell surface phenotype determined by FACS analysis. The tumor cells express high levels of class I MHC antigens, B220, AA4,and frequently GF1 antigens. They do not express detectable quantities of class II antigens nor the T-cell antigens Thy-1, Ly 1 or Ly 2, nor do they express the myeloid marker Mac-1. From these results we conclude that FARF-induced tumors are of the pre-B cell phenotype. Examination of immunoglobulin gene arrangement is currently in progress.

Table 4 Tumorigenicity of FARF Virus

Mouse (age)	A-MuLV (M-MuLV)	FARF (M-MuLV)	FARF (F-MuLV)
BALB/c (1-10d)	11/11	20/20	7/7
BALB/c (60d)	9/9	9/9	23/23
C57BL/6 (1-10d)	8/8	11/11	9/9
C57BL/6 (60d)	0/7	0/14	0/13

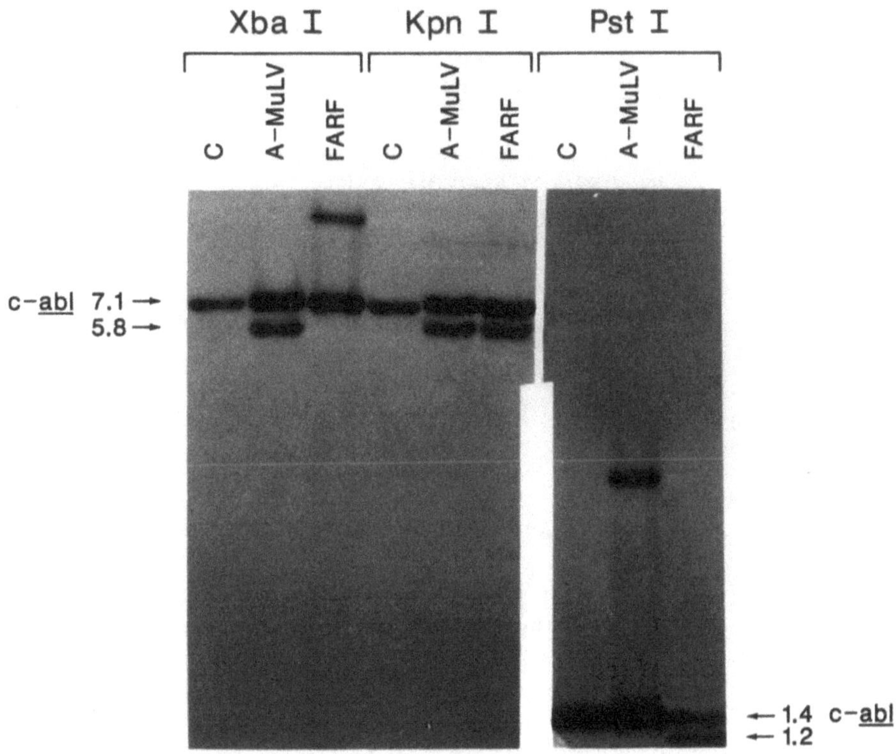

Fig. 4. Restriction Maps of LTR Sequences of A-MuLV and FARF Tumors

One possible explanation for these results is that FARF genomes have recombined with M-MuLV or endogenous MuLV genomes to generate viruses more like the original A-MuLV. To test that possibility we took advantage of restiction site polymorphisms that distinguish A-MuLV from F-MuLV U3 sequences. Both A-MuLV and FARF contain a unique KpnI site in R and therefore cleavage with that enzyme will yield a genome size 5.8 kb fragment. F-MuLV lacks an Xba I site , whereas A-MuLV contains an Xba I site in U3. Cleavage of A-MuLV proviruses will yield a 5.8 genome-size fragment, whereas cleavage of genomic DNA containing a FARF provirus and hybridization with an abl-specific probe will yield a fragment larger than 6.4 kb. A-MuLV lacks a Pst I site in U3 whereas FARF contains one. Cleavage of genomic DNA containing A-MuLV or FARF and hybridization with an appropriate probe will yield a fragment greater than 1.7 kb and exactly 1.2 kb, repectively. These predicted patterns are precisely those observed when genomic DNA from an A-MuLV or a FARF induced tumor was analyzed (Fig. 4). Parallel results were observed with each of the 8 FARF tumors analyzed. Therefore tumors induced by FARF contain the

F-MuLV U3 sequences joined to v-*abl* sequences as predicted. From these results we conclude that substitution of F-MuLV U3-R sequences dramatically alters the *in vitro* transforming activity of A-MuLV but does not alter its *in vivo* tissue tropism.

IN VITRO TRANSFORMATION
BY HELPER-FREE A-MuLV

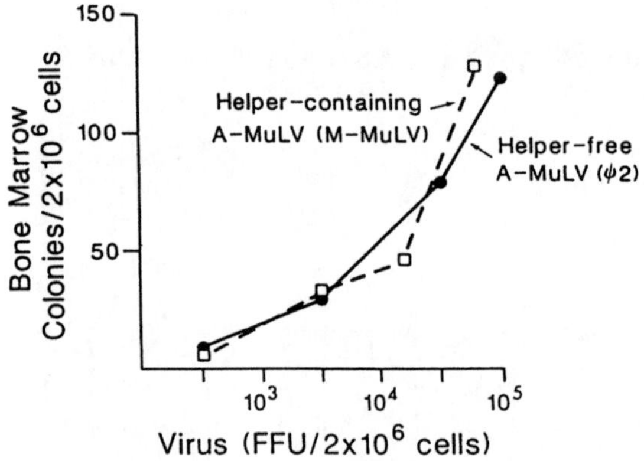

IN VIVO TUMOR INDUCTION
BY HELPER-FREE A-MuLV

	LYMPHOMAS/TOTAL	
VIRUS DOSE	A-MuLV(M-MuLV)	A-MuLV(ψ2)
10^4 FFU	15/16	2/17
$3x10^2$ FFU	19/20	

Fig. 5. Activity of Helper-Free A-MuLV

ACTIVITY OF HELPER-FREE A-MuLV

A-MuLV is defective for replication and therefore preparations of A-MuLV used for infection have invariably contained helper virus, usually M-MuLV. Using the psi-2 helper cell of Mann et al (1983) we have prepared helper-free pools of A-MuLV. We transfected psi-2 cells with a molecular clone of an A-MuLV provirus recovered from a tumor cell line, and selected transformed foci. Virus was prepared from supernatants of A-MuLV transformed psi-2 cells and titered on NIH3T3 cells for transforming activity and XC plaque forming activity. Of the 5 pools of helper-free A-MuLV prepared, 3 lacked detectable helper virus and had titers of transforming virus of 10^3 to 5×10^4 FFU/ml. These pools were then used to infect BALB/c bone marrow cells or newborn BALB/c mice.

We found that the *in vitro* transforming activity of A-MuLV for mouse bone marrow cells was as efficient as that of helper containing A-MuLV (Fig. 5). When helper-free A-MuLV was injected into mice however it was much less efficient at tumor induction. Of 17 mice injected as newborns two developed macroscopic growths :one with slight lymphadenopathy and the other with slight cranial enlargement. Attempts to culture either growth *in vitro* were unsuccessful, and it is not clear that either was truly malignant. This is in contrast to tumors induced by helper-containg A-MuLV from which cell lines are readily established. Based on these results we conclude that helper-free A-MuLV is as efficient as helper-containing A-MuLV in bone marrow transformation but differs significantly from helper-containing A-MuLV in its *in vivo* activity. This may simply reflect the relative inefficiency of *in vivo* infection or it may reflect some actual effect of helper virus on the course of disease *in vivo*.

ACTIVITY OF VIRAL ONCOGENES IN IL-3 DEPENDENT PRE-B CELL LINES

Previous studies have demonstrated that infection of mast cells or myeloid precursor cells with A-MuLV results in the establishment of IL-3-independent tumorigenic cell lines. Recently McKearn , McCubrey and Fagg (1985) have reported the establishment of IL-3 dependent cell lines that have the capacity to differentiate *in vitro* into IgM-secreting cells. We have studied the response of those lines to infection with oncogenic retroviruses and have found that A-MuLV infection does indeed lead to IL-3 independence.

To carry out these experiments we infected G/G1.12 cells, an IL-3-dependent pre-B cell line identical to the FL5.12 of McKearn et. al. (1985), with oncogenic retroviruses in the absence of IL-3. We then washed the cells in medium and cultured them overnight in the presence of IL-3 to allow for cell division. Cells were then washed three times in medium lacking IL-3 and resuspended at 5×10^4 cells/0.1 ml in medium containing fetal calf serum (5%) in the absence of IL-3. Colonies of dividing cells were scored at 14 days post-infection. Colonies were picked and cells cultured in the absence of IL-3. Eleven colonies infected with A-MuLV or helper-free A-MuLV were picked and each was successfully established into cells lines in the absence of IL-3. Examination of the DNA of the lines indicated that each carried an A-MuLV provirus. Proviruses were located in different cellular sequences in the different cell lines. Examination of v-*abl* p160 expression indicated that each line was positive for oncogene expression. Colonies that arose following Ha-MSV infection could not be established in the absence of IL-3 following their initial burst of growth immediately after infection. Infection with M-MuLV, MLV-src or M-MSV did not result in colony formation although infectious center assays indicated the cells were infected. A-MuLV IL-3-independent G/G1.12 cells have been tested for their growth in nude mice, and tumors developed at 2-3 weeks post-infection. We conclude that A-MuLV infection of these IL-3-dependent pre-B cell lines does render them independent of growth factor for continued proliferation *in vitro*, and tumorigenic in nude mice.

Table 5 Activity of Oncogenic Retroviruses in IL-3-dependent Pre-B Cells

Virus	Oncogene	Efficiency of Infection[1] X 10-2	IL-3 independent[2] colonies per infected cell
M-MuLV	none	.5	.00001
A-MuLV	v-*abl*	.6	.06
MLV-src	v-*src*	2	.0001
M-MSV	v-*mos*	13	.000005
Ha-MSV	v-*ras*^{H}	3.3	.01

1 Cells were irradiated 24 hrs post-infection and plated on susceptible NIH3T3 cells to score the number of cells producing focus-forming virus or XC plaque-forming virus per 10^5 total cells.

2 Cells were plated 24 hrs post-infection at 5 $X10^4$ cells per 0.1 ml in medium lacking IL-3 in microtiter wells. Colonies were scored 14 days later.

DISCUSSION

Our results indicate that A-MuLV tumors arise from a minority of infected cells. Although infection of mice is clearly polyclonal the tumors that emerge are monoclonal or oligoclonal in origin. It is also apparent that many clones of cells capable of some growth *in vitro* are present in A-MuLV infected mice. It could be that clonal dominance is largely a kinetic phenomenon in that the first cell transformed is the one that finally emerges as the dominant population in the tumor. Data from one mouse suggest that such may be the case. Agarose colonies recovered from that mouse at 10 days post-infection already show clonal dominance. It is also apparent , however, that the growth properties of cells from colonies of pre-leukemic mice differ from those of tumor cells. Each of eight tumors tested could readily grow continuously *in vitro* when plated in microtiter wells, whereas of 29 colonies picked from agarose colonies of pre-leukemic bone marrow only 2 showed that capability. We have also demonstrated the presence of an additional activated non-*abl* transforming gene in the DNA of primary A-MuLV tumors. It will indeed be interesting to determine if that gene is invoIoved in the greater growth potential of A-MuLV tumor cells. There is also some suggestion that the presence of helper virus may influence the course of disease *in vivo*, in that to date we have not been able to culture the growths induced by helper-free A-MuLV. It is apparent, however, that helper virus is not necessary for the induction of bone marrow colonies by A-MuLV.

The tissue tropism of A-MuLV is of considerable interest, and the first interpretation of our results would be that the v-abl oncogene is the major determinant of that property. This conclusion is based on the observation that A-MuLV carrying the F-MuLV U3 sequences induces pre-B cell tumors by serological criteria. In vitro the activity of the virus appears quite different from that of A-MuLV in that only rare diffuse colonies are induced by FARF. As yet we do not know the cell type comprising these colonies , however morphologically it is not the type of lymphocyte found in standard A-MuLV induced colonies. Once again the role of in vivo selection may be the major determinant of the outcome of infection of mice with FARF viruses. It should also be noted that only the F-MuLV U3 recombinant has been tried and others, particularly those with fibrotropic host range, will have to be tested before firm conclusions can be drawn about the tissue tropism of A-MuLV.

Our results with IL-3 dependent lines confirm those of Cook et al (1985) and Pierce et al (1985). We found that infection of an IL-3 dependent cell line relieved its dependence on IL-3. The efficiency of transformation to IL-3-independence was not equal to the efficiency of infection but rather was lower by a factor of about 20. This is somewhat different from what was found by previous workers but could be explained by the long periods of culture used by them before selection of IL-3 independent lines. It is interesting to note that other oncogenic viruses do not appear to have this capability. The role of IL-3 in A-MuLV disease however is far from clear. In an attempt to culture agarose colonies from pre-leukemic bone marrow we supplemented their cultures with supernatant from WEHI-3B or ANN-1 cells, and did not observe any improvement in in vitro growth. It could be that several genes or factors are necessary for the final emergence of A-MuLV tumor cells.

ACKNOWLEDGMENTS

This work was supported by PHS grant R01-CA41302 to R.R. and PHS grants 1 P30 CA07175 and PHS grant P32-CA-09135 to the McArdle Laboratory.

REFERENCES

Abelson HT, Rabstein LS (1970) Lymphosarcoma: virus-induced thymic-independent disease in mice. Cancer Res 30:2213-2222

Chatis PA, Holland CA, Hartley JW, Rowe WP, Hopkins N (1983) Role for the 3' end of the genome in determining disease specificity of Friend and Moloney murine leukemia viruses. Proc Natl Acad Sci USA 80:4408-4411

Cook WD, Metcalf D, Nicola N, Burgess AW, Walker F (1985) Malignant transformation of a growth factor-dependent myeloid cell line by Abelson virus without evidence of an autocrine mechanism. Cell 41:677-683

Lane M-A, Neary D, Cooper GM (1982) Activation of a cellular transforming gene in tumors induced by Abelson murine leukemia virus. Nature 300:659-661

Mann R, Mulligan RC, Baltimore D (1983) Construction of a retrovirus packaging mutant and its use to produce helper-free defective retrovirus. Cell 33:153-159

McKearn J, McCubrey J, Fagg B (1985) Enrichment of hematopoietic precursor cells and cloning of multipotential B-lymphocyte precursors. Proc Natl Acad Sci USA 82:7414-7418
Pierce JH, DiFiore PP, Aaronson SA, Potter M, Pumphrey J, Scott A, Ihle JN (1985) Neoplastic transformation of mast cells by Abelson-MuLV: abrogation of IL-3 dependence by a nonautocrine mechanism. Cell 41:685-693
Reynolds FH, Sacks, TL, Deobagkar DN, Stephenson JR (1978) Cells nonproductively transformed by Abelson murine leukemia virus express a high molecular weight polyprotein containing structural and non-structural components. Proc Natl Acad Sci USA 75:3974-3978
Risser R, Kaehler D, Lamph WW (1985) Different genes control the susceptibility of mice to Moloney or Abelson murine leukemia viruses. J Virol 55:547-553
Risser R, Potter M, Rowe WP (1978) Abelson virus-induced lymphomagenesis in mice. J Exp Med 148:714-726
Rosenberg N, Baltimore D (1976) A quantitative assay for transformation of bone marrow cells by Abelson murine leukemia virus. J Exp Med 143:1453-1463
Scher CD, Siegler R (1975) Direct transformation of 3T3 cells by Abelson murine leukemia virus. Nature (London) 253:729-731
Wang JYJ, Ledky F, Goff S, Lee R, Groner Y, Baltimore D (1984) The mouse cabl locus. Cell 36:349-356
Whitlock CA, Ziegler SF, Witte ON (1983) Progression of the transformed phenotype in clonal lines of Abelson virus-infected lymphocytes. Mol Cell Biol 3:596-604
Witte ON, Goff S, Rosenberg N, Baltimore D (1980) A transformation-defective mutant of Abelson murine leukemia virus lacks protein kinase activity. Proc Natl Acad Sci USA 77:4993-4997
Witte ON, Rosenberg N, Paskind M, Shields A, Baltimore D (1978) Identification of an Abelson murine leukemia virus-encoded protein present in transformed fibroblast and lymphoid cells. Proc Natl Acad Sci USA 75:2488-2492

An *In Vitro* Model for Tumor Progression in Murine Lymphoid Cells

Richard C. Schwartz, Lawrence W. Stanton*, Kenneth B. Marcu* and Owen N. Witte

Department of Microbiology and Molecular Biology Institute, University of California, Los Angeles, CA 90024

*Biochemistry Department, State University of New York, Stony Brook, N.Y. 11794

INTRODUCTION

Histopathological observations of the development of tumors have led to the concept that oncogenesis proceeds through the sequential acquisition of independent growth-related phenotypic characteristics (Foulds 1975). This process of tumor progression occurs through events involving the expression of specific genes affecting the regulation of cellular growth (recently reviewed in Weinberg 1985; Klein and Klein 1985; Bishop 1985). The requirement of two complementing oncogenes for the *in vitro* transformation of primary rat embryo firbroblasts provides a useful *in vitro* experimental model of tumor progression. Ha-*ras* (EJ) and v-*myc* or Ha-*ras* (T24) and *E1A* can act together to transform primary fibroblasts, while neither oncogene acting alone is capable of causing efficient transformation (Land et al. 1983; Ruley 1983) unless expressed at a high level (Spandidos and Wilkie 1984).

Tumor Progression and B Cell Neoplasia

Burkitt's lymphoma and murine plasmacytoma are B cell tumors that display a progression in their development (reviewed in Klein and Klein 1985). Infection with Epstein-Barr virus appears to be the primary event in the development of African Burkitt's lymphoma (Klein 1979). Subsequent to infection with Epstein-Barr virus, the *myc* proto-oncogene is activated by a chromosomal translocation event (reviewed in Perry 1983; Klein 1983; Leder et al. 1983). At least one Burkitt's lymphoma has an activated N-*ras* oncogene in addition to *myc* (Murray et al. 1983). The induction of murine plasmacytoma is preceded by the development of an intraperitoneal granuloma through the application of mineral oil (reviewed in Potter et al. 1984). Like Burkitt's lymphoma, murine plasmacytomas have undergone chromosomal translocations activating the *myc* proto-oncogene (reviewed in Klein 1983; Perry 1983). One plasmacytoma, additionally, displays activation of the c-*mos* oncogene by insertion of an intracisternal A particle (Rechavi et al. 1982; Canaani et al. 1983). Infection with Abelson leukemia virus in conjunction with application of mineral oil accelerates the process of tumor induction (reviewed in Potter et al. 1984). The induction of B cell neoplasia may require the activation of several oncogenes.

RESULTS

V-myc and v-Ha-ras Act in Synergy

An *in vitro* culture system in which to observe the affects of multiple oncogenes in the genesis of B cell neoplasia has been

Current Topics in Microbiology and Immunology, Vol. 132

lacking. We have utilized the long term B cell culture system of Whitlock and Witte (1982) to examine the transforming activity of recombinant murine retroviruses expressing the v-myc (OK10) and v-Ha-ras oncogenes (Schwartz et al. 1986). Freshly explanted bone marrow of BALB/c mice was either singly or doubly infected with these vectors and then cultured as in Whitlock and Witte (1982). While infection with the v-myc retroviruses had no apparent effect on culture establishment and growth, infection with the v-Ha-ras vector alone or co-infection with both v-Ha-ras and v-myc vectors resulted in the appearance of growth stimulated cell populations. The populations arising from co-infection grew to densities between 1 and 4×10^6 cells/ml, while populations arising from infection with the v-Ha-ras vector generally grew to densities between 1 and 4×10^5 cells/ml.

The Growth Stimulated Populations are Clonal Pre-B Cells that Retain and Express the Viral Oncogenes

The cell populations that grew out from these experiments were pre-B cells. These cells expressed the B-cell specific B220 surface antigen and were rearranged at their immunoglobulin heavy chain loci, but did not expresss μ-chain and retained a germ line configuration at their K light chain loci (Schwartz et al. 1986). Hybridization and serological analyses revealed that the v-Ha-ras oncogene was retained and expressed in all the populations studied with the additional retention and expression of v-myc in doubly infected populations. Each population possessed single retroviral integration sites indicating their clonal or pauci-clonal nature (Schwartz et al. 1986). Thus in doubly infected populations, both v-myc and v-Ha-ras are expressed in the same cell.

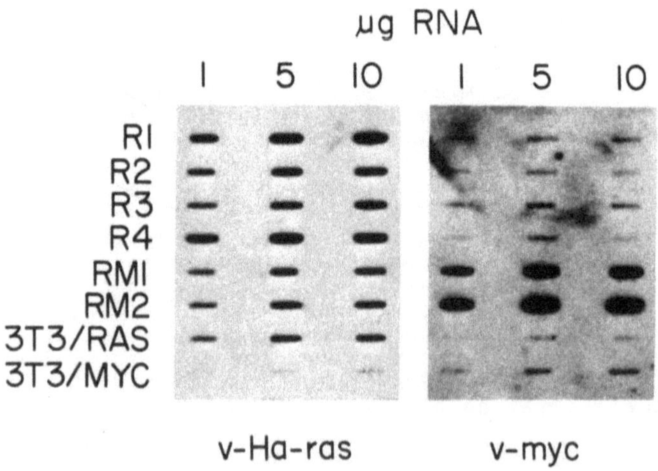

Fig. 1. Slot blot analysis of cytoplasmic RNA. RNA prepared by the method of Schwartz et al. (1981) was hybridized to either a Ha-ras specific probe or a v-myc specific probe. R1, R2, R3 and R4 refer to pre-B cell lines expressing v-Ha-ras alone. RM1 and RM2 refer to pre-B cell lines expresssing both v-Ha-ras and v-myc.

We examined the level of expression of the viral oncogenes in order to determine whether that level was consistent with the transformed phenotype. A slot blot analysis of graded amounts of cytoplasmic RNA (Fig. 1) revealed that the viral oncogenes were expressed at levels equivalent or above that expressed in the transformed NIH 3T3 cells that produced the virus stocks used in these experiments.

Cells Expressing both V-Ha-ras and v-myc Show a Dramatic Increase in their Transformed Phenotype Compared to Cells Expressing v-Ha-ras Alone

Cell lines expressing both v-Ha-ras and v-myc had a more pronounced transformed phenotype than cell lines expressing v-Ha-ras alone. They were capable of growth in the absence of an adherent layer of feeder cells, while cells expressing v-Ha-ras alone were not (Schwartz et al. 1986). Cells expressing both v-Ha-ras and v-myc could grow in soft agar medium whereas cells expressing only v-Ha-ras could not (Figure 2). This growth was dependent on the presence of an underlayer of adherent feeder cells. Although highly transformed, the cell lines expressing v-Ha-ras and v-myc do not represent an endpoint in neoplastic progression.

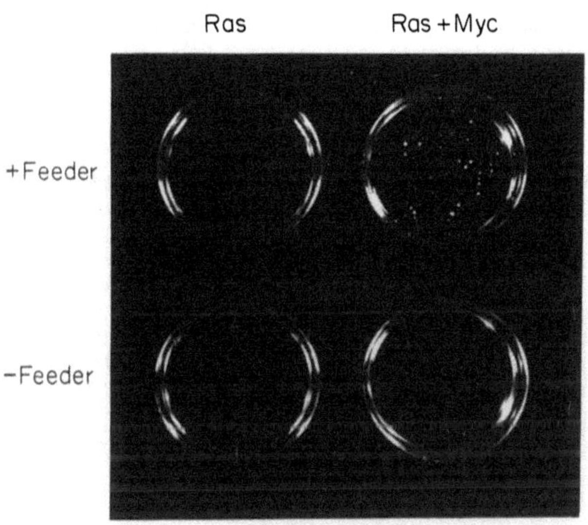

Fig. 2. Plating in soft agar. 1000 cells of a representative pre-B cell line expressing v-Ha-ras alone or a cell line expressing both v-Ha-ras and v-myc were plated in soft agar medium as described in Whitlock et al. (1983). Platings were performed with and without an underlaying feeder of adherent bone marrow stromal cells.

Tumor challenges were performed by the intraperitoneal injection of cells into syngeneic animals (Fig. 3). Cell lines expressing both v-Ha-ras and v-myc almost invariably formed subcutaneous tumors with metastases throughout the lymph nodes and spleen. Cell lines expressing v-Ha-ras alone formed tumors infrequently over the maximum 10 week period with the typical animal showing no signs of illness.

Ras
2 X 10⁶ cells (R1) injected IP
Sacrificed at 70 days

Ras + Myc
2 X 10⁶ cells (RM1) injected IP
Sacrificed at 38 days

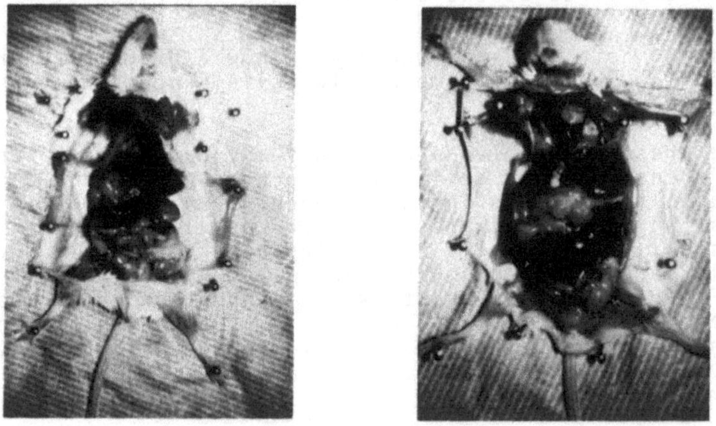

Fig. 3. Tumor challenges. BALB/c mice, 4 tO 10 weeks old, were injected intraperitoneally with 2 x 10^6 cells. Animals were observed for a maximum of 10 weeks post-injection. R1 is a pre-B cell line expressing v-Ha-ras alone and RM1 is a pre-B cell line expressing both v-Ha-ras and v-myc.

Similar results were obtained in athymic nude mice. In this case, 5 week old animals received 1 x 10^6 cells intraperitoneally. Of three mice injected with a cell line expressing both v-Ha-ras and v-myc, all became moribund within three weeks with subcutaneous tumors and lymphatic metastases. Of 12 mice injected with four different v-Ha-ras expressing cell lines (three animals each), only three mice developed lymphatic tumors by six weeks. This suggests that the differences in tumorigenic potential correlated best with the proliferative potential of the cell lines rather than differential antigenicity.

CONCLUSIONS AND FUTURE GOALS

We have demonstrated a synergy between v-myc and v-Ha-ras oncogenes in the in vitro neoplastic progresson of murine pre-B lymphoid cells. The replacement of either agent in this synergy with other oncogenes should prove useful in defining the activities of these oncogenes in lymphoid transformation. In particular, the replacement of v-myc (OK 10) with human or murine c-myc and mutant derivatives may provide a structure and function analysis of the myc oncogene in lymphoid transformation.

The cell lines derived from these experiments represent intermediate transformed phenotypes. The experimental manipulation of these cell lines through the introduction of additional oncogenes may provide useful experimental models of lymphoid tumor progression. The examination of tumors derived from cells of a pre-neoplastic phenotype (cells expressing v-Ha-ras alone) may provide an in vivo correlate to such in vitro manipulations.

ACKNOWLEDGEMENTS

This work was supported by a grant from the National Cancer Institute and a Faculty Scholar Award from the American Cancer Society to O.N.W. R.C.S was supported by a felllowship from the Cancer Research Coordinating Committee of the University of California. The authors thank M. Newman for technical assistance and C. Crookshank for secretarial assistance.

REFERENCES

Bishop JM (1985) Viral oncogenes. Cell 42: 23-38

Canaani E, Dreazen O, Klar A, Rechavi G, Ram D, Cohen JB, Givol D (1983) Activation of the c-mos oncogene in a mouse plasmacytoma by insertion of an endogenous intracisternal A-particle genome. Proc Nat Acad Sci USA 80: 7118-7122

Foulds L (1975) Neoplastic development, Vol 2. Academic Press, London

Klein G (1979) Lymphoma development in mice and humans: diversity of initiation is followed by convergent cytogenetic evolution. Proc Nat Acad Sci USA 76: 2442-2446

Klein G (1983) Specific chromosmal translocations and the genesis of B-cell-derived tumors in mice and men. Cell 32: 311-315

Klein G, Klein E (1985) Evolution of tumours and the impact of molecular oncology. Nature 315: 190-195

Land H, Parada LF, Weinberg RA (1983) Tumorigenic conversion of primary embryo fibroblasts requires at least two cooperating oncogenes. Nature 304: 596-602

Leder P, Battey J, Lenoir G, Moulding C, Murphy W, Potter H, Stewart T, Taub R (1983) Translocations among antibody genes in human cancer. Science 222: 765-771

Murray MJ, Cunningham JM, Parada LF, Daultry F, Lebowitz P, Weinberg RA (1983) The HL-60 transforming sequence: a ras oncogene coexisting with altered myc genes in hematopoietic tumors. Cell 33: 749-757

Perry, RP (1983) Consequences of myc invasion of immunoglobulin loci: facts and speculation. Cell 33: 647-649

Potter M, Wiener F, Mushinski JF (1984) Recent developments in plasmacytomagenesis in mice. Viral Oncology 4: 139-162

Rechavi G, Givol D, Canaani E (1982) Activation of a cellular oncogene by DNA rearrangement: possible involvement of an IS-like element. Nature 300: 607-622

Ruley HE (1983) Adenovirus early region 1A enables viral and cellular transforming genes to transform primary cells in culture. Nature 304: 602-606

Schwartz RC, Soneshein GE, Bothwell A, Gefter ML (1981) Multiple expression of Ig λ-chain encoding RNA species murine plasmacytoma cells. J Immunol 126: 2104-2108

Schwartz RC, Stanton LW, Riley SC, Marcu KB, Witte ON (1986) Synergism of v-myc and v-Ha-ras in the in vitro neoplastic progression of murine lymphoid cells. Submitted

Spandidos DA, Wilkie NM (1984) Malignant transformation of early passage rodent cells by a single mutated human oncogene. Nature 310: 469-475

Weinberg RA (1985) The action of oncogenes in the cytoplasm and nucleus. Science 230: 770-776
Whitlock CA, Witte ON (1982) Long-term culture of B lymphocytes and their precursors from murine bone marrow. Proc Nat Acad Sci USA 79: 3608-3612
Whitlock CA, Ziegler SF, Treiman LJ, Stafford, JI, Witte ON (1983) Differentiation of cloned populations of immature B cells after transformation with Abelson murine leukemia virus. Cell 32: 903-911

Structural Modification of c-*abl* in Lymphoma and Leukemia

Yinon Ben-Neriah* and David Baltimore

Whitehead Institute for Biomedical Research, Nine Cambridge Center, Cambridge, MA 02142 and Massachusetts Institute of Technology, Department of Biology, Cambridge, MA 02139

*Present Address: Department of Immunology, The Hebrew University, Hadassah Medical School, Jerusalem 91010 Israel

INTRODUCTION

Vertebrate DNA contains a gene, named c-abl, that was disclosed by a rapidly oncogenic retrovirus, Abelson murine leukemia virus (A-MuLV). A-MuLV carries a portion of c-abl (Goff et al., 1980) including a region encoding a protein-tyrosine kinase which is essential to the oncogenic activity of A-MuLV (Prywes et al., 1983). The cellular protein product of c-abl, like that of v-abl, is an active protein kinase (Konopka et al., 1985; Ben-Neriah et al., 1986a).

The c-abl gene is expressed in every tissue studied so far (Muller et al., 1982; Wang and Baltimore, 1983). Its mRNAs usually separate into two size classes after electrophoresis: 5.3 and 6.5 kb in the mouse and 6 and 7 kb in man. The mature testis shows an extra band of 4.2 kb (Muller et al., 1982; Ponzetto and Wolgemuth, 1985; Ben-Neriah et al., 1986b). Analysis of c-abl cDNA clones revealed no heterogeneity at the 3'-end of the mRNA but showed that 5' heterogeneity is responsible for the size variation both in mice and in man (Ben-Neriah et al., 1986b; E. Canaani, personal communication). In the mouse we identified at least 4 types of c-abl mRNA, two of which have been also found in human cells (E. Canaani, personal communication). The four murine and two equivalent human mRNA types (the equivalent of murine c-abl, types I and IV) have a common core sequence consisting of the eleven 3' exons (Fig. 1), but diverge at a common site corresponding to a genomic splice junction. S1 nuclease analysis has shown that the addition of alternative 5' exons by splicing is the origin of the 5' heterogeneity. The splicing pattern of c-abl involves multiple splicing events occurring at a single splice junction flanking the first common c-abl exon. In the Philadelphia chromosome found in human chronic myelogenous leukemia cells, the same junction attracts exons of a different gene translocated to the proximity of the c-abl locus from another chromosome (described below). In some cases these foreign exons are spliced to abl at the common splice junction from a distance of at least 97 kb (Grosveld et al., 1986).

The unique splicing pattern of c-abl is not specific to any tissue. The two major splice forms of c-abl, types I and IV, are present in every tissue examined in constant proportions of about 2:1, respectively. S1 nuclease analysis suggests that these two major c-abl types represent about 70% of the total abl mRNA; the rest consists, in part, of types II and III and perhaps of other mRNA types yet to be identified.

Current Topics in Microbiology and Immunology, Vol. 132

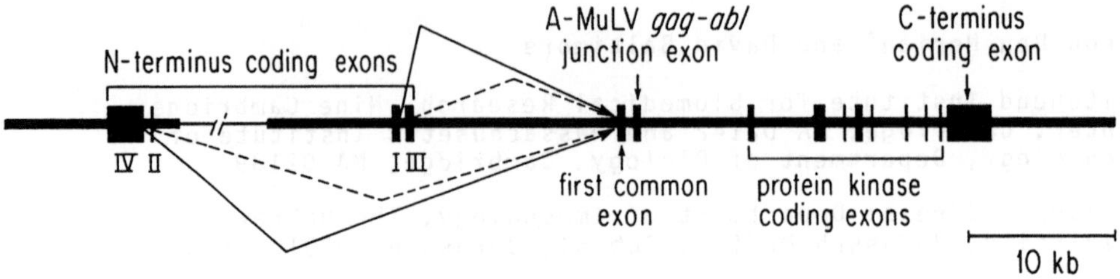

Fig. 1. Organization and splicing in the mouse c-abl locus. Vertical bars represent individual exons; horizontal thickened lines represent introns. The N-terminal coding exons II and IV have not been linked yet to the rest of the c-abl region; this is indicated by a break in the horizontal axis. Major splicing events are indicated with solid arrows, minors are indicated with dashed arrows. The map was constructed according to Wang et al. (1984) and A. Bernards et al. (unpublished).

The c-abl protein has a molecular weight of approximately 150 kd in the mouse, 140 kd in man, and 140 kd in the rat. The predicted number of amino acids of the protein made from the different splice products of the c-abl locus are 1117 to 1142, suggesting a closely uniform size for the c-abl proteins in mice and humans. The different mRNA types, if indeed translated in vivo, will differ only at the N-terminal lengths of 20 to 45 amino acids. Nevertheless, using v-abl and c-abl specific antibodies we have observed some molecular weight heterogeneity in certain mouse tissues, perhaps due to post-translational modification. Comparison of the different N-terminal sequences indicate 3 unrelated hydrophilic and one hydrophobic amino acid sequence. None of these sequences display the typical primary structure of a signal sequence or membrane-spanning region. The N-terminal sequence predicted from the type IV cDNA starts with met-gly-gln in common with the gag N-terminus of v-abl. v-abl, v-src and c-src are all myristylated on a glycine residue found next to the N-terminal methionine residue suggesting the possibility that the type IV c-abl protein may be likewise myristylated and anchored to the internal side of the plasma membrane. c-abl would thereby have two protein forms, one cytoplasmic and one membrane-bound, although neither form would have any other characteristics of a receptor or a transmembrane protein.

abl IN RETROVIRUSES

c-abl is contained within the genome of two acutely transforming retroviruses, Abelson murine leukemia virus (A-MuLV) and Hardy-Zukerman-2 feline sarcoma virus (HZ-2FeSV) (Besmer et al., 1983). A-MuLV was isolated from a steroid treated Balb/c mouse infected with a replication competent Moloney murine leukemia virus (Abelson and Rabstein, 1970). The infecting virus presumably recombined with the mouse genome at the cellular abl locus and as a result produced a replication defective retrovirus containing part of the c-abl gene and capable of rapid transformation of mouse cells both in vivo and in vitro (Baltimore et al., 1979). The structure of A-MuLV is shown schematically in Fig. 2. The virus retains most of the sequences common to all the c-abl mRNA types and is truncated at the 5'-end. The recombination between the viral gag and abl occurred in the middle of the second common exon (junction exon in Fig. 1). The viral genome shares with c-abl a short sequence, "TACA", which is found at the recombination site and might have facilitated the recombination event (Wang et al., 1984). A-MuLV encodes a 160 kd gag-abl fusion protein in which the N-terminus is derived from Moloney virus gag sequence (including p15, p12 and part of P30), replacing about 125 N-terminal amino acids of the predicted normal c-abl protein. The viral fusion protein has a strong protein tyrosine kinase activity, evident by autophosphorylation (Witte et al., 1980) and by phosphorylation of tyrosine-containing peptides (Foulkes et al., 1985).

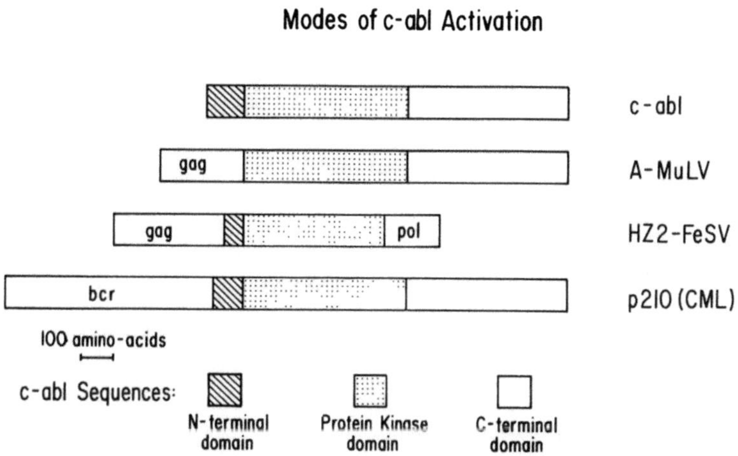

Fig. 2. Schematic illustration of the structure of c-abl and its different transforming variants. gag, pol, and bcr are non-abl sequences involved in the transforming activation of c-abl by retroviruses or as a consequence of the Philadelphia chromosome translocation in CML - [P210(CML)], A-MuLV = Abelson murine leukemia virus. HZ2-FeSV = Hardy-Zuckerman 2 feline sarcoma virus.

Only a small portion of the A-MuLV genome is necessary for transforming fibroblasts in vitro. The minimal transforming region determined so far is composed of the 14 first amino acids of gag (the p15 region) and the 400 N-terminal amino acids of the transduced abl. Somewhat more of the gag sequences are needed

required IL3 for proliferation whereas the cells infected with the recombinant gag-Δ5' c-abl virus proliferated in the absence of IL3. We have infected NIH/3T3 cells with three viral constructs and have assayed the cells for morphological transformation in vitro. Only the gag-Δ5' c-abl virus induced morphological changes, similar to those induced by A-MuLV P160 virus. Thus, the replacement of the normal type I N-terminus with A-MuLV gag was sufficient to induce properties of transformed cells both in fibroblasts and lymphocytes. Other alterations in the gene structure are apparently not required for transformation.

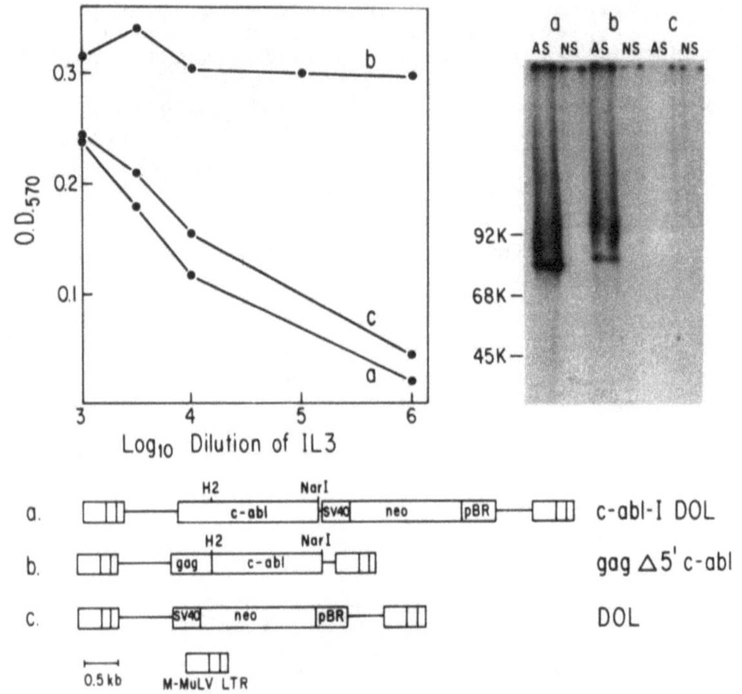

Fig. 3. Expression of an N-terminally modified c-abl is associated with characteristics of transformation. Ba/F3 lymphocytes (gift of Dr. R. Palacios, Basel Institute) were infected with viral constructs containing c-abl fragments assayed for proliferation. Proliferation was measured by a colorimetric method adapted from Mosmann (1983) and based on the capacity of proliferating cells to reduce a tetrazolium dye MTT (4,5 dimethyl-thiazol-2-yl) 2,5-diphenyl tetrazolium bromide. A schematic representation of the viral constructs are given below. DOL is a retroviral expression vector developed by Dr. Alan Korman (Whitehead Institute). H2, NarI: restriction enzyme sites HincII and NarI, indicating the origin of the c-abl fragments (Ben-Neriah et al., 1986b). The experiments described in this figure were done in collaboration with Dr. Gary Nabel (Whitehead Institute).

for transformation of lymphocytes in vitro (Prywes et al., 1983). The additional p15 sequences stabilize the protein in a lymphocyte cell line.

v-abl is among the very few viral oncogenes that transform lymphocytes efficiently both in vitro and in vivo. The specificity for lymphocyte transformation is probably provided by the kinase domain of v-abl. Experiments with src-abl hybrid retroviruses (Mathey-Prevot et al., 1985) showed that the gag N-terminus of v-abl could be replaced by the N-terminus of src and retain lymphocyte transforming specificity, whereas a gag-src virus was capable of transforming fibroblasts, but not lymphocytes.

The c-abl gene was transduced by a retrovirus in another species -- the cat (Besmer et al., 1983). The c-abl containing retrovirus, Hardy Zukerman 2 feline sarcoma virus (HZ-2FeSV), was isolated from a cat fibrosarcoma tumor. Its structure is shown in Fig. 2; it shares several characteristics with A-MuLV (Goff et al., 1980). It is truncated at both the 3'-end and at the 5'-end with respect to c-abl. HZ-2 FeSV also codes for a fusion protein in which the N-terminus is coded by the feline leukemia virus gag. Recombination in this case occurred in the middle of the first common abl exon where a hexanucleotide sequence is shared between c-abl and FeLV (P. Besmer, personal communication).

The structure of the transforming variants of c-abl (Fig. 2) suggests that the modification of the N-terminus may be important for the activation of c-abl to a transforming oncogene; however, there may be other alterations which are necessary for its activation (e.g., point mutation elsewhere in c-abl). To address this issue, we created a chimeric construct between v-abl and c-abl and studied its expression in fibroblasts and lymphocytes in comparison to a 3' truncated c-abl.

The three viral constructs used to study abl transformation are shown in Fig. 3. c-abl fragments were expressed in retroviral expression vectors under a M-MuLV LTR promoter. Construct (a) contains the 5'-end of the c-abl including the type I N-terminus and the entire kinase domain as well as a neo resistance gene driven by the SV40 promoter; construct (b) contains the gag fragment of v-abl joined in frame to the tyrosine kinase coding region of c-abl at a site close to the fusion point of gag and abl in A-MuLV; (c) the vector used for construction of (a) was used as a control. The three constructs were transfected into the ψ2 mouse 3T3 cell line which contains an integrated Moloney genome able to provide the viral packaging proteins (Mann et al., 1982). Transient virus was harvested after 18 hr and used to infect a lymphocyte cell line, Ba/F3, which is dependent on interleukin 3 (IL3) for growth. After three days of culture, the infected cells were selected either for neo (G418) resistance or for IL3 independence. Cells infected with constructs (a) or (c) could be selected in the presence of G418, but not without IL3; whereas cells infected with construct (b) could be maintained without IL3, but were sensitive to G418. Selected cells were cloned and when established in culture were tested for expression of the exogenous abl gene (Fig. 3 inset) and tested again for IL3 dependent proliferation. Cells infected with (a) or (b) expressed an active protein kinase. Both the control cells (c) and the Ba/F3 cells infected with the type I-c-abl virus (a)

Inset: In vitro kinase assay on immunoprecipitates from virus infected Ba/F3 cells using v-abl antiserum (gift of Dr. J.Y.J. Wang). Protein A-Sepharose immunoprecipitates were processed for in vitro kinase assay as described (Ben-Neriah et al., 1986a). Lane codes (a-c) match the codes for the viral constructs. (a) lanes were loaded with five-fold equivalent more cellular extract than in (b) lanes. AS = Antiserum; NS = Normal serum control.

ACTIVATION IN LEUKEMIA

The 9:22 translocation found in the Philadelphia chromosome is the most consistent translocation associated with human cancer (Rowley, 1973). It occurs in over 95% of chronic myelogenous leukemia (CML) cases. A karyotype containing the Philadelphia chromosome is present in all the lineage of hematopoietic origin, although the proliferating cells are usually granulocytes. This cytogenetic hallmark is molecularly characterized by the translocation of the abl oncogene from chromosome 9 to the break-point cluster region (bcr) of chromosome 22. The recombination site of the two chromosomal sequences in the Philadelphia chromosome usually occurs within the c-abl locus at a variable length 5' to the common abl exon and is clustered around two of the exons of the bcr gene normally localized on chromosome 22 (Heisterkamp et al., 1985). In some cases, as in K562 cells, the translocation occurred over 97 kb upstream of the common abl exon (Grosveld et al., 1986). In K562 cells, both the abl and the bcr sequences on the 22(q-) chromosome are amplified four-fold. Thus the amplification unit covers over 140 kb of chromosome 9 sequences. If the translocation in K562 had occurred within the c-abl locus, c-abl sequences residing on the reciprocal chromosome 9(q+) might not have been amplified. We have analyzed different regions of the c-abl gene for amplification on Southern blots and found that the type IV exon is not part of the bcr-abl amplification unit (Bernards et al., unpublished). Therefore, the translocation in K562 occurred between the type IV 5' c-abl exon and the type I 5' exon, interrupting the c-abl gene.

As a consequence of the translocation event, Philadelphia chromosome-positive CML cells express an aberrant c-abl transcript of 8.5 kb. This transcript was studied by Shtivelman et al. (1985) by cDNA cloning and was found to be a fusion transcript of bcr and c-abl. The fusion results from splicing of exons located in the genomic region denoted bcr to the first common c-abl exon. This genomic region contains 6 exons, 3 of which could match the c-abl reading frame if spliced at the common abl splice junction. In fact, two of these exons have been found to join the abl exon in a series of 12 CML cases; one predominates over the other in a ratio of 2:1 (E. Canaani, personal communication). It is possible that the observation of the break-point clustering (Groffen et al., 1984) is in part due to selection of productive splice products, resulting in leukemia.

In addition to the 8.5 kb bcr/abl transcript, CML cells express another novel product -- a 210 kd phosphoprotein recognized by v-abl specific antisera (Konopka et al., 1984). With the aid of site-specific antibodies against c-*abl* and *bcr* peptides predicted from the cDNA structure of the 8.5 kb transcript, we have shown that P210 is the product of the CML specific 8.5 kb transcript (Ben-Neriah et al., 1986a). P210 contains all the precicted *abl* sequences up to the common exon junction and, similarly to v-*abl*, the normal N-terminus of c-*abl* is replaced by the translocated *bcr* sequences (Fig. 2). P210 is overexpressed with respect to c-*abl* in leukemic cells derived from patients at the late stage of CML. It is present in cells from the chronic phase of the disease although its level of expression in these cells may be variable (O.N. Witte, personal communication); the 8.5 kb transcript, however, is clearly over-expressed in all stages of the disease (E. Canaani, personal communication). The expression of P210 is not restricted to myeloid cells, being expressed in hybrids of CML cells and mouse fibroblasts (Kozbor et al., 1986) and in ERBV immortalized Philadelphia positive lymphocytes from CML patients. However, in these non-myeloid cells it is expressed at low levels even in comparison to the normal c-*abl* protein (Konopka et al., 1986. This pattern of expression suggests that the presence of the Philadelphia chromosome in a cell is not sufficient to elicit the malignant phenotype typical for myeloid cells in CML. It will be important to determine whether the expression levels of P210 correlate with the cell type specificity and the aggressiveness of the disease.

It is probable that P210 is expressed from the *bcr* gene promoter; however, the expression of the 8.5 kb *bcr*/*abl* transcript in the Philadelphia positive K562 cells greatly exceeds the concomitant expression of the normal *bcr* allele (Shtivelman et al., 1985). Furthermore, rearrangement of the *bcr* locus was seen in CML in the absence of a 9:22 chromosomal translocation (Bartram, 1985). It is therefore possible that the activation of the *bcr* locus precedes the translocation event in CML. Transcriptional activation of the *bcr* locus associated with an open chromatin configuration may promote the recombination of *bcr* and *abl* sequences in a manner similar to the mating type switch mechanism in the yeast (Klar et al., 1984) and the immunoglobulin rearrangement process in lymphocytes (Yancopoulos et al., 1986). Under the influence of an activated *bcr* promoter the translocation event results in overexpression of the *bcr*/*abl* transcript gene. Overexpression of P210 may release the CML granulocytes from their dependence on a certain limiting growth factor leading to their excessive proliferation. In this respect the effect of the *bcr*/*abl* oncogene may be equivalent to the v-*abl* effect on various hematopoietic cell lines *in vitro* (see above).

In conclusion, the examples shown above indicate that structural modification of c-*abl* is critical to its function. The replacement of the normal N-terminus with certain viral or cellular structures, perhaps concomitant with overexpression of the fusion product, may result in an aberrant growth of cells. However, structural variation of the N-terminus of *abl* is characteristic of the normal c-*abl* protein. The N-terminal variation of c-*abl* is generated by a unique RNA splicing pattern. In the presence of the Philadelphia chromosomal translocation, the same splicing mechanism may select a transforming N-terminal variant of *abl* resulting in leukemia.

ACKNOWLEDGEMENTS

We are grateful to Drs. E. Canaani, P. Besmer and O.N. Witte for the communication of valuable unpublished data. We thank G.Q. Daley for reading of the manuscript and Ginger Pierce for typing the manuscript. Y.B.-N. was supported by a Fogarty International Fellowship Award. This work was supported by a Program Project Grant (CA 38497) from the National Cancer Institute.

REFERENCES

Abelson HT and Rabstein LS (1970) Lymphosarcoma: virus induced thymic independent disease in mice. Cancer Res 30:2213-2222.

Bartram CR (1985) bcr rearrangement without juxtaposition of c-abl in chronic myelocytic leukemia. J Exp Med 162:2175-2179.

Ben-Neriah Y, Daley GQ, Mes-Masson AM, Witte ON and Baltimore D (1986a, to be published) The chronic myelogenous leukemia specific P210 protein is the product of the bcr/abl hybrid gene. Science.

Ben-Neriah Y, Bernards A, Paskind M, Daley GQ and Baltimore D (1986b) Alternative 5' exons in c-abl mRNA. Cell 44:577-586.

Besmer P, Hardy WD Jr, Zuckerman EE, Bergold D, Lederman L and Snyder HW Jr. (1983) The Hardy Zuckerman 2-FeSV a new feline retrovirus with oncogene homology to Abelson-MuLV. Nature 303:825-828.

Cross FR, Garber EA, Pellman D and Hanafusa H (1984) A short sequence in the p60src N terminus is required for p60src myristylation and membrane association and for cell transformation. Mol Cell Biol 4:1834-1842.

Foulkes JG, Chow M, Gorka C, Frackelton R Jr and Baltimore D. (1985) Purification and characterization of a protein-tyrosine kinase encoded by the Abelson murine leukemia virus. J Biol Chem 260:8070-8077.

Goff SP, Gilboa E, Witte ON and Baltimore D (1980) Structure of the Abelson murine leukemia virus genome and the homologous cellular gene: studies with cloned DNA. Cell 22:777-785.

Groffen J, Stephenson JR, Heisterkamp N, de Klein A, Bartram CR and Grosveld G (1984) Philadelphia chromosomal breakpoints are clustered within a limited region bcr on chromosome 22. Cell 36:93-99.

Grosveld G, Verwoerd T, Van-Agthoven T, de Klein A, Ramachandran KL, Heisterkamp N, Stam K and Groffen J (1986) The chronic myelocytic cell line K562 contains a breakpoint in bcr and produces a chimeric bcr/c-abl transcript. Mol Cell Biol 6:607-616.

Heisterkamp N, Stam K, Groffen J, de Klein A and Grosveld G (1985) Structural organization of the bcr gene and its role in the Ph' translocation. Nature 315:758-761.

Klar AJS, Strathern JN and Abraham JA (1984) Involvement of double strand chromosomal breaks for mating type switch in saccharomyces cerevisiae. Cold Spring Harbor Symp Quant Biol 49:77-88.

Konopka JB, Watanabe SM and Witte ON (1984) An alteration of the human c-abl protein in K562 leukemia cells unmasks associated tyrosine kinase activity. Cell 37:1035-1042.

Konopka JB and Witte ON (1985) Detection of c-abl tyrosine kinase activity in vitro permits direct comparison of normal and altered abl gene products. Mol Cell Biol 5:3116-3123.

Kozbor D, Giallongo A, Sierzega ME, Konopka J, Witte O, Showe LC and Croce CM (1986) Expression of a translocated c-abl gene in hybrids of mouse fibroblasts and chronic myelogenous leukemia cells. Nature 319:331-333.

Mann, R, Mulligan RC and Baltimore D (1983) Construction of a retrovirus packaging mutant and its use to produce helper-free defective retrovirus. Cell 33:153-159.

Mathey-Prevot B and Baltimore D (1985) Specific transforming potential of oncogenes encoding protein tyrosine kinases. EMBO J 4:1769-1774.

Mossman T (1983) Rapid colorimetric assay for cellular growth and survival: application to proliferation and cytotoxicity assays. J Immunol Methods 65:55-63.

Muller R, Salmon DJ, Tremblay JM, Cline MJ and Verma IM (1982) Differential expression of cellular oncogenes during pre- and post-natal development of the mouse. Nature 299:640-643.

Ponzetto C and Wolgemuth DJ (1985) Haploid expression of a unique c-abl transcript in the mouse male germ line. Mol Cell Biol 5:1791-1794.

Prywes R, Foulkes JG, Rosenberg N and Baltimore D (1983) Sequences of A-MuLV needed for fibroblast and lymphoid cell transformation. Cell 34:569-579.

Rowley JD (1975) Nonrandom chromosomal abnormalities in hematologic disorders of man. Proc Nat Acad Sci USA 72:152-156.

Sefton BM, Trowbridge IS, Cooper JA and Scolnick EM (1982) The transforming proteins of Rous sarcoma virus, Harvey sarcoma virus and Abelson virus contain tightly bound lipid. Cell 31:465-474.

Shtivelman E, Lifshitz B, Gale RP and Canaani E (1985) Fused transcript of abl and bcr genes in chronic myelogenous leukemia. Nature 315:550-554.

Wang JYJ and Baltimore D (1983) Cellular RNA homologous to the Abelson murine leukemia virus transforming gene: expression and relationship to the viral sequence. Mol Cell Biol 3:773-779.

Wang JYJ, Ledley F, Goff S, Lee R, Groner Y and Baltimore D (1984) The mouse c-abl locus: molecular cloning and characterization. Cell 36:349-356.

Witte ON, Dasgupta A and Baltimore D (1980) Abelson murine leukemia virus protein is phosphorylated *in vitro* to form phosphotyrosine. Nature 238:826-831.

Witte ON, Rosenberg NE and Baltimore D (1979) A normal cell protein cross reactive to the major Abelson murine leukemia virus gene product. Nature 281:396-398.

Yancopoulos GD, Blackwell K, Suh H, Hood L and Alt FW (1986) Introduced T cell receptor variable region gene segments recombine in pre-B cell: evidence that B and T cells use a common recombinase. Cell 44:251-259.

Transposable Elements and Cancer

E. Arman, N. Katzir, G. Rechavi* and D. Givol

Department of Chemical Immunology, The Weizmann Institute of Science Rehovot, Israel.
*Institute of Hematology, Sheba Medical Center, Tel Hashomer, Israel.

INTRODUCTION

Tumor progression is accompanied by many chromosomal aberrations and DNA rearrangements which contribute to the aggressiveness of the tumor. It is possible that active transposition of DNA elements play a role in these events. Approximately one third of the mammalian genome is composed of repetitive sequences (10^3 - 10^5 copies). This includes endogeneous retrovirus-like elements as well as short (SINE) and long (LINE) interdispersed DNA elements (Singer 1982; Singer 1982). The features of these elements is given in Fig. 1. Some of these features may suggest that they can behave as mobile elements and therefore may be adequate candidates for transposition in tumors. By integration near oncogenes or related genes these elements may affect the activity of such genes. One example for such an event was provided by the transposition of the intracisternal A-particle genome near the oncogene c-mos in mouse plasmacytoma (Rechavi et al 1982; Kuff et al 1983; Canaani et al 1983). Since then several additional examples of IAP transposition near cellular genes were described (Table 1). As a result of these transpositions the expression of the cellular genes was affected (Table 1) and in the case of c-mos the activated gene transformed NIH 3T3 cells. These examples prompted us to look in various tumors for oncogenes rearrangement and to search if other repetitive elements may also be transposed.

The canine transmissible venereal tumor (TVT) is a naturally occurring tumor that affects the external genitalia of both sexes and is transmitted during coitus (Cohen D 1985). The etiologic agent that originally induced this tumor is unknown but cytogenetic and immunologic studies strongly suggest that the tumor is transmitted by transplantation from one animal to another (Cohen D 1985). The uniqueness of this tumor lies in the fact that it is the only naturally occurring tumor which is transmitted by cell transplantation. TVT was first described 110 years ago (Novinsky 1876) and was later defined by Sticker (Sticker 1906) as lymphosarcoma, although the final definition of the cell type in the tumor is not yet clear (Cohen D 1985). Because of its long persistence in dogs and its extensive chromosomal aberrations we chose this tumor to look for oncogene rearrangements. We found that c-myc was rearranged due to the insertion of LINE (KpnI element) sequence upstream to c-myc. This provides evidence for the possible

Current Topics in Microbiology and Immunology, Vol. 132

behavior of LINE as mobile elements and enabled us also to prove the common cellular origin of this tumor in dogs from various geographical distribution.

RESULTS

The analysis of c-myc in DNA digest from normal and TVT tissues of various dogs is shown in Fig. 2. The HindIII digest shows one band of approximately 20 kbp of c-myc which is identical in all samples. The EcoRI digest shows a band of 7.5 kbp which corresponds to a part of exon 3 of c-myc, and a 15 kbp band which corresponds to exon 1 and 2 and part of exon 3 of c-myc. In addition a 16.5 kbp (arrow) rearranged c-myc can be observed in all tumor tissues, but not in normal DNA (Fig. 2). We cloned the 15 kbp EcoRI fragment (c-myc) and the 16.5 kbp rearranged gene (rc-myc) in Charon 4A. The analysis of c-myc and rc-myc demonstrated that rc-myc contains an insert of 1.5 kbp DNA approximately 4 kbp upstream to exon 1 of c-myc. The physical maps of the rearranged c-myc and the inserted 1.5 kbp DNA is given in Fig. 3.

In order to understand the nature of the DNA insert in rc-myc of TVT we sequenced the inserted piece according to the strategy shown in Fig. 3. In Fig. 4 we give the partial sequence of the novel DNA element inserted between the two PstI sites (Fig. 3), as compared to that of c-myc in this region. The results showed that c-myc and rc-myc are identical at both 5' and 3' ends. However rc-myc contains an insert of approximately 1.5 kbp which is absent in c-myc. The sequence of this insert showed 62% homology to that of the monkey KpnI (LINE) element (Fig. 4). The homology is to a 3' region of the KpnI element (between nucleotides 5079 and 4663, (M. Singer personal communication)). In addition the insert is bounded by a 10bp direct repeat (boxed) resulting from duplication of the target site, similar to that present in integration sites of transposable elements or retroviruses. The insert also contains a 3' tail of an A-rich sequence (60 bp) which includes the structure $A_7(TA_4)_7$, similar to that of other LINE or SINE elements (Rogers 1985). These features may classify the inserted DNA in rc-myc as a retroposon (Rogers 1983) or retrotransposon (Baltimore 1985), suggesting its origin from mRNA which reintegrate via a mechanism involving reverse transcription. These results demonstrate that the KpnI element can transpose somatically in a tumor tissue and integrate nearby to an oncogene. To further verify the repetitive nature of the DNA insert we used the BglII-PstI fragment of the insert (Fig. 3) as a probe to hybridize a blot of EcoRI digest of canine DNA. The results showed that the probe hybridized strongly to the entire blot indicating that this sequence is represented in multiple copies in canine DNA (Katzir et al 1985).

The inserted DNA can also be used as a marker to probe the origin of TVT in various dogs. We asked whether the same insert is present in the DNA of tumors from various geographical location. In order to do this we compared the Southern blots of HindIII digested DNA from tumors obtained from various dogs in Israel and USA. If we use the KpnI-HindIII fragment of c-myc (Fig. 3) as a probe we should obtain in a HindIII digest a 3.6 kpb hybridizing band in TVT whereas in normal tissue we should obtain a band larger than 5 kbp since there is not second HindIII site upstream to the one present in cmyc (Fig. 3). The result (Fig. 5) demonstrates that all DNA from TVT tumors of various geographical distribution contain 3.6 kbp and 4.3 kbp hybridizing bands which are absent in DNA from the normal dog tissues. On the other hand the normal tissue as well as tumor DNA contains a 6.3 kbp band which must be derived from the cellular DNA upstream to c-myc. Since the insert in rc-myc is of 1.5 kbp we expect a corresponding hindIII fragment in TVT to be of 7.8 kbp (6.3 + 1.5). The two hybridizing bands in TVT (3.6 + 4.3 kbp, Fig. 5) are in good agreement with this and are due to the presence of a HindIII site in the insert (Fig. 3). The fact that TVT tumors from different geographical distribution contain the same additional bands indicates that they contain the same insert in c-myc. This result indicates a common cellular origin for TVT in dogs from various location and support the hypothesis that TVT was spread between dogs by cell transplantation from a single original tumor.

SUMMARY

We have presented evidence that cellular repetitive DNA elements can behave as a mobile element. It seems logical that DNA transposition will be more frequent in tumor tissues. We found that in the canine RVT a 1.5 kbp DNA element was transposed upstream to c-myc. The transposed insert is bounded by a 10 bp direct repeats and contains a 3' A-rich region. This suggest its insertion via reverse transcription and its classification as retroposon (Rogers 1983). The sequence showed 62% homology to the monkey LINE 1 (Kpn I) element and indicates the possibility of transposition of this family of repeated interdispersed DNA. We have used a probe from the insertion region, upstream to c-myc, to probe whether the same insert is present in TVT from dogs of various geographical distribution. Our results showed that tumor from individual dogs in Israel and USA contain the same size insert in c-myc. Hence there is a common cellular origin for TVT in different dogs.

REFERENCES

Baltimore D (1985) Retroviruses and retroposons: The role of reverse transcription in shaping the eukaryotic genome. Cell 40: 481-482

Canaani E, Dreazen O, Klar A, Rechavi G, Ram D, Cohen JB, Givol D (1983) Activation of the c-mos oncogene in a mouse plasmacytoma by insertion of an endogenous intracisternal A-particle genome. Proc. Natl. Acad. Sci. USA 80: 7118-7122

Cohen D (1985) The canine transmissible venereal tumor: A unique result of tumor progression. Adv. in Can. Res. 43: 75-112

Cohen JB, Unger T, Rechavi G, Canaani E, Givol D (1983) Rearrangement of the oncogene c-mos in mouse myeloma NSI and hybridomas. Nature (London) 306: 797-799

Greenberg R, Hawley R, Marcu KB (1985) Acquisition of an intracisternal A-particle element by a translocated c-myc gene in a murine plasma cell tumor. Mol. and Cell Biol. 5: 3625-3628

Hawley RG, Shulman MJ, Hazumi N (1984) Intracisternal A-particle genes: A family of copia-like transposable elements in Mus musculus. Cancer Cells 2: 273-279

Katzir N, Rechavi G, Cohen JB, Unger T, Simoni F, Segal S, Cohen D, Givol D (1985) "Retroposon" insertion into the cellular oncogene c-myc in canine transmissible venereal tumor. Proc. Natl. Acad. Sci. USA 82: 1054-1058

Kuff EL, Feenstra A, Lueders K, Rechavi G, Givol D, Canaani E (1983) Homology between an endogenous viral LTR and sequences inserted in an activated cellular oncogene. Nature (London) 302: 547-548

Novinsky MA (1876) Zur frage uber die impfung der krebsigen geschulste. Zentralbl. Med. Wiss. 14: 790-791

Rechavi G, Givol D, Canaani E (1982) Activation of a cellular oncogene by DNA rearrangment: possible involvement of an Is-like element. Nature (London) 300: 607-611

Rogers JH (1983) Retroposons defined. Nature (London) 301: 460.

Rogers JH (1985) The structure and evolution of retroposons. Int. Rev. Cytol. 93: 231-279

Shen-Ong GLC, Keath EJ, Piccoli SP and Cole MD (1982) Novel myc oncogene RNA from abortive immunoglobulin gene recombination in mouse plasmacytomas. Cell 31: 443-452

Singer MF (1982) Highly repeated sequences in mammalian genomes. Int. Rev. Cytol. 76: 67-112

Singer MF (1982) Sines and Lines: Highly repeated short and long interspersed sequences in mammalian genomes. Cell 28: 433-434

Sticker A (1906) Transplantables rundzellensarkom des hundes, ein beitrag zur lehre der krebsubertragbarkeit. Z. Krebforsch 4: 227-314.

Ymer S, Tucker QJ, Sanderson CJ, Hapel AJ, Cambell HD, Young IG (1985) Constitutive synthesis of interleukin-3 by leukemia cell line WEHI-3B is due to retroviral insertion near the gene. Nature (London) 317: 255-258

Table 1: Transposition of IAP nearby to cellular genes in mouse genome.

Cellular gene	Cell line	IAP location	Effect on transcription	Reference
c-mos	XRPC-24	5'	increase	Rechavi et al
c-mos	NSI	5'	"	Cohen et al
c-myc	j558	3'	no effect	Greenberg et al
IgK	IgK-20	IVS1	decrease	Hawley et al
IgK	Sp603	IVS2	"	Hawley et al
IL-3	WHEI-3B	5'	increase	Ymer et al

REPETITIVE DNA SEQUENCES AS RETROPOSONS

A. Endogeneous retrovirus-like elements

1. Two LTR
2. Flanked by direct repeats.
3. $\sim 10^3$ copies, e.g. IAP in mouse, RTVL-H in man.
4. Expressed in early embryo, thymus, some tumors.

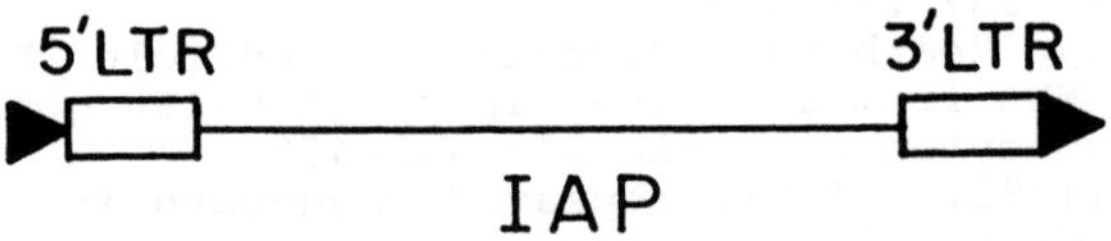

B. Short (SINE) and Long (LINE) interdispersed elements.

1. Conserved sequence.
2. PolyA at 3' end (origin from mRNA).
3. Flanked by direct repeats.
4. Expressed as heterogeneous mRNA.
5. Long open reading frame.
6. Truncation (5' region) rearrangements, deletions.
7. $\sim 10^4$ copies, e.g. Alu $\sim$500 bp (SINE), KpnI family $\sim$6 kbp (LINE).

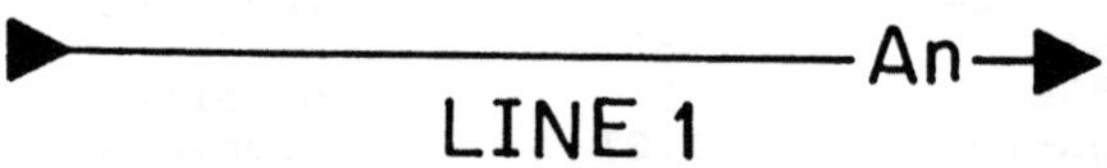

Figure 1: Features of repetitive DNA elements in mammals.

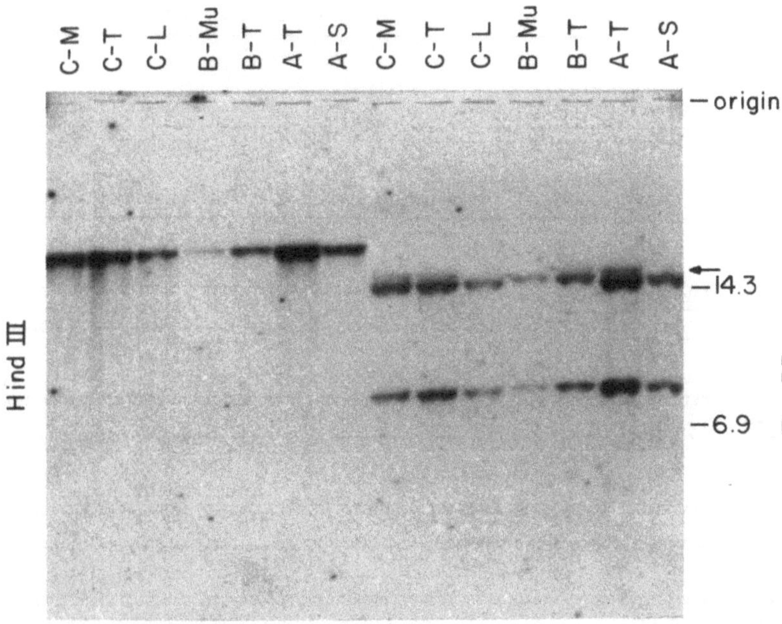

Fig. 2: Rearrangement of c-myc in canine TVT. Aliquots (10ug) of tumor or normal tissue DNA was digested with either HindIII or EcoRI, electrophoresed on 0.7% agarose and after blotting onto nitrocellulose was hybridized to the radiolabeled mouse *myc* probe pM104BH (17) which corresponds to exon 2 and 3. Only in the EcoRI digest *myc* rearrangement (arrow) was observed. A,B,C- tissues from different dogs. L, liver; M, metastatic tumor; Mu, muscle; S, spleen; T, TVT.

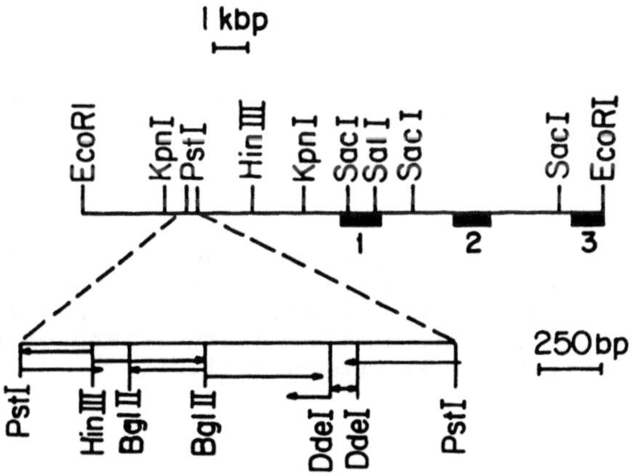

Fig. 3: Physical map of rc-*myc*. Upper line shows the map of c-*myc*. Lower line show the map and sequence strategy of the 1.5 kbp insert between the two PstI sites. The exons of c-*myc* are marked by black rectangles.

```
         PstI                                                                        70
rc-myc   CTGCAGCATA GGGGTGGGGC AGGGAGACAA CATTTTAAAA ACAATGCATT TTTAAAAATG CACCAAGATT
 c-myc   ---------- ---------- ---------- ---------- ---------- ---------- ----------
                        . . . .
                                                                                    140
rc-myc   TTCTTCACTG CCTTTTTTTT TTATCATTCC TACGAATGAA TGATTGGCCA GATTTCGTCT GCTCGTCTGC
 c-myc   ---------- ---------- ---------- ---------- ---------- ---------- ----------

                                                                                    210
rc-myc   TGAAGAGCTT CCCAGTGTTC CTCTCACTGG GACACATGGT TAGCACAGGA AATACTGGTG AGGCTTTCCC
 c-myc   ---------- ---------- ---------- ---------- ---------- ---------- ----------

                                                                        HinIII      280
rc-myc   ATCCTTTAAC [ATTCTCTGGC] TGTCTTCGAC CCCCGCCGAC TGTATCCTTT GCTGTGCAAA AGCTTCTTAT
 c-myc   ----------
 Kpn I                          --C--GT-CA -T-T-AT-GT A--T--T--- --------G- ----CT---G

                                                                                    350
rc-myc   CTTGATGAAG TCCCAATAGT TCATTTTTGC TTTTGTTTCT TTTGCCTTCG TGGATGTATC TTGCAAGAAG
 c-myc
 Kpn I   T--A--T-GA -----T-T-- CA-----G-- -------C-C A----T--T- GA-T-T--GA CATG---TCT

                                                                                 417BglII
rc-myc   TTACTATGGC CGAGTTCAAA AAGGGTGTTG CCTGTGTTCT TCTCTAGGAT TTTGATGGAA CCTTGCC...
 c-myc
 Kpn I   --G-CCAT-- -T-TG--CTG --T---A--- ---AG---T- CT------G- ---T----T- TTAG-T-

                                                                                    510
rc-myc   TGAAGTGTAT GGTGAAAGAG AGTGGTCTAG TTTCATTCTT TCTGCATGTG GATGTCCAAT TTCCCAGCAC
 c-myc
 Kpn I   -TTT--A--A ----T---GA --G-A--C-- -----G---- ---A-T-A-- -C--C-A-T- ----------

                                                                                    580
rc-myc   CATTTATTGA GAGCAATGTC TTTCTTCCAA TGGATAGTCT TTCCTCCTTT ATCGAATATT AGTTGCCCAT
 c-myc
 Kpn I   --------A- ATAGGGAA-- C--TCC---T -TCT-GT--C -CT-AGG--- G--A--G--C --A--GTTG-

                                                            635
rc-myc   AAAGTTCAGG TCCACTTCTG GATTCTCTAT TCTGTTGGAC TGATCTATGT GTCTG.....~1.4 kbp..
 c-myc
 Kpn I   -G-TG-GT-- -TT-T----- GAAG----G- ------CC-T --G-----A- -----

                                                                                   2070
rc-myc   TGTTCATCTG TATGTTAGTA AATTGAACAC CAATAAAAAT AAAATAAAAT AAAATAAAAT AAAATAAAAT
 c-myc

                                                                                   2140
rc-myc   AAAAAAAAAA AATAA[ATTC TCTGGC]CGCC TTGGTTTTGA ATCTCATGGC CCTTCTTTCA AAATGATCTT
c-myc                  ---- ---------- ---------- ---------- ---------- ----------
            PstI
rc-myc   TCTGCAG
 c-myc   -------
```

Fig. 4: Partial sequence of the DNA insert in rc-myc. The sequence shows the beginning and end of the insert and the junction with c-myc sequence. Direct repeats are boxed. The sequence of the insert is compared with that of the complementary strand of the monkey KpnI element (M. Singer, personal communication).

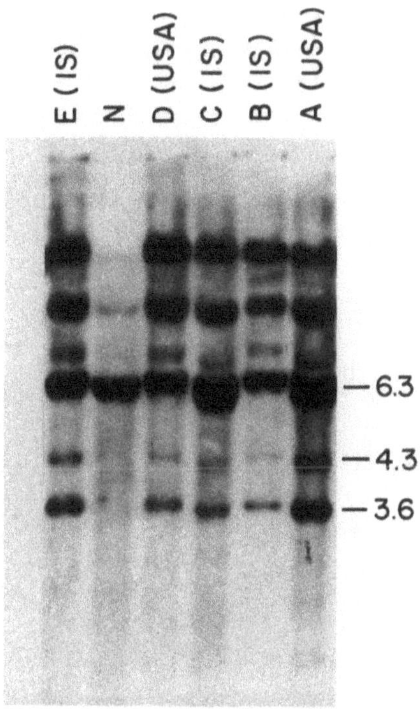

Fig. 5: Analysis of KpnI element insert in tumors from various geographical location. DNA (10ug) of TVT or normal spleen DNA was digested with HindIII, electrophoresed on 0.7% agarose and blotted onto nitrocellulose. Hybridization was with the KpnI-HindIII fragment of c-*myc* (see Fig. 3). Normal canine DNA shows a major hybridizing band of 6.3 kbp. TVT yields additional two hybridizing bands (3.6 kbp and 4.3 kbp) which if contain the same insert should be together 7.8 kb (6.3 kbp + 1.5 kbp insert, see text).

Alpha-type B Cell Growth Factor and Complement Component C3: Their Possible Structural Relationship

Waldemar Lernhardt*, William C. Raschke*, and Fritz Melchers**

*Cancer Research Center, La Jolla Cancer Research Foundation, La Jolla, California 92037 USA

**Basel Institute for Immunology, CH 4058 Basel, Switzerland

INTRODUCTION

The third component of complement C3 has been found to control the entry of activated B cell blasts into the S-phase of the cell cycle (Erdei et al., 1985; Melchers et al., 1985). In its activity as a synergistic growth factor, it therefore replaces α-type B cell growth factors (BCGF; Corbel and Melchers, 1984) which have been found to act at the same temporal point (restriction point) in the cell cycle (Melchers and Lernhardt, 1985). Furthermore, soluble C3d inhibits the synergistic action of α-type BCGF (Melchers et al., 1985). These results have suggested that both C3 and α-type BCGF act by signalling through the C3d-specific complement receptor CR2 (Fearon, 1984). The growth regulating properties of the CR2 receptor for B cells have also been implied in studies which demonstrated stimulating activities of CR2-specific, monoclonal antibodies with human B cells (Nemerow et al., 1985). These results have prompted us to investigate whether a structural relationship exists between C3 and α-type BCGF.

RESULTS

Alpha-type BCGFs have been found to be produced by normal macrophage colonies and established macrophage cell lines such as P388D1. They are furthermore produced by a variety of cell lines established from B and T cell tumors and by T and B cell hybridomas (Corbel and Melchers, 1984). One T cell hybridoma has previously been identified as producing B cell growth factors with apparent molecular weights of 80-90 Kd and 20-30 Kd which do not induce maturation to immunoglobulin secretion (Lernhardt et al., 1982) and therefore appear to be different from BCGFII (Swain et al., 1983; Harada et al., 1985).

Synthesis of mRNA Hybridizing to C3 cDNA in Cell Lines Producing α-type BCGF

The T cell hybridoma A32-26 and the T cell lymphoma EL-4 produce detectable levels of α-type BCGF only when stimulated with concanavalin A. Messenger RNA was analyzed by Northern blotting after gel electrophoresis on formaldehyde/agarose gels (Thomas, 1980) and hybridization to a radiolabelled cDNA probe containing more than 80% of the coding sequence of C3 (pMLC3/7, kindly provided by Dr. G. Fey, Dept. of Immunology, Scripps Research Institution, La Jolla, CA; Domdey et al., 1982; Wetsel et al., 1984; Lundvall et al., 1984). Two major bands with sizes of 4.2 and 1.8 kb, respectively, were detected in all four preparations (Fig. 1). The size of mRNA coding for the complete C3 molecule was expected to be 5.6 kb as detected in liver RNA (Domdey et al., 1982) or the C3-producing macrophage line, WEHI 3 (Fig. 2, right panel). This cell line, after stimulation with lipopolysaccharide for 12 and 24 hours, shows three species of mRNA hybridizing to C3 cDNA; the 5.6 kb species, however, is in large excess (Fig. 2). WEHI 3 produces barely detectable levels of α-type BCGF (Corbel and Melchers, 1984). The T cell hybridomas V215 BW1 and V215 BW2, known to produce α-type BCGF, and the T helper line OI6 produce the 1.8 kb mRNA

Current Topics in Microbiology and Immunology, Vol. 132

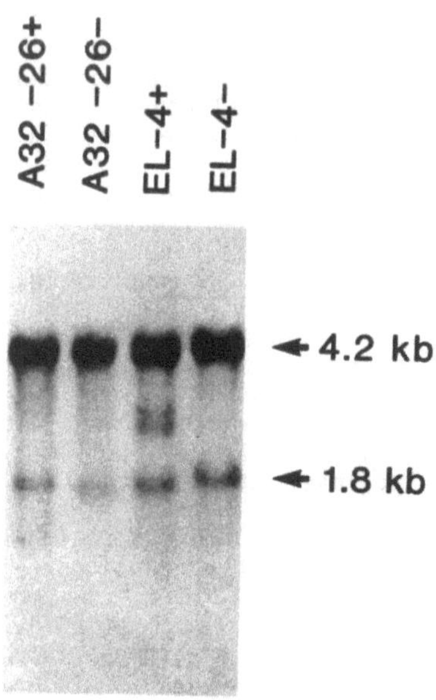

Fig. 1. The cell lines indicated were grown in Iscove's medium (Iscove and Melchers, 1978) and cytoplasmic RNA from induced (+) cells (concanavalin A, 5 µg/ml for 24 h, 10^6 cells per ml) or uninduced cells (-) was prepared and, after poly A selection, subjected to Northern blot analysis using the C3 cDNA probe pMLC3/7 as described in the legend to Fig. 2.

species only (Fig. 3). The α-type BCGF-negative cell line, BW 5147, L cells, and a subline of EL-4 selected for the loss of α-type BCGF production fail to show detectable hybridization signals with the C3 cDNA probe (Fig. 2, right panel, and Fig. 3). These results suggest a correlation between α-type BCGF production and the transcription of mRNA(s) hybridizing to C3 cDNA.

Failure to Detect IL-1α-specific mRNA Sequences in α-type BCGF-producing Cell Lines

The Northern blot shown in Figure 2, right panel, was reprobed with an IL-1α-specific radioactively labelled oligonucleotide after boiling-off of the C3 cDNA probe to provide an independent RNA size and integrity control and to concurrently investigate whether α-type BCGF-producing cell lines produce IL-1. Figure 2, left panel, shows that only WEHI 3 produces IL-1α mRNA of the appropriate size (Lomedico *et al.*, 1984), whereas neither BW 5147 nor the concanavalin A-induced lines A32-26 and EL-4 show detectable IL-1α mRNA. The upper faint band at 5.6 kb is attributed to incomplete boiling-off of the C3 cDNA probe. The experiments have been repeated with both IL-1α and IL-1β cDNA probes kindly provided by Dr. P. Grey, Genentech, South San Francisco, CA (data not shown). Again, only WEHI 3 showed IL-1α- and β-specific mRNAs. These results indicate that these cell lines do not contain IL-1 mRNA at any detectable level.

Translation of mRNA into α-type BCGF Activity

We have previously shown that mRNA from the α-type BCGF-producing cell line A32-26, but not from the T cell lymphoma BW 5147, can be translated into α-type BCGF activity after injection into *Xenopus laevis* oocytes (Lernhardt *et al.*, 1984). Injection of mRNA from A32-26 size-fractionated by sucrose gradient centrifugation into *Xenopus* oocytes resulted in the resolution of two peaks of

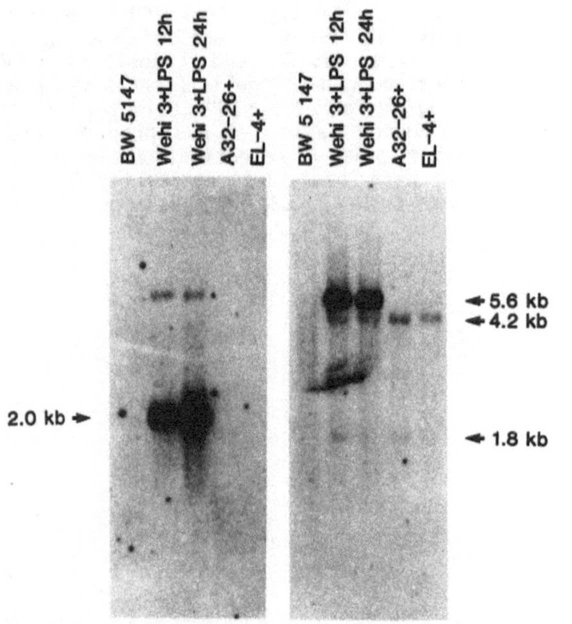

Fig 2. The cell lines indicated were grown in Iscove's serum substituted medium (Iscove and Melchers, 1978) except WEHI 3 which was grown in DMEM + 10% fetal calf serum. WEHI 3 cells were treated with lipopolysaccharide (2 µg/ml) for 12 and 24 h, respectively. The other cell lines were induced with concanavalin A (5 µg/ml) for 24 h at 10^6 cells/ml except for BW 5147. Poly A^+ RNA (5 µg/lane) was incubated at 65° C for 5 min. in 50% formamide, 2.2 M formaldehyde, 0.02 M marpholinopropansulfonic acid, 5 mM sodium acetate, 1 mM EDTA, pH 7.0, and electrophoresed on 1% agarose gels containing 2 M formaldehyde. The RNA was blotted onto nitrocellulose paper and hybridized to the nick-translated C3 cDNA probe pMLC3/7 (right panel) (specific activity 3 x 10^8 cpm/µg) as described by Thomas (1980). After exposure, the nitrocellulose filter was boiled in H_2O for 10 min. and reprobed with an IL-1α-specific oligonucleotide end-labelled with polynucleotide kinase (specific activity 10^7 cpm/µg) (left panel).

activity of 12s and 24s (Fig. 4). These mRNA sizes roughly correspond to the mRNA sizes of 1.8 kb and 4.2 kb detected in Northern blot analysis using a C3 cDNA probe. These results demonstrate a correlation between the sizes of mRNA translatable into growth factor activity and the sizes of mRNA showing homology to C3.

DISCUSSION

The results presented in this report indicate that there is a correlation between the production of α-type BCGF and the synthesis of mRNA hybridizing to C3 cDNA. The cell lines producing α-type BCGF show either both the 4.2 and 1.8 kb mRNA species or the 1.8 kb species only, whereas cell lines which score negative in our cellular assays for α-type BCGF production do not show detectable hybridization signals with the C3 cDNA probe. The macrophage line WEHI 3 shows the genuine C3 mRNA of 5.6 kb and the 4.2 and 1.8 kb species, albeit to a much lesser extent. The low α-type BCGF activity produced by this cell line might be due to the inhibitory nature of the genuine soluble C3 molecule (Erdei et al., 1985).

Interleukin-1 has been implicated in B lymphocyte growth control (Howard et al., 1983; Pike and Nossal, 1985), and since it is produced by macrophage and macrophage cell lines, the question has been raised whether this interleukin is responsible for α-type BCGF activity. Therefore, the cell lines used in this study have also been probed for the presence of IL-1 mRNAs. As expected, WEHI 3 showed the 2 kb mRNA species reported for IL-1α (Lomelico et al., 1984). However, none of the other cell lines producing α-type BCGF contained detectable mRNA hybridizing to an IL-1α-specific oligonucleotide (Fig. 2). These results

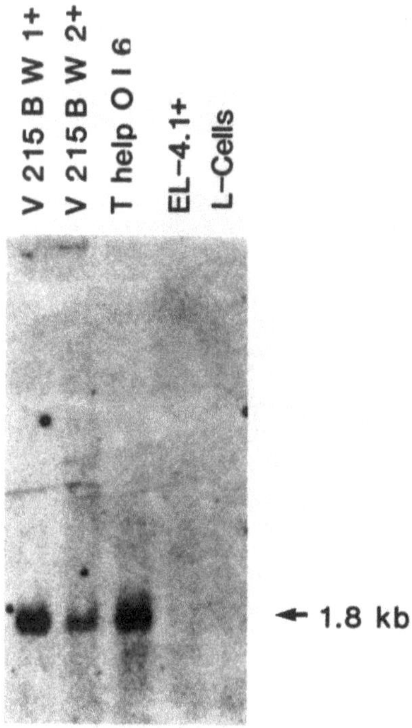

Fig. 3. RNA from the induced (concanavalin A, 5 µg/ml, 24 h) T cell hybridomas V215 BW1, V215 BW2, the T cell lymphoma EL-4, the uninduced T helper cell line OI6 and from L cells were subjected to Northern blot analysis using the C3 cDNA probe pMLC3/7 as described in Fig. 2.

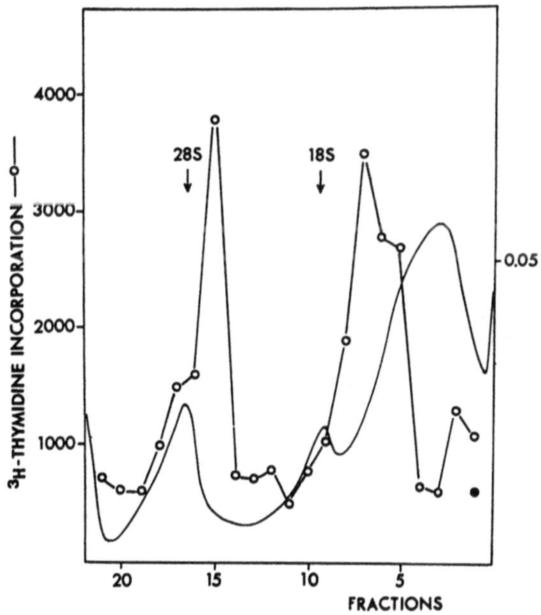

Fig. 4. Poly A^+ RNA from the concanavalin A-induced T cell hybridoma A32-26 was centrifuged through a sucrose gradient of 15-30% sucrose in 10 mM Tris-HCl, pH 7.4, 1 mM EDTA, and 0.1% SDS for 17 h at 27,000, and spun in a SW41 rotor. RNA in each fraction was precipitated and injected into Xenopus laevis oocytes. Oocytes were incubated in Barth's medium for 48 h at 22° C. The supernatants were then assayed for α-type BCGF activity on lipopolysaccharide-activated B cell blasts (10^5/ml), purified by velocity sedimentation (Miller and Phillips, 1969) in the presence of 25 µg/ml lipopolysaccharide in Iscove's medium (Iscove and Melchers, 1978). Under these conditions, the proliferation of B cell blasts is dependent on α-type BCGF (Corbel and Melchers, 1984). Proliferation was assessed by ^{3}H-thymidine uptake (4 h, 1 µCi/0.2 ml culture).

were confirmed by using cDNA probes for both IL-1α and β (data not shown). We therefore conclude that neither A32-26 nor EL-4 α-type BCGF preparations contain IL-1. The question remains to be answered whether IL-1 acts directly on B lymphocytes in a growth-controlling fashion or whether it elicits other interleukins such as α-type BCGF from contaminating T lymphocytes, which in turn act directly on B lymphocytes.

The mRNA sizes determined by Northern analysis roughly coincide with the size of mRNA which can be translated into α-type BCGF activity by injection into Xenopus laevis oocytes. This size correlation might be taken as evidence that α-type BCGF is in fact encoded by sequences with homologies to complement component C3. The results indicating that two mRNA species can be translated into full α-type BCGF activity independently of each other is supported by the finding that the T cell hybridomas 215 BW1 and 215 BW2 only show the 1.8 kb mRNA species, and nevertheless, the level of α-type BCGF produced by these lines is comparable to that of A32-26 and EL-4. The existence of two mRNA species both coding for α-type BCGF might explain the heterogeneity in protein sizes previously determined for this BCGF activity. The apparent molecular weights found were 80000-90000 dalton and 20000-30000 dalton (Lernhardt et al., 1982). The mRNA species described here could code for proteins of these sizes. The physiological implications of having two mRNAs and therefore two protein species with apparently the same function, as well as their structural interrelationship, are not clear at this point. The molecular characterization of the two growth factor species by cDNA cloning and sequence analysis should reveal their relationship.

Should the α-type BCGF mRNAs in fact prove to be derived from C3 sequences, a viable mode for their generation would be through alternative splicing patterns from a primary C3 transcript. Such a putative mechanism is supported by the finding that only one C3 gene exists (Wiebauer et al., 1982). Furthermore, our own results (not included here) showed that an oligonucleotide specific for the C3d region containing the sequences responsible for binding to CR2 (Lambris et al., 1985) hybridizes to both mRNA species, lending support to the idea that both species are generated from a common precursor through alternative RNA processing. An increasing number of cases are currently being reported which demonstrate the generation of several mRNA species from an individual gene through alternative RNA processing mechanisms. Our own laboratory has shown that the different polypeptide forms of the lymphocyte surface glycoprotein T200 (Ly 5) arise due to alternative splicing mechanisms (Raschke, submitted for publication). It is conceivable that similar mechanisms are involved in the generation of the α-type BCGF mRNAs.

It can be assumed that α-type BCGF acts through the complement receptor CR2 based on the findings that soluble C3b and C3d inhibit α-type BCGF activity (Erdei et al., 1985), and both α-type BCGF and cross-linked C3b and C3d act upon the same restriction point in the G_1 phase of the cell cycle of B cell blasts (Melchers et al., 1985). As mentioned above, both mRNA species contain the sequence elements required for binding to CR2. However, the question remains as to how the soluble α-type BCGF molecules convey this growth promoting effect, since cross-linking of CR2 is considered a requirement for the transduction of the growth-stimulating signal. Cross-linking of CR2 can be achieved by aggregated C3b or C3d, whereas, the inhibitory action of C3d and C3b is considered to result from their failure to cross-link this receptor. The structural analysis through cDNA cloning of these two mRNA species and expression of these cDNAs in suitable expression systems will yield α-type BCGF proteins in large quantities and in pure form which in turn will allow us to address this question.

ACKNOWLEDGEMENT

The authors wish to thank Drs. G. Fey, Dept. of Immunology, Scripps Research Institution, La Jolla, CA, and Dr. P. Grey, Genentech, South San Francisco, CA, for generously providing cDNA probes. We thank Diana Lowe for helping to prepare this manuscript. This work was supported by NSF grant DCB 8316700 and NIH grant CA 37344. The Basel Institute for Immunology was founded and is supported by F. Hoffmann-LaRoche & Co., Ltd.

REFERENCES

Corbel C, Melchers F (1984) The synergism of accessory cells and of soluble α-factors derived from them in the activation of B cells to proliferation. Immunol Rev 78: 51-74

Domdey H, Wiebauer K, Kazmaier M, Muller V, Odink K, Fey G (1982) Characterization of the mRNA and cloned cDNA specifying the third component of mouse complement. Proc Natl Acad Sci (USA) 79: 7619-7623

Erdei A, Melchers F, Schulz TF, Dierich M (1985) The action of human C3 in soluble or cross-linked form with resting and activated murine B lymphocytes. Eur J Immunol 15: 184-188

Fearon DT (1984) Cellular receptors for fragments of the third component of complement. Immun Today 5: 105-110

Harada N, Kikuchi Y, Tominaga A, Takaki S, Takatsu K (1985) BCGFII activity on activated B cells of a purified murine T cell-replacing factor (TRF) from a T cell hybridoma (B151K12). J Immunol 134: 3944-3951

Howard M, Mizel SB, Lachman L, Ansel J, Johnson B, Paul WE (1983) Role of Interleukin I in anti-immunoglobulin induced B cell proliferation. J Exp Med 157: 1529-1543

Iscove NN, Melchers F (1978) Complete replacement of serum by albumin, transferrin and soybean lipid in cultures of LPS-reactive B lymphocytes. J Exp Med 147: 923-933

Lambris JD, Vishwas SG, Hirani S, Muller-Eberhard HJ (1985) Mapping of the C3d receptor (CR2)-binding site and a neoantigenic site in the C3d domain of the third component of complement. Proc Natl Acad Sci (USA) 82: 4235-4239

Lernhardt W, Corbel C, Wall R, Melchers F (1982) T cell hybridomas which produce B lymphocyte replication factor only. Nature 300: 355-357

Lernhardt W, Corbel C, Melchers F, Wall R (1984) Functional and molecular characterization of murine B cell replication factor derived from a T cell hybridoma. In: Cantor H, Chess L, Sercarz E (eds) Regulation of the immune system. Alan R. Liss, Inc, New York, pp 573-581

Lomedico PT, Gubler U, Hellmann CP, Dukowich M, Giri JG, Yu-ching EP, Collier K, Semionbw R, Chua AO, Mizel SB (1984) Cloning and expression of murine interleukin-1 cDNA in E. coli. Nature 312: 458-462

Lundvall A, Wetsel RA, Domdey H, Tach BF, Fey GH (1984) Structure of murine complement component C3. I. Nucleotide sequence of cloned complementary and genomic DNA coding for the β chain. J Biol Chem 259: 13851-13856

Melchers F, Lernhardt W (1985) Three restriction points in the cell cycle of activated murine B lymphocytes. Proc Natl Acad Sci (USA) 82: 355-357

Miller RG, Phillips RA (1969) Separation of cells by velocity sedimentation. J Cell Physiol 73: 191-202

Nemerow GR, McNaughton ME, Cooper NR (1985) Binding of monoclonal antibody to the Epstein Barr Virus (EBV)/CR2 receptor induces activation and differentiation of human B lymphocytes. J Immunol 135: 3068-3073

Pike BL, Nossal GJV (1985) Interleukin I can act as a B-cell growth and differentiation factor. Proc Natl Acad Sci (USA) 82: 8153-8157

Swain SL, Howard M, Kappler J, Marrack P, Watson J, Booth R, Wetsel GD, Dutton R (1983) Evidence for two distinct classes of murine B-cell growth factors with activities in different functional assays. J Exp Med 158: 822-835

Thomas PS (1980) Hybridization of denatured RNA and small DNA fragments transferred to nitrocellulose. Proc Natl Acad Sci (USA) 77: 5201-5205

Wetsel RA, Lundvall A, Davidson F, Gibson T, Tach BF, Fey GH (1984) Structure of murine complement component C3. II. Nucleotide sequence of cloned complementary DNA coding for the α chain. J Biol Chem 259: 13857-13862

Wiebauer K, Domdey H, Diggelmann H, Fey G (1982) Isolation and analysis of genomic DNA clones encoding the third component of mouse complement. Proc Natl Acad Sci (USA) 79: 7077-7081

A Growth-Factor Dependent B-Cell Hybridoma

P.M. Lansdorp, L.A. Aarden, J. Calafat*, and W.P. Zeiljemaker

Central Laboratory of the Netherlands Red Cross Blood Transfusion Service and Laboratory for Experimental and Clinical Immunology, University of Amsterdam, and *Netherlands Cancer Institute, Amsterdam, The Netherlands

INTRODUCTION

Injection of pristane (2,6,10,14 tetramethylpentadecane) into the peritoneal cavity of Balb/c mice has been used to induce plasmacytomas (1) and to induce a microenvironment that will support the growth of transplanted plasmacytomas derived from primary hosts (2) and B-cell hybridomas (3). In vitro growth of primary plasmacytomas (4) and B-cell hybrids immediately after fusion (5) requires the addition of "feeder" cells to the culture medium. In previous studies we have shown that this feeder-cell requirement of B-cell hybrids can be overcome by the addition of the supernatant of human endothelial cell cultures to the culture medium (6,7). The characterization of this growth-promoting activity has been hampered by the lack of rapid and reproducible assay.

We now describe a stable B-cell hybridoma cell line, B13.29, that is, for its survival and growth, dependent on exogenous growth-factor. With these cells a rapid and convenient assay for "hybridoma growth factor" (HGF) was developed. The isolation and partial characterization of HGF produced by human peripheral blood monocytes has been reported elsewhere (8).

MATERIALS AND METHODS

Cells

The factor dependent hybridoma cell line B13.29 was obtained from a fusion of Sp2/0Ag14 cells (9) with spleen cells from a Balb/c mouse immunized with human peripheral blood leukocytes. The cells are maintained in Iscove's modified Dulbecco's medium (IMDM, Gibco, Paisley, Scotland) supplemented with 10% (v/v) fetal calf serum (FCS, Flow Laboratories, Irvine U.K.), penicillin (100 U/ml), streptomycin (100 μg/ml) and 5.10^{-5} M 2-mercaptoethanol (IMDM-FCS) and an appropriate source of HGF such as 1% (v/v) peripheral blood mononuclear cell conditioned medium (8). The FCS was selected from 5 different lots for its growth-promoting activity on Sp2/0Ag14 cells seeded at low cell densities. B13.29 cells produce an IgG_1 antibody reactive with a determinant expressed selectively on mature human granulocytes. Antibody production was assayed by an ELISA technique as described (11). Cultures of B13.29 cells and factor independent subclones of this line were tested for mycoplasma contamination by a sensitive assay based on adenosine-phosphorylase activity of mycoplasma (12). On various occasions the cells were found to be negative in this assay. Chromosome preparations were prepared as described by Worton and Duff (13).

Conditioned Media

Culture of endothelial cells and production of conditioned medium from these cells was performed as described (6,7). Cultures of smooth muscle cells were prepared from umbilical cord arteries as described by Ross (14). Conditioned medium of typical smooth-muscle-cell cultures obtained after several passages was used. No contamination with other cell types of the umbilical cord was detectable (Dr. Ph. G. de Groot, personal communication). Medium conditioned by human fibroblasts was prepared from cultures of fetal-skin-biopsy fragments as described (15). Fibroblast-like cells were also grown from bone-marrow cells of a patient with myeloma. Human-placenta-conditioned-medium was prepared according to Schlunk and Schleyer (16) and was a gift from Dr. P. Baines (University of Wales, Cardiff U.K.). HGF was prepared as described (8). Medium conditioned by mouse fibroblastoid L929 cells and mouse myelomonocytic WEHI-3B cells were gifts from Dr. L. Mets (National Cancer Institute, Amsterdam, The Netherlands) and Dr. P. Baines, respectively. Medium conditioned by adherent cells from long-term cultures of mouse bone-marrow and P388D cell line cells were kindly provided by Dr. R. Gisler and Dr. N. Iscove (Basel Institute for Immunology, Basel, Switzerland). To prepare thymocyte conditioned medium, thymocytes obtained from 6-week-old Brown Norway were cultured for 2 days at a concentration of 10^6/ml in IMDM-FCS.

Growth-Factor Assay

B13.29 cells from cultures at densities between 2-10 x 10^5/ml were harvested by centrifugation, washed 2x in IMDM-FCS, and adjusted to a concentration of 5 x 10^5/ml in IMDM-FCS. Volumes of 100 μl IMDM-FCS, with or without (diluted) test sample, were pipetted into the wells of flat-bottom tissue-culture plates (Costar, Cambridge, Mass., USA). To each well, a 10 μl volume of cell suspension was added. After various time intervals of culture, cells were labeled with .2 μCi ^{3}H-labeled thymidine (^{3}H-TdR, Radiochemical Centre, Amersham, UK; spec. act. 2 Ci/mMol). Cultures were harvested 4 hours after the addition of ^{3}H-TdR and the incorporation into DNA was measured as described (17). The dilution of a test sample resulting in half-maximal ^{3}H-TdR incorporation is used to express the activity in units/ml.

Cell-Cycle Analysis

B13.29 cells, cultured with or without growth factor (1% HGF), were harvested by centrifugation after fixed time intervals. The cells ($\pm$ 10^6 cells) were resuspended in 1 ml ice-cold phosphate buffered saline (PBS) and added dropwise to 2 ml of 96% (v/v) ethanol (-20° C) under continuous stirring. After fixation for several hours, the cells were treated with RNAse (analytical grade, 100,000 units/mg; Serva, Heidelberg, FRG) for 15 minutes at room temperature (1 mg of RNAse/ml PBS), washed and resuspended in PBS containing propidium iodide (Calbiochem-Behring Corp., La Jolla, CA, USA) 10 μg/ml. The cells were allowed to stain for at least 15 minutes prior cytofluorometric analysis on a FACS-II (Beckton-Dickinson, Oakland, CA, USA). After background correction, DNA histograms were analysed as described by Schultz et. al. (18). This program yields the composition of the cell population expressed as the cumulative percentage of cells in the G_1, S and G_2+M phases of the cell cycle.

Electron Microscopy

B13.29 cells and B13.29-M9 cells (see Results) were harvested by centrifugation, and the pellets fixed with 2.5% glutaraldehyde in 0.1 M cacodylate buffer, pH 7.2 and postfixed for 1 h with 1% (w/v) osmium tetroxide in the same buffer. After fixation, the pellets were dehydrated and embedded in a mixture of Epon and Araldite. Thin sections were stained with uranyl acetate and lead hydroxide, and examined with Philips electron microscopes EM-300 and EM-301.

RESULTS

Isolation of a Growth Factor Dependent Hybridoma Cell Line

The hybridoma clone B13.29 was selected from a cell fusion experiment aimed at the production of antibodies against human cell-surface antigens (10). After fusion the cells were grown in the presence of the culture supernatant of human endothelial cell cultures (HECS) as described (6). The growth of B13.29 cells was, and remained, dependent on the presence of HECS. Dose-response curves obtained with different batches of HECS are shown in Fig. 1a. For this experiment the thymidine incorporation of 5 x 10^3 B13.29 cells, cultured with various concentrations of HECS, was measured at day 2. As little of 0.5% (v/v) of each batch was sufficient to maximally stimulate thymidine incorporation. The time-response of 5 x 10^3 B13.29 cells are shown in Fig. 1b. Although no differences between cultures with or without HECS were measured after 8 h of culture, a dramatic difference in ^{3}H-TdR incorporation was observed after 24-48 h. For further experiments the ^{3}H-TdR incorporation of 5 x 10^3 B13.29 cells at 48 h of culture was used to quantitate HGF activity.

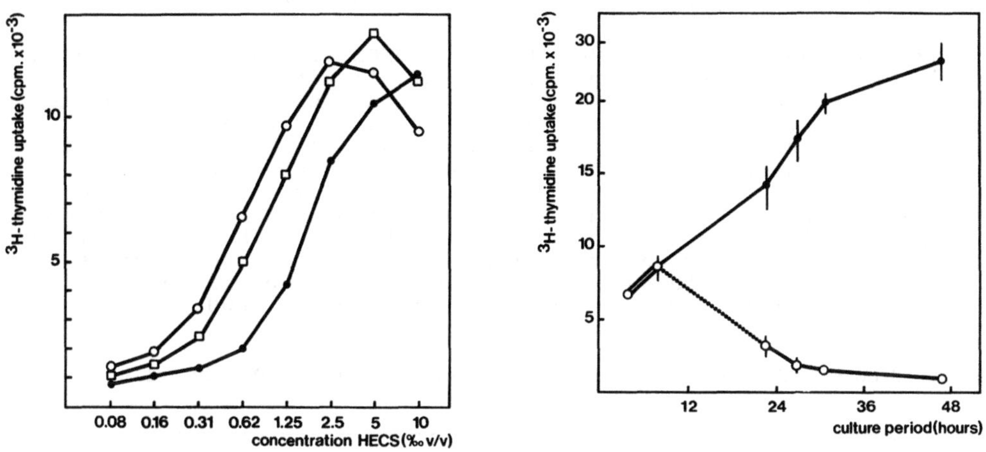

Fig. 1a (left). Dose-response of 3 different batches of HECS tested with B13.29 cells.
Fig. 1b (right). Thymidine incorporation of 5 x 10^3 B13.29 cells cultured for various time intervals with (o--o) or without (o--o) 0.5% (v/v) HECS.

Different Cell Types Produce Growth Factor Activity

Once a rapid and reproducible assay for growth-factor activity of HECS was established, other conditioned media were screened for growth-factor activity. The results are summarized in Table 1. Media conditioned by Sp2/0Ag14, WEHI-3B or L929 cells did not support the growth of B13.29 cells, whereas media conditioned by cultures of P388D cells, long-term mouse bone-marrow cultures, human leukocytes, placenta, smooth muscle cells, fibroblasts or rat thymocytes, all had growth-factor activity.

Table 1. Sources of growth-factor activity (units/ml) required by B13.29 cells

Origin	Cell Type	Species	HGF Activity
Sp2/OAg14	Hybrid plasmacytoma	mouse	0
WEHI-3B	Myelomonocytic cell line	Mouse	0
L929	Fibroblastoid	Mouse	0
P388D	Macrophage cell line	Mouse	200
Long-term bone marrow culture	Unknown	Mouse	10000
Thymus	Unknown	Rat	2000
Placenta	Unknown	Human	800
Peripheral blood	Monocytes	Human	4000
Umbilical cord	Smooth muscle cells	Human	800
Fetal skin	Fibroblast	Human	80
Bone marrow from a myeloma patient	Fibroblast-like	Human	20000

Selection of Growth-Factor Independent Subclones of B13.29 Cells

We previously observed that the effect of HECS is most noticeable on hybridomas not yet fully adapted to culture in vitro (6). It was suspected that such adaptation may involve the selection of growth-factor-independent hybrid cells, and we therefore tried to select factor-independent subclones of B13.29 cells. To this end, B13.29 cells were cultured at various cell numbers without growth-factor in microtiter plates. Although the large majority of B13.29 cells did not survive this procedure, individual clones of viable cells became visible after 3-4 days in most cultures (Table 2). The number of such factor-independent subclones was proportional to the number of cells added at day 0. From these results, the frequency of factor independent revertants was calculated to be about 1:4000.

Table 2. Growth-Factor Dependency is not an Absolute Trait of B13.29 Cells

Number of Cells/Well at Day 0	Number of Wells Seeded	Number of Clones at Day 4	Calculated Frequency
10×10^3	14	38	1:3684
5×10^3	18	23	1:3930
2×10^3	18	10	1:3600
1×10^3	21	4	1:5250

The supernatants of five factor-independent subclones and B13.29 cells were tested for anti-granulocyte antibody in an ELISA technique. All supernatants contained antibody (titers > 1:1000). One factor-independent subclone (B13.29-M9) was used as a control in further studies. No growth-factor activity was found in undiluted or concentrated supernatants of these cells. When the line was tested for antibody-production after a few months in culture, no antibody was detected in the supernatant. Loss of antibody production of the original B13.29 cells has not been observed over a period of more than one year in continuous culture.

Chromosome Analysis

The hybrid nature B13.29 cells was verified by chromosome analysis. A metaphase spread of B13.29 cells is shown in Fig. 2. The mean number of chromosomes (plus range and number of metaphases studied) found in spreads of B13.29, B13.29-M9 and Sp2/0Ag14 cells was 103 (81-118, n = 13), 99 (91-108, n = 12) and 76 (70-80, n = 10) respectively.

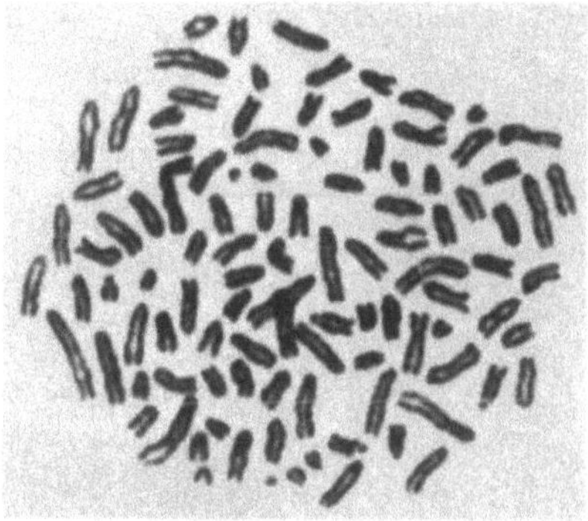

Fig. 2. A metaphase spread of B13.29 cells

Cell-Cycle Analysis

To test whether the requirement for growth-factor could be allocated to some phase of the cell cycle, DNA histograms of B13.29 cells, grown with or without growth-factor for various times were prepared. From these histograms the percentage of cells in G_1, S and G_2+M was calculated. The results of these experiments (Fig. 3), show that without growth-factor cells accumulate in G_1. Apparently B13.29 cells require growth-factor in order to enter the S-phase of the cell cycle.

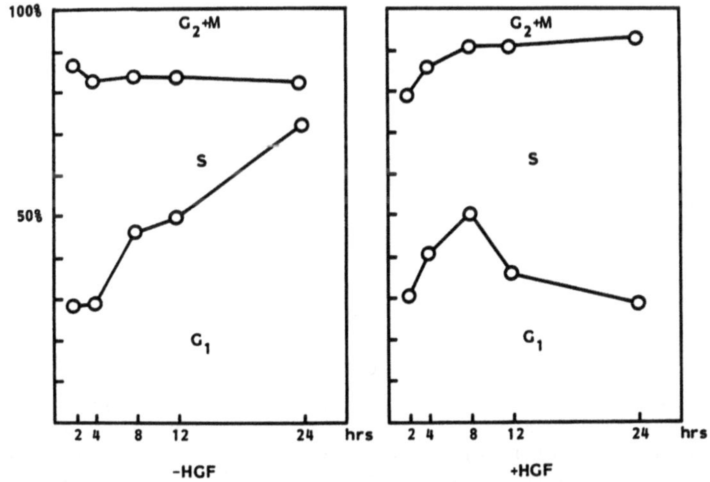

Fig. 3. Cell-cycle analysis of B13.29 cells cultured with or without growth-factor for various time intervals. Results are expressed as the cumulative percentage of cells in the G_1, the S or the G_2+S phase of the cell cycle.

Electron Microscopy

B13.29 (Fig. 4) and B13.29-M9 cells showed similar morphology. The nucleus was of irregular shape with peripheral chromatin condensation; separate nuclear masses were often seen in one cell section. The cytoplasma contained abundant free ribosomes, with significant amounts of rough endoplasmatic reticulum (RER) mainly in the areas with clusters of intracisternal type-A particles. The cisternae of the RER were distended to a variable extend. Many mitochondria and a multifocal Golgi apparatus were present. Various degrees of cytoplasmatic vacuolation frequently occurred. In both cell lines large numbers of intracisternal type-A particles were present (Fig. 4). Often, more than two clusters of these particles were found budding from the membrane of RER in a cell section. Intracisternal type-A particles with an average diameter of 70 nm were located inside the cisternae of RER and consisted of two concentric shells, the inner, more electron dense, surrounding an electron-lucent core.

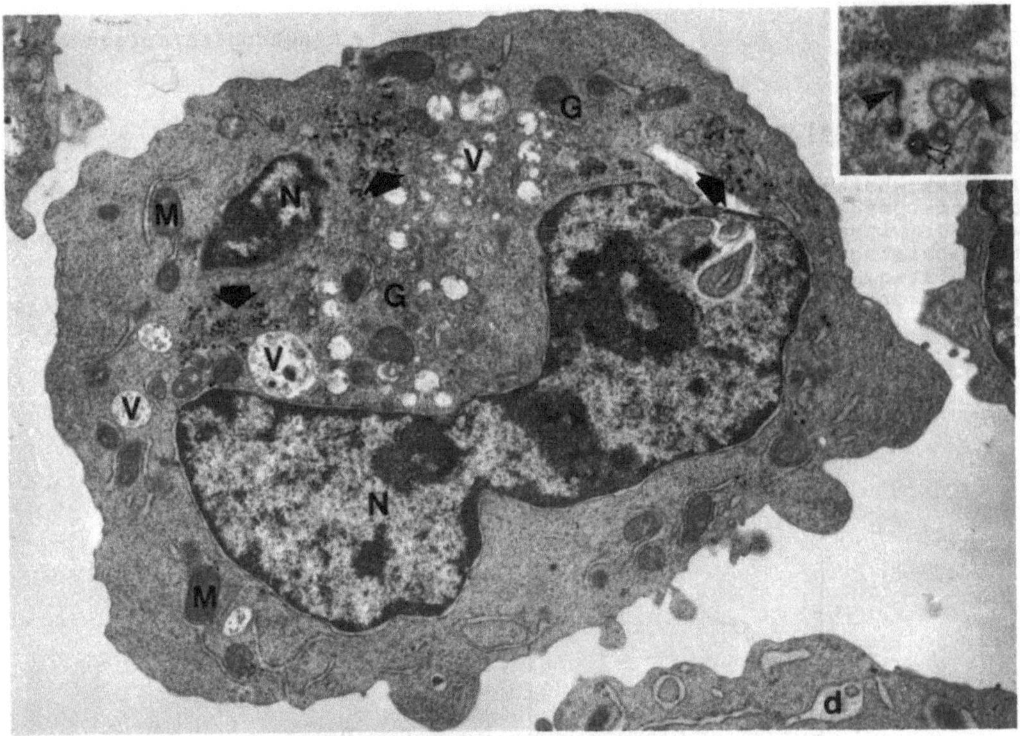

Fig. 4. Thin section of B13.29 cells. Magnification x9000. Two nuclear lobes (N) with chromatin condensation are seen. In the cytoplasm, Golgi apparatus (G), vacuoles (V), abundant mitochondria (M), free ribosomes and rough endoplasmatic reticulum with distended (d) cisterna are present in some areas. Note: the clusters of abundant intracisternal type-A particles (arrows). Inset: higher magnification (x57000) showing budding intracisternal type-A particles (arrowheads) and a free particle in the cisternae of rough endoplasmatic reticulum consisting of an outer shell (1) and a more electron-dense inner shell (2)

A few immature C-type particles were seen in the B13.29 cell line. In B13.29-M9 cells, however, more C-type particles were observed, mainly in intracytoplasmatic vacuoles (Fig. 5) and sometimes outside the cell. The mature C-type particle had a diameter ranging from 85 to 110 nm and consisted of an envelope surrounding an electron-dense nucleoid.

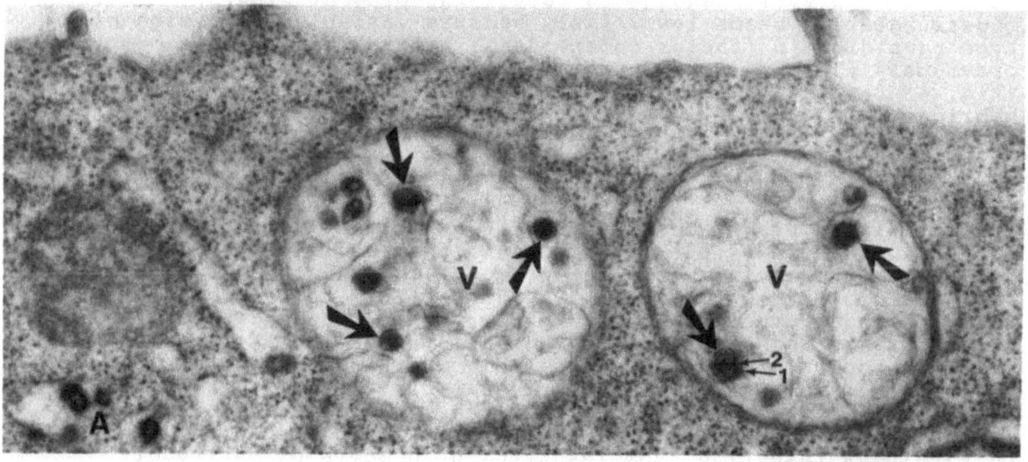

Fig. 5. Thin section of B13.29-M9 cells showing an area of the cytoplasm containing intracisternal type-A particles (A) and vacuoles (V) with mature C-type particles (arrows) consisting of an envelope (1) and an electron dense nucleoid (2). x47500

DISCUSSION

In this report we have described some properties of a growth-factor dependent B-cell hybridoma. We have shown that in addition to human endothelial cells several other cell types from human, rat and mouse origin were capable of growth-factor production. From human monocyte-conditioned medium, growth-factor activity has been purified by a combination of gel filtration, ion-exchange chromatography and SDS-polyacrylamide gel electrophoresis (8). Activity was eluted from SDS-gels at two peaks, corresponding to isolated protein bands with apparent molecular weight of 21 kD (major band) and 25 kD (minor band) as revealed by silver staining of the gels. Analysis by chromatofocussing of partially purified material also yielded two peaks of activity at pI = 4.9 and pI = 5.1. At this stage, it is not possible to conclude whether HGF produced by human monocytes is identical with the growth-factor(s) produced by the other cell types. This and possible similarities of HGF to factors that enhance the growth of primary plasmacytomas (19,20) and normal B cells (21) are subject to further study.

The finding that growth-factor-independent subclones could be obtained indicates that the observed factor-dependency is not absolute. Because these subclones also produced antibody, a relation between antibody specificity and factor-dependency seems unlikely. On the other hand, antibody production has been a stable characteristic of the factor-dependent cells, whereas a factor-independent subclone did not produce antibody, when tested after a few month in culture.

Further study is needed to determine if growth-factor requirement is linked to the secretion of immunoglobulins, as e.g. proposed by Potter and Cancro (4).

An interesting finding was the increased expression of C-type particles in a growth-factor independent subclone of B13.29 cells (Fig. 5). More growth-factor-independent subclones need to be examined to clarify a possible relation of C-type particle expression to the mechanism(s) leading to factor-independent growth. A direct causal relation seems less likely because variable expression of C-type particles in (factor-independent) hybridomas has been described previously (22,23). The expression of intracisternal type-A particles (Fig. 4) has been a consistent finding in plasmacytomas and B-cell hybridomas (22,23).

It has been shown that the induction of plasmacytomas in mice by intraperitoneal injection of mineral oil or other non-metabolizable materials involves at least two steps and requires a genetic susceptibility (4). According to the selection theory proposed by Potter and Cancro (4), the peritoneal oil granuloma acts as an abnormal micro-environment that promotes the growth of rarely occuring "mutated preplasmacytoma cells". Part of this tumor-promoting effect could be the production of growth-factors as required by B13.29 cells. Apart for studies of plasmacytomagenesis, these cells could be valuable tools for studies of the molecular mechanisms that regulate the growth of normal and neoplastic B cells. Finally, the use of hybrid cell lines to study growth-factors, as described in this report, can be considered in other studies of cell biology to overcome difficulties resulting from insufficient numbers or purity of responding cell populations.

ACKNOWLEDGEMENT

Expert technical assistance was given by Frida Oosterhof and Els de Groot. Mycoplasma tests were performed by Elisabeth Stricker. Media conditioned by human endothelial cells, smooth muscle cells and fetal-skin fibroblasts were provided by Joke Zandbergen. The preparation of DNA histograms and computer analysis of these histograms was performed by Anton Martens and Frank Schultz from the Radiobiological Institute TNO, Rijswijk, The Netherlands.

REFERENCES

1. Anderson, PN and M Potter (1969) Nature 222:994
2. Potter, M, Pumphrey, JG and JL Walters (1972) J Natl Cancer Inst 49:305
3. Brodeur, BR, Tsang, P and Y Larose (1984) J Immunol Methods 71:265
4. Potter M and M Cancro (1978) in : Cell Differentiation and Neoplasia. GF Saunders (Ed) Raven Press, New York, pp 145-161
5. Fazekas de St Groth, S and D Scheidegger (1980) J Immunol Methods 35:1
6. Astaldi, GCB, Janssen MC, Lansdorp PM, Willems, C, Zeijlemaker and F Oosterhof (1980) J Immunol 125:1411
7. Astaldi GCB, Janssen MC, Lansdorp PM, Zeijlemaker WP and C Willems (1981) J Immunol 126:1170
8. Aarden LA, Lansdorp PM and E de Groot (1985) in: Lymphokines, vol 10, Academic press, pp 175-185
9. Shulman M and G Kohler (1978) Nature 276:269

10. Tetteroo PAT, Lansdorp PM, Geurts van Kessel, AH, Hagemeijer A and AEGKr von dem Borne (1984) in: Human Leucocyte Differentiation Antigens, H Gotze (Ed) Springer-Verlag Heidelberg, pp 419-423
11. Lansdorp, PM, Astaldi GCB, Oosterhof, F, Janssen MC, and WP Zeijlemaker (1980) J Immunol Meth 39:393
12. Uytendaal MP, de Bruyn CHMM, Hatanaka M and P Hosli (1979) In Vitro 15:103
13. Worton and Duff (1979) in: Methods in Enzymology, vol 58 Jacoby WB and IH Pastan (Eds) Academic Press, New York, pp 322-344
14. Ross, R (1971) J Cell Biol 50:172
15. De Groot, PhG, Strijland A, Kalsbeek, R, Meera Khan P, Westerveld A, Hamers MN and JM Tager (1980) Exp Cell Res 126:207
16. Schlunk T and M Schleyer (1980) Exp Hematol 8:179
17. Du Bois, MJGJ, Meinesz, A, Bierhorst, A, Groenewoud, M, Schellekens PThA and VP Eijsvoogel (1974) Tissue Antigens 4:458
18. Schultz FW, Mulder JA and P Sonneveld (1986) Anal Quant Cytometry (in press)
19. Namba, Y and M Hanaoka (1972) J Immunol 109:1193
20. Metcalf D (1974) J Immunol 113:235
21. Moller G (Ed) (1984) Immunol Rev 78, Munksgaard Copenhagen
22. Weiss RA (1982) Immunol Today 3:292
23. Rudolph, M, Karsten, U and M Micheel (1983) Immunol Today 4:185

A Growth Factor Required by Plasmacytoma Cells *In Vitro*

R.P. Nordan[1], L.M. Neckers[2], S. Rudikoff[1] and M. Potter[1]

[1]Laboratory of Genetics and [2]Laboratory of Pathology, National Cancer Institute, National Institutes of Health, Bethesda, Maryland 20892

INTRODUCTION

In BALB/c mice, plasmacytomas (PCT) arise and proliferate in the granulomatous tissue that forms in response to the intraperitoneal administration of pristane (Potter and Boyce, 1962; Anderson and Potter, 1969). Studies by Cancro and Potter (1976) suggest that the oil granuloma provides a special microenvironment which is necessary for the growth of early PCT's. Although the specific contributions of this microenvironment are unknown, in vitro studies suggest that PCT's that have not been adapted previously to cell culture require added factors for in vitro growth and proliferation. Namba and Hanaoka (1972) described a 50 kDa macrophage-derived protein that was required for the in vitro growth of the MOPC104E PCT. Metcalf (1974) demonstrated that mouse serum or peritoneal macrophages supported the clonal growth of PCT's in soft agar. Recently, Corbel and Melchers (1984) reported that "alpha factor-containing" supernatant from the P388D1 cell line also supported the in vitro growth of several PCT's. We have recently reported the establishment of PCT cell lines that are totally dependent on a factor for survival and proliferation in vitro (Nordan and Potter, 1986). We discuss here our initial biological and biochemical characterizations of this factor.

FACTOR DEPENDENT PCT CELL GROWTH IN VITRO

Factor dependent PCT cell lines were initially established by adding 48 hour supernatants from nonstimulated rat spleen cells to primary cultures of ascites-derived PCT cells. In the presence of the spleen cell supernatant, small colonies of proliferating PCT cells were nursed into cell lines that were totally dependent on a factor which we call plasmacytoma growth factor (PCT-GF). We now use an induced supernatant (SN) from the P388D1 murine macrophage cell line as a source of PCT-GF for the establishment and maintenance of factor dependent PCT cell lines.

The growth of two factor-dependent cell lines, T1165tc and T2027tc is shown in Figure 1. In the presence of P388D1 SN (see below) the cells grow logarithymically; however, without the P388D1 SN the cells cease to proliferate and die within 24 (T1165tc) and 72 (T2027tc) hours.

Current Topics in Microbiology and Immunology, Vol. 132

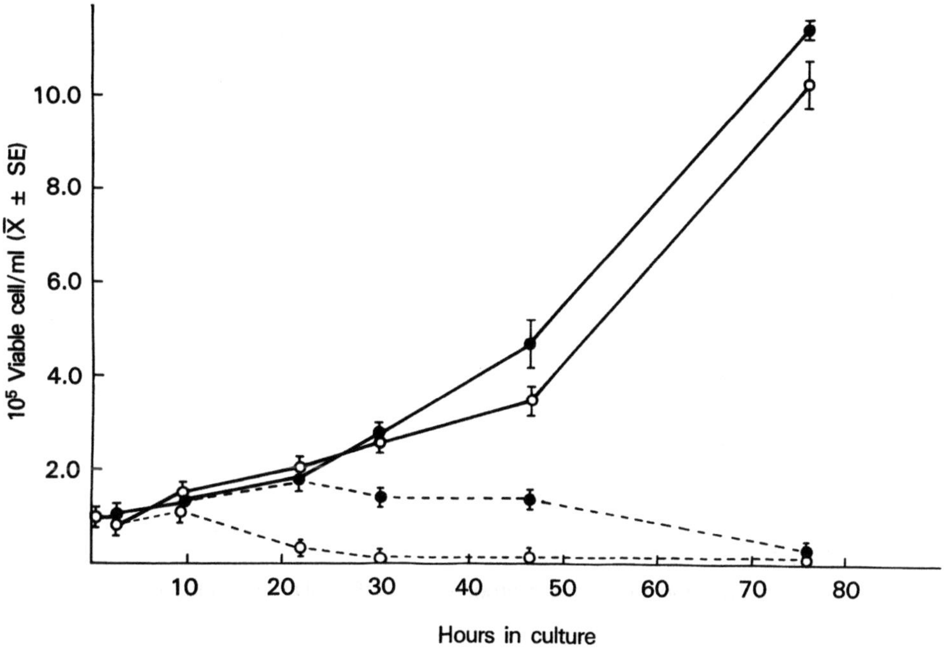

Fig. 1. Growth of T1165tc (O) and T2027tc (●) PCT cells in the presence (——) and absence (----) of 10 U/ml P388D1 SN. Results are expressed as the mean ± SE of triplicate cultures. Data from Nordan and Potter (1986).

Table 1. Synchronization of Factor-Dependent PCT Cells Following Removal of PCT-GF

Cells	PCT-GF[a]	Percent of cells in cycle phase[b]		
		G1	S	G2 + M
T1165tc	ON	58%	15%	27%
	OFF 15 hr	74%	9%	14%
T2027tc	ON	40%	25%	35%
	OFF 50 hr	82%	17%	11%
	OFF 50 hr, ON 15 hr	27%	63%	11%

[a] Cells in the ON group were grown in medium supplemented with P388D1 SN (10 U PCT-GF/ml). OFF cells were transferred into control medium (no PCT-GF) and then analyzed at the indicated time.

[b] Flow cytometry was used to evaluate the DNA content of propidium-iodide stained cells.

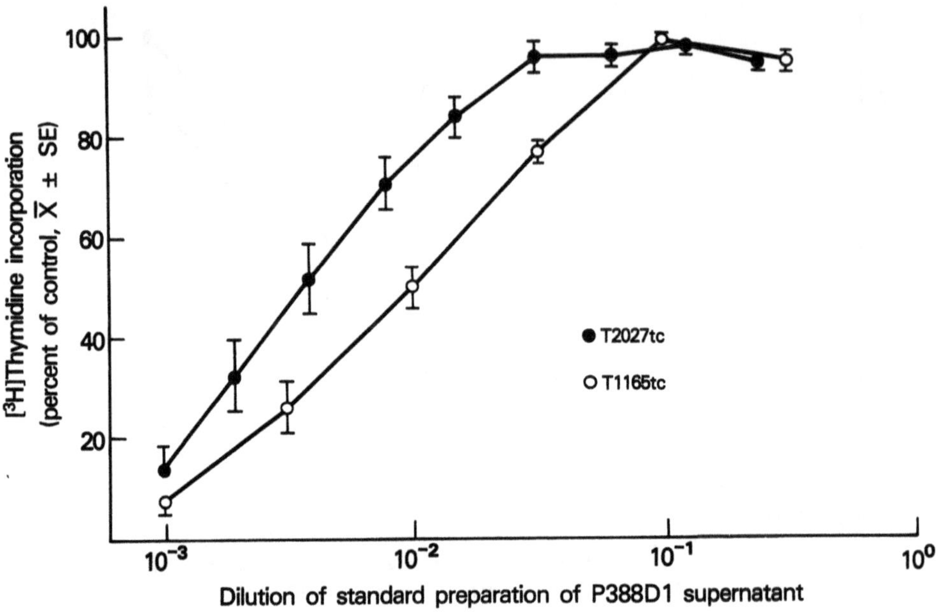

Figure 2. Response of T1165tc and T2027tc PCT cells to decreasing amounts of PCT-GF. Cells (1×10^4) were cultured with limiting dilutions of a standard P388D1 SN in triplicate wells of 96 well plates. After 24 (T1165tc) or 72 (T2027tc) hours the cultures were pulsed for 2 hours with 0.5 µCi [^{3}H]-thymidine, harvested over glass fiber filters and counted. Units of activity are defined as the reciprocal of the dilution which gives 1/2 maximal [^{3}H]-thymidine incorporation relative to a control preparation of P388D1 SN.

To determine where in the cell cycle PCT-GF acts, we examined the cell cycle parameters of the T1165tc and T2027tc cell lines before and after removal from PCT-GF-containing P388D1 SN (Table 1). Removal of PCT-GF resulted in a synchronization of cells in the G1 phase of the cell cycle. Furthermore, re-addition of the factor resulted in the synchronous movement of cells into S phase within 15 hours. These results indicated that PCT-GF relieved a block in the G1 phase of the cell cycle.

In order to measure the level of PCT-GF in various preparations a sensitive bioassay was developed which utilized [^{3}H]-thymidine incorporation by the T1165tc and T2027tc cell lines (Fig. 2). One unit of activity was defined as the concentration of PCT-GF that elicited a half maximal response with the T1165 cell line in this assay. With this assay we proceeded to characterize PCT-GF production by various cells and to examine the relationship of PCT-GF to previously characterized factors.

Table 2. PCT-GF Activity Found in Various Supernatants

Supernatant	PCT-GF, U/ml
Expt A	
P388D1 SN, day 2	6
day 4	27
day 6	66
day 4 + LPS	22
P388D1 LPS-SN, day 2	63
day 4	198
day 6	310
Expt B	
Pristane-induced APC-SN	22
Normal Resident APC-SN	<0.1

[a] P388D1 cells were harvested from log phase spinner cultures growing in RPMI 1640, 10% FCS. The cells were washed, resuspended in serum-free RPMI 1640 at 1 x 10^6/ml and seeded into tissue culture flasks. LPS was added to the indicated cultures at a concentration of 5 μg/ml.

[b] Peritoneal cells (APC) were collected from untreated (resident) and 30 day pristane-primed BALB/c AnPt mice. 1 x 10^6 monocyte-macrophages were seeded into 16 mm culture wells and allowed to adhere for 2 hours at 37°C. The adherent cells were then incubated at 37°C in low serum medium (RPMI 1640, 1% FCS). After 5 days the supernatants were collected and dialyzed against fresh medium.

PRODUCTION OF PCT-GF BY P388D1 AND BY PERITONEAL MACROPHAGES

It is important to note that proliferating P388D1 cells (RPMI 1640, 10% FCS) produce little or no PCT-GF; however, P388D1 cells can be induced to produce PCT-GF by subculturing cells at high density into fresh medium containing little or no serum. PCT-GF levels in the low serum P388D1 supernatant (P388D1 SN) usually peak within 5-6 days (Table 2A). Furthermore, the cells must be adherent in order to produce PCT-GF. The addition of LPS to the low serum cultures results in a 2 to 4 fold increase in the production of PCT-GF. This increase is not due to a synergism with LPS since the addition of LPS to non-LPS induced P388D1 SN has no additional effect. We have observed a large variation in PCT-GF production by different P388D1 sublines.

The *in vivo* requirement by PCT's for the oil granuloma led us to compare the *in vitro* production of PCT-GF by normal and pristane-induced adherent peritoneal cells (Table 2B). Pristane-induced adherent peritoneal cells produced more than 50 fold higher levels of PCT-GF than did normal control adherent peritoneal cells, suggesting an association between elevated levels of this factor and the induction of PCT's in pristane-primed BALB/c AnPt mice.

RELATIONSHIP OF PCT-GF TO PREVIOUSLY CHARACTERIZED FACTORS

Since P388D1 produces substantial amounts of interleukin 1 (IL-1) (Lachman et al. 1977; Mizel et al. 1978), we examined the possibility that IL-1 was responsible for PCT-GF activity. An ammonium sulphate precipitated preparation of P388D1 SN was chromatographed on a Pharmacia chromatofocusing column. PCT-GF and IL-1 were easily separated on the basis of their isoelectric points indicating that these two molecules were distinct entities. PCT-GF was found in two peaks at pH 6.4 and 6.2 whereas IL-1 activity was found at pH 5.1 and 4.8.

A number of well-characterized lymphokines and other biologically active molecules (see Nordan and Potter, 1986, for factor references) were then tested for activity in the PCT-GF assay (Table 3). PCT-GF activity was not exhibited by any of the factors tested suggesting that PCT-GF is distinct from those molecules.

SUMMARY AND CONCLUSIONS

1. We have established PCT cell lines that are totally dependent on a growth factor, PCT-GF, for survival and proliferation *in vitro*. PCT-GF acts by releasing a block in the G1 phase of the cell cycle.

2. A high level of PCT-GF production *in vitro* is associated with cells, presumably macrophages, obtained from the peritoneal oil granuloma. It is tempting to speculate that elevated levels of PCT-GF may be involved in the establishment and maintenance of PCT's *in vivo*; however, information on the *in vivo* production of PCT-GF and its possible effect on normal B lymphocytes is necessary before such a conclusion can be reached.

3. PCT-GF appears to be distinct from a number of other well characterized factors including IL-1, IL-2, BSF-1, BCGF II, EGF, TGF_{β}, α- and β-IFN, C3b and thymosin fraction V. PCT-GF has apparent isoelectric points of 6.4 and 6.2 and preliminary data indicates a molecular weight of 24 kDa.

Table 3. PCT-GF activity found in characterized factors

	Source	Amount tested per milliliter	PCT-GF activity U/ml
Pure factors			
IL-1, human	J. Schmidt	0.5 to 5,000 U	0
rIL-2, human	Biogen	0.3 to 1,000 U	0
IL-3, mouse	J. Ihle	0.3 to 350 U	0
BSF-1, mouse	J. Ohara	0.1 to 560 U	0
EGF, mouse	R. Asoian	6 pg to 20 ng	0
TGF_{β}, human w/2.5 ng EGF	R. Asoian	6 pg to 20 ng	0
γ-IFN, mouse	G. Spitalny	0.1 to 500 U	0
β-IFN, mouse	P. Lengyel	0.1 to 1,000 U	0
C3b, human	L. Fries	5 pg to 5 μg	0
Partially purified factors			
BCGF-II, mouse	S. Swain	0.1 to 50 U	0
Mϕ-CSF, mouse	S. Vogel	1 to 10,000 U	0
Thymosin V	A. Goldstein	5 pg to 500 μg/ml	0
Other reagents			
Con A		5 pg to 50 μg	0
LPS		5 pg to 50 μg	0

REFERENCES

Anderson PN, Potter M (1969) Induction of plasma-cell tumours in BALB/c mice with 2,6,10,14-tetramethylpentadecane (pristane). Nature (London) 222:994-995

Cancro M, Potter M (1976) The requirement of an adherent substratum for the growth of developing plasmacytoma cells in vivo. J Exp Med 144:1554-1566

Corbel C, Melchers F (1984) The synergism of assessory cells and of soluble α-factors derived from them in the activation of B cells to proliferation. Immun Rev 78:51-74

Lachman LB, Hacker MP, Blyden GT, Handschumacher RE (1977) Preparation of lymphocyte-activating factor from continuous murine macrophage cell lines. Cell Immunol 34:416-423

Metcalf D (1974) The serum factor stimulating colony formation in vitro by murine plasmacytoma cells: response to antigens and mineral oil. J Immunol 113:235-243

Mizel SB, Oppenheim JJ, Rosenstreich DL (1978) Characterization of lymphocyte-activating factor (LAF) produced by the macrophage cell line, P388D1. I. Enhancement of LAF production by activated T lymphocytes. J Immunol 120:1497-1503

Namba Y, Hanaoka M (1972) Immunocytology of cultured IgM-forming cells of mouse. I. Requirement of phagocytic cell factor for the growth of IgM-forming tumor cells in tissue culture. J Immunol 109:1193-1200

Nordan RP, Potter M (1986) A macrophage-derived factor required by plasmacytomas for survival and proliferation in vitro. Science (in press)

Potter M (1962) Induction of plasma-cell neoplasms in strain BALB/c mice with mineral oil and mineral oil adjuvants. Nature (London) 193:1086-1087

Genes Affecting the Production or Action of B Cell-Active Lymphokines

C. L. Sidman

The Jackson Laboratory, Bar Harbor, Maine 04609

INTRODUCTION

Lymphokines are soluble polypeptides that appear to play important roles in controlling the immune system. The activation, proliferation, and differentiation of many cell types, including B lymphocytes (for reviews, see Moller 1984), are affected by these molecules *in vitro*. Tumor B cells differ from their nontransformed counterparts by virtue of their heightened proliferation and transplantability. Nevertheless, different activities of specific tumor B cell lines can still be regulated by lymphokines or other signals. A discussion of lymphokines is thus pertinent to the topic of B cell neoplasia in three ways. First, understanding the operation of lymphokines that regulate B cell development and function may yield insights into the cell populations giving rise to B cell neoplasia or the circumstances under which this occurs. Second, lymphokines may be important in controlling the fate and activity of transformed B cells in a tumor-bearing animal. Third, deliberate manipulation of the lymphokine system may eventually offer one or more modes of treatment for patients with B cell neoplasia.

Genes affecting B cell-active lymphokines are important for at least two reasons. First, as in other areas of biology, a genetic approach should prove valuable in understanding the basic mechanisms of lymphokine control of B cell development and function. Some categories of genes affecting lymphokine activity might include structural genes for the lymphokines themselves, genes whose products regulate lymphokine production, structural genes for lymphokine receptors, and other genes involved in the transduction of lymphokine signals from cell surface receptors to the interior of responding cells. A second reason for considering lymphokine related genes is that much progress is currently being made in understanding the specific genetic changes involved in the generation of B cell neoplasia, as can be seen from a large number of papers in this volume. Since lymphokines may be critical elements in controlling B cell activity, alterations in lymphokine-related genes might be primary factors in the development of certain B cell tumors. Alterations in receptor genes or other genes affecting signal transmission would be the most likely candidates in this regard.

A modified copy of the mouse gene map, with genes affecting the operation of the immune system marked in bold symbols, is shown in Fig. 1. Most of the immunological loci indicated were defined by the occurrence of specific mutations, and were mapped by classical genetic analyses. The primary genes and gene products involved are not known, nor are the nature of the specific mutations leading to the recognizably altered phenotypes. With the advent of recombinant DNA technology, immunological genes are now also being defined by the cloning of DNA fragments without the prior recognition of naturally

Current Topics in Microbiology and Immunology, Vol. 132

occuring variants. A number of lymphokines (IL-1 [Lomedico et al. 1984], IL-2 [Kashima et al. 1985], IL-3 [Fung et al. 1984], IL-4 [Noma et al. 1986], CSF [Gough et al. 1984], and IFN-gamma [Gray and Goeddel 1983]), and a lymphokine receptor (the IL-2 receptor [Leonard et al. 1984]), have been cloned and are thus included on the map.

B CELL MATURATION FACTORS (BMFs)

For several years our lab has been investigating a number of lymphokines that promote B cell maturation from the immunocompetent, resting, non-Ig-secreting state to active Ig secretion (reviewed by Sidman et al. 1984b, 1986a). To signify that these molecules induce not just any B cell changes (all of which could be termed differentiation), but specifically those leading to B cells' primary functional destiny of antibody production, we have termed these molecules B cell Maturation Factors (or BMFs). Three distinct BMF species have been resolved to date. Gamma interferon and one non-interferon species are derived from helper T lymphocytes, and another non-interferon species is produced by B cells. The activity of all three of these BMFs has been assayed *in vitro* at the level of Ig-secreting cells (the polyclonal anti-Ig-Protein A reverse plaque forming cell [PFC] assay [Gronowicz et al. 1976]), and by studying Ig metabolism at the molecular level (Sahr et al. 1986). Studied biochemically, the various BMFs enhance Ig production by different combinations of effects at the following levels of Ig metabolism: transcription, post-transcriptional RNA processing, mRNA frequencies and pool sizes, polypeptide synthesis, and post-translational steps regulating protein degradation vs. secretion. BMFs appear to be equally active on all populations of B cells isolated from normal and most mutant mice, and also on the B cell tumor line WEHI-279. Purified BMFs have no detectable influence on B cell proliferation (Sherris and Sidman 1986). It thus appears that B cell proliferation has no obligate role in maturation to Ig secretion, at least as driven by BMFs. Whether the state of B cell proliferation can modulate the effects of BMFs, or whether BMF-driven maturation to Ig secretion has any influence on B cell proliferation, are important questions that have not yet been resolved.

The remainder of this paper will discuss two genetic systems which have contributed to our understanding of BMFs and B cell responses to these molecules. These two systems are: 1) an autoimmune mutant mouse whose polyclonal B cell activation and Ig secretion is associated with, and may be due to, an extraordinary *in vivo* production of two B cell-active lymphokines, and 2) a mouse strain whose B cells are specifically unresponsive to BMFs *in vitro*.

OVERPRODUCTION OF BMF

Mice homozygous for either of the allelic Chromosome 6 recessive mutations "Motheaten" (symbol *me*)(Green and Shultz 1975) or "Viable Motheaten" (symbol *me*^{v})(Shultz et al. 1984) show the most severe immunodeficiency coupled with autoimmunity documented in mice, living an average of only 3 or 9 weeks, respectively. (The locus was named "Motheaten" because of the patchy appearance of the coat, which is due to accumulations of granulocytes displacing hair follicles in the skin.) Besides being almost totally unresponsive, on both humoral and cellular levels, to deliberate immunization, me/me and me^v/me^v homozygotes show massive polyclonal B cell activation, multiple species of autoantibodies, and serum Ig levels 10-20 times those of control littermates (genotype +/-). The Ig classes most elevated in me^v/me^v mice are IgM followed by IgG3 followed by IgA, all of which show unexpectedly high levels (up to 40%) of lambda light chains (Sidman et al. 1986c).

Associated with and perhaps the cause of polyclonal B cell activation and antibody secretion are two lymphokines affecting B cell maturation which are found in the serum of these animals. The B cell-derived BMF (BMF-B)(Sidman et al. 1984a), and another molecule (called the "potentiator"), which lacks direct BMF activity but which enhances the potency of a given amount of BMF by up to three orders of magnitude (Sidman et al. 1985), are both active on normal and WEHI-279 tumor B cells in vitro. The observations that 1) me^v/me^v serum or supernatant equally enhance membrane-type and secretory-type IgM production (Sahr et al. 1986), and 2) that large amounts of BMF-B plus potentiator actually inhibit PFC formation (Sidman et al. 1985), may explain the finding in me^v/me^v tissues of so-called "Mott" cells (Shultz et al. 1984, 1986). These atypical plasma cells, which have been seen previously in situations of chronic immune stimulation, are non-Ig-secreting B cell derivatives with massive deposits and even crystals of Ig within their endoplasmic reticulum.

Analysis of B cell surface antigens using a fluorescence-activated cell sorter has revealed that most of the B cells from me^v/me^v mice belong to a lineage of cells that is a relatively minor component in normal animals (Sidman et al. 1986c). The phenotype of these B cells is a high amount of surface IgM, a low amount of surface IgD, and a detectable level of the Ly-1 marker (which is present in much higher amounts on most T cells). The predominance of these B cells in me^v/me^v mice, coupled with their production of an autostimulatory lymphokine (BMF-B) and a restricted pattern of Ig isotypes (especially IgM, IgG3, IgA, and lambda light chains), suggests that different subsets of B cells may play distinct roles in the immune system. Possibilities relevant to B cell neoplasia include the preferential production of autocrine factors or favored genetic rearrangements in particular B cell subsets.

Among other murine genetic models of autoimmunity, only the polygenic NZB strain is similar to me^v/me^v mice in having high levels of Ly-1(+) B cells and circulating BMF. Since the motheaten locus does not appear to be one of the many genes contributing to autoimmunity in NZB mice (NZB mice do not complement me^v/me^v mice and yield phenotypically "motheaten" offspring), one can conclude that different genetic pathways can lead to similar immunoregulatory abnormalities. A comparable conclusion regarding multiple paths to the same end may pertain to the generation of B cell tumors as well.

NONRESPONSIVENESS TO BMFs

B cells from the DBA/2Ha mouse strain are unresponsive to all three recognized species of BMF in vitro, but respond normally to the mitogen LPS (Sidman et al. 1986b). These B cells are thus capable of maturing to active Ig secretion, but have a specific lesion in their responses to BMFs. In our laboratory colony, DBA/2Ha mice show average viability, and have normal serum Ig levels. Questions currently being investigated with these mice are what role (if any) BMFs might play *in vivo*, and whether there are alternate means for achieving these ends if BMFs cannot act.

Genetic analyses have shown that two genes together account for the unresponsiveness of DBA/2Ha B cells to BMFs (Sidman et al. 1986b). At both loci, responsiveness is largely dominant over nonresponsiveness. The major gene determining B cell responsiveness to BMFs is termed B cell maturation factor responsiveness-1 (*Bmfr-1*), and is located on Chromosome 4 at a distance of 13 centimorgans distal to the brown locus. From birth until puberty, homozygotes for the nonresponder allele of *Bmfr-1* are BMF-nonresponsive, while heterozygotes and responder homozygotes are BMF-responsive. After puberty, a second locus, termed *Bmfr-2* and located on Chromosome 9 near the dilute locus, also affects BMF responsiveness. *Bmfr-2* determines whether mice previously unresponsive to BMFs due to *Bmfr-1* will convert to BMF responsiveness or remain nonresponsive. The *Bmfr-2*-determined conversion of BMF-nonresponder mice into BMF-responders may involve the operation of steroid sex hormones. An interesting feature of *Bmfr-1* and *Bmfr-2* is that they are each linked to paralogous phosphoglucomutase loci, and may thus represent descendants of an ancestral gene whose regulation has diverged since gene duplication. Whether the *Bmfr-1* and *Bmfr-2* genes represent cell surface BMF receptors or components of the signal transduction mechanism has not yet been determined.

CONCLUSIONS

Examples of structural genes for lymphokines and lymphokine receptors have been identified by molecular cloning, while genes regulating lymphokine production and responsiveness have been identified and mapped by phenotypically recognizable mutations and classical genetic analyses. In the coming years, functional mutations of already cloned genes will be sought, and cloning of the phenotypically identified mutant genes will be actively pursued. These studies should yield important insights into the biology of both normal and neoplastic lymphocytes.

ACKNOWLEDGEMENTS

I thank the many colleagues whose efforts and discussions contributed to the work reviewed here, M. Davisson and T. Roderick for permission to use their mouse gene map, and M. Davisson and R. Evans for critical reading and comments on the manuscript. The author is supported by grants CA-35845 and AI-20232 from the National Institutes of Health. The Jackson Laboratory is fully accredited by the American Association for Accreditation of Laboratory Animal Care.

REFERENCES

Fung MC, Hapel AJ, Ymer S, Cohen DR, Johnson RM, Campbell HD, Young IG (1984) Molecular cloning of cDNA for murine interleukin-3. Nature 307:233-237

Gough NM, Gough J, Metcalf D, Kelso A, Grail D, Nicola NA, Burgess AW, Dunn AR (1984) Molecular cloning of cDNA encoding a murine haematopoietic growth regulator, granulocyte-macrophage colony stimulating factor. Nature 309:763-767
Gray PW, Goeddel DV (1983) Cloning and expression of murine immune interferon cDNA. Proc Natl Acad Sci USA 80:5842-5846
Green MC, Shultz LD (1975) Motheaten, an immunodeficient mutant of the mouse. I. Genetics and pathology. J Hered 66:250-258
Gronowicz E, Coutinho A, Melchers F (1976) A plaque assay for all cells secreting Ig of a given type or class. Eur J Immunol 6:588-590
Kashima N, Nishi-Takaoka C, Fujita T, Taki S, Yamada G, Hamuro J, Taniguchi T (1985) Unique structure of murine interleukin-2 as deduced from cloned cDNAs. Nature 313:402-404
Leonard WJ, Depper JM, Crabtree GR, Rudikoff S, Pumphrey J, Robb RJ, Kronke M, Svetlik PB, Peffer NJ, Waldmann TA, Greene WC (1984) Molecular cloning and expression of cDNAs for the human interleukin-2 receptor. Nature 311:626-631
Lomedico PT, Gubler U, Hellmann CP, Dukovich M, Giri JG, Pan YE, Collier K, Semionow R, Chua AO, Mizel SB (1984) Cloning and expression of murine interleukin-1 cDNA in Escherichia Coli Nature 312:458-462
Moller G (1984) B Cell Growth and Differentiation Factors. Imm Rev 78:1-224
Noma Y, Sideras P, Naito T, Bergstedt-Lindquist S, Azuma C, Severinson E, Tanake T, Kinashi T, Matsuda F, Yaoita Y, Honjo T (1986) Cloning of cDNA encoding the murine IgG1 induction factor by a novel strategy using SP6 promoter. Nature 319:640-646
Sahr KE, Wang X-F, Calame KL, Sidman CL (1986) Lymphokines Affect IgM Metabolism in B Lymphocytes at the Transcriptional and Post-Transcriptional Levels. submitted
Sherris DI, Sidman CL (1986) Distinction of B Cell Maturation Factors from Lymphokines Affecting B Cell Growth and Viability. J Immunol 136:994-998
Shultz LD, Coman DR, Bailey CL, Beamer WG, Sidman CL (1984) "Viable Motheaten", A New Allele of the Motheaten Locus. I. Pathology. Am J Pathol 116:179-192
Shultz LD, Coman DR, Lyons BL, Sidman CL, Taylor S (1986) Development of Plasmacytoid Cells with Russell Bodies in Autoimmune "Viable Motheaten" Mice. submitted
Sidman CL, Marshall JD, Masiello NC, Roths JB, Shultz LD (1984a) A Novel B Cell Maturation Factor from Spontaneously Autoimmune Viable Motheaten Mice. Proc Natl Acad Sci USA 81:7199-7202
Sidman CL, Paige CJ, Schreier MH (1984b) B Cell Maturation Factors. Lymphokines 10:187-200
Sidman CL, Shultz LD, Evans R (1985) A Serum Derived Molecule from Autoimmune Viable Motheaten Mice Potentiates the Action of a B Cell Maturation Factor. J Immunol 135:870-872
Sidman CL, Sahr KE, Sherris DI (1986a) Lymphokines Affecting B Cell Maturation. In: Singhal SK, Delovitch TL (eds) Mediators of Immune Regulation and Immunotherapy. Elsevier NY, p 151
Sidman CL, Marshall JD, Beamer WG, Nadeau JH, Unanue ER (1986b) Two Loci Affecting B Cell Responses to B Cell Maturation Factors. J Exp Med 163:116-128
Sidman CL, Shultz LD, Hardy R, Hayakawa K, Herzenberg L (1986c) Production of Immunoglobulin Isotypes by Ly-1 B Cells in Viable Motheaten and Normal Mice. Science, in press

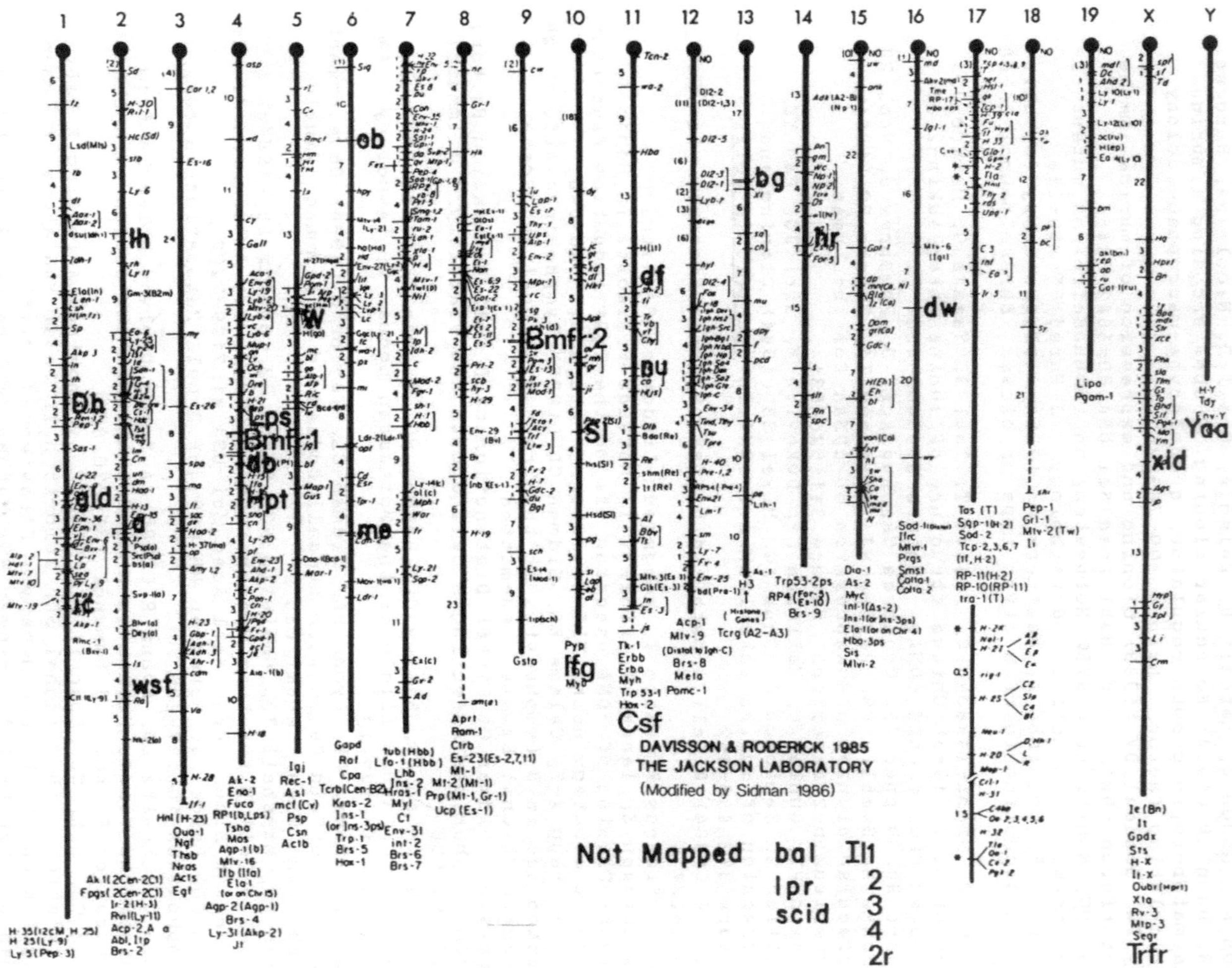

Fig. 1: The immunological gene map of the mouse.

Lymphokine Regulation of Murine IgE Production

Robert L. Coffman

DNAX Research Institute of Molecular and Cellular Biology,
901 California Avenue, Palo Alto, California 94304

INTRODUCTION

Many studies during the last 15 years have clearly established that IgE responses are regulated by T lymphocytes and that IgE production can be regulated independent of the production of other immunoglobulin isotypes (Ishizaka 1976; Itaya and Ovary 1979; Katz 1980). The mechanisms by which T cells effect this isotype-specific regulation of IgE, however, has not as yet been clearly defined. Much recent work has centered on the role of IgE-binding potentiator and suppressor factors in this regulation (Ishizaka 1984; Suemura et al. 1981; Young et al. 1984). In this report, we summarize evidence that B cell stimulatory factor-1 (BSF-1) and interferon-γ (IFN-γ) can also regulate IgE production in a relatively isotype-specific manner.

MATERIALS AND METHODS

Preparation and culture of mouse T-depleted spleen cells (B cells) and isotype-specific assays for supernatant immunoglobulin levels were performed as described previously (Coffman and Carty 1986). B cells were stimulated with lipopolysaccharide (LPS) on day 0 of culture and T cell supernatants and lymphokines were added on day 1. Culture supernatants were harvested on day 7 and frozen until assayed. Purified recombinant IFN-γ and Interleukin-2 (IL-2) were provided by Dr. Paul Trotta, Schering Research, Bloomfield, NJ. Purified BSF-1 (Ohara et al. 1985) and monoclonal anti-BSF-1 (Ohara and Paul 1985) were supplied by Drs. Junichi Ohara and William Paul, National Institutes of Health, Bethesda, MD.

RESULTS AND DISCUSSION

IgE Regulation by T Cell Supernatants

This series of experiments began with our inability to stimulate IgE production by activating B cells with mitogens such as LPS (Coffman and Carty 1986). LPS stimulated significant, and, in some cases, very large responses of all other secreted isotypes but consistently failed to stimulate measurable IgE responses (Table 1). The addition of concanavalin-A stimulated supernatants from some, but not all, cloned helper T cell (TH) lines caused a profound enhancement of the IgE response (Table 1). D9.1 is our prototype of this subset of TH line, but many other lines have been isolated which produce the same activities (Mosmann et al. 1986). These same supernatants also cause a 5- to 10-fold increase in IgG1 and IgA levels and a 5- to 10-fold decrease in IgG3 levels in the same cultures (Table 1). The levels of IgG2a, IgG2b and IgM, as well as total immunoglobulin levels remain relatively unchanged. This report will focus on factors which specifically affect IgE and IgG1 production relative to IgM production. The effect of these factors on the remaining isotypes have been published elsewhere (Coffman and Carty 1986; Coffman et al. 1986a,b).

Table 1. Effect of T_H supernatants on isotype expression

	Immunoglobulin Levels (ng/ml)						
Day 1 Additions	IgE	IgA	IgG1	IgG2a	IgG2b	IgG3	IgM
Medium	<1	104	1,300	38	267	2,380	58,400
3% D9.1	145	727	12,200	46	191	574	73,900
10% LB2-1	<1	182	620	86	115	295	23,300
3% D9.1 + 1% LB2-1	<1	308	760	52	100	312	25,500

Supernatants from many other TH lines, such as LB2.1, did not cause an increase in IgE or any other isotype and, in fact, often caused some inhibition of all isotypes (Table 1). The addition of small amounts of LB2.1 supernatant to B cell cultures stimulated with LPS and D9.1 supernatant resulted in a total inhibition of the D9.1 enhanced IgE and IgG1 levels with no more than a two-fold inhibition of any other isotype (Table 1).

IgE Enhancing Activity is Mediated by BSF-1

Several types of evidence demonstrate that the IgE enhancing activity found in supernatants of D9.1 and similar TH lines is mediated by the lymphokine BSF-1. The IgE enhancing activity has proven inseparable from BSF-1 by a number of biochemical fractionation techniques (Coffman et al. 1986a). It likewise cannot be separated from a novel T cell and mast cell growth factor activity that has also been shown to be mediated by BSF-1 (Mosmann et al. submitted for publication). Highly purified BSF-1 from the EL-4 lymphoma cell line (Ohara et al. 1985) can stimulate IgE production to the same extent as D9.1 supernatant (Table 2a). Furthermore, a monoclonal antibody to BSF-1 that inhibits BSF-1 function can totally inhibit IgE enhancement by D9.1 supernatant (Table 2a). In a similar set of experiments, Vitetta et al.(1985) demonstrated that IgG1 enhancing and IgG3 inhibiting activities are also mediated by BSF-1 and we have confirmed those results. The 5- to 10-fold enhancement of IgA obtained with these same supernatants is not, however, mediated by BSF-1 (Coffman et al. 1986a,b) and appears to be mediated by a molecule which is easily separated from BSF-1 (unpublished observations).

Table 2. Effect of purified and recombinant BSF-1 and anti-BSF-1 on IgE and IgG1 expression

	Immunoglobulin Levels (ng/ml)		
Day 1 Additions	IgE	IgG1	IgM
A.			
Medium	<2	1,060	43,000
D9.1 supernatant	102	19,700	41,500
200 units/ml BSF-1 (EL-4)	99	8,790	23,700
D9 + rat anti-BSF-1 (5 μg/ml)	<2	1,460	48,400
D9 + rat IgG1 control (5 μg/ml)	120	15,500	51,300
B.			
Medium	<1	1,410	24,900
D9.1 supernatant	47	13,300	28,000
COS-BSF-1	48	13,700	7,400

The recent cloning of the gene for mouse BSF-1 provides the most convincing demonstration that BSF-1 can preferentially enhance IgE production by LPS-stimulated B cells (Lee et al. 1986). Supernatants of monkey COS-7 cells transfected with the gene for mouse BSF-1 can specifically enhance IgE and IgG1 (Table 2b) and can significantly inhibit IgG2b and IgG3 levels in B cell cultures (Coffman et al. 1986b).

It is not obvious how this very specific enhancement of only two of seven isotypes can be mediated by a molecule which can activate nearly all B cells (Noelle et al. 1984; Rabin et al. 1985). D9.1 supernatant (Coffman and Carty 1986) and recombinant BSF-1 (unpublished observations) stimulate IgE and IgG1 responses even in LPS-stimulated cultures of rigorously purified small B cells. This argues against the possibility that BSF-1 acts by stimulating the production of isotype-specific molecules by non-B cells. It has been suggested that BSF-1 affects IgG1 production by promoting a switch to IgG1 rather than by selectively expanding IgG1 producing cells (Isakson et al. 1982). It seems reasonable to postulate that it enhances IgE responses by the same mechanism. If this proves correct, it would mean that BSF-1 plays a central role in the initiation of the atopic state.

The SJA/9 congenic mouse strain may provide a useful model in which to examine the role of BSF-1 in vivo. SJA/9 mice do not make significant IgE responses either to antigens or to helminth parasite infections under normal immunization conditions. (Kumagai,et al. 1983; Hirano et al. 1983). However, SJA/9 B cells can produce as much IgE as Balb/c B cells when stimulated with LPS and a source of BSF-1 (Coffman and Carty 1986).

IFN-γ Inhibits the BSF-1-Mediated Enhancement of IgE

As was shown in Table 1, the majority of TH supernatants which do not enhance IgE production by LPS-stimulated B cells can instead inhibit the enhancement mediated by BSF-1. We observed a very strong correlation between the production of IFN-γ and IL-2 by a TH line and its ability to inhibit IgE production. Using purified recombinant IL-2, we found that IL-2 concentrations from 5 ng/ml to 5 μg/ml (10-10,000 units/ml) had little on no effect on BSF-1 stimulated IgE or IgG1 levels (unpublished observations). However, as little as 1 ng/ml (2-4 antiviral units/ml) of recombinant IFN-γ could totally inhibit BSF-1 stimulated IgE production and reduce IgG1 production to below the levels obtained with LPS stimulation alone (Table 3). This action of IFN-γ is also quite isotype-specific since these concentrations produce less than a two-fold inhibition of IgM (Table 3) or of other isotypes (Coffman and Carty 1986). The relative specificity of this inhibition may simply reflect the ability of IFN-γ to inhibit the action of BSF-1. Other known activities of BSF-1 on B cells, such as Ia induction and anti-μ costimulation, can also be inhibited by IFN-γ (Mond et al. 1985; Mond, personal communication).

Table 3. Inhibition of the IgE and IgG1 response by recombinant IFNγ

	Immunoglobulin Levels (ng/ml)		
Day 1 Additions	IgE	IgG1	IgM
Medium	<1	2,100	36,200
D9.1 supernatant	144	15,800	56,100
D9.1 supernatant + 0.25 mg/ml IFNγ	29	11,200	26,200
D9.1 supernatant + 1.0 mg/ml IFNγ	<1	7,700	25,600
D9.1 supernatant + 4.0 mg/ml IFNγ	<1	2,200	21,000

The observation that BSF-1 and IFN-γ, which have profound but opposite effects on IgE responses, are produced by separate subsets of TH cells (Mosmann et al. 1986) suggests a mechanism for the regulation of IgE responses. The magnitude of an IgE response may well reflect the relative activation of the BSF-1 producing TH cells, which would stimulate IgE production, and the IFN-γ producing subset, which would antagonize that stimulation.

It is not known whether the activation requirements of these two subsets are different, but after testing many antigen and Ia specific TH clones, we have found that only BSF-1 producing clones can provide "help" for a secondary IgE response in vitro (Coffman and Mosmann, unpublished observations).

REFERENCES

Coffman RL, Carty J (1986) A T cell activity that enhances polyclonal IgE production and its inhibition by interferon-γ. J Immunol 136:949-955

Coffman RL, Ohara J, Bond MW, Carty J, Zlotnik A, Paul WE (1986a) B cell stimulatory factor-1 enhances the IgE response on LPS-activated B cells, in press.

Coffman RL, Lee F, Yokota T, Arai, K and Mosmann T (1986b) The effect of BSF-1 and IFNγ on mouse immunoglobulin isotype expression. In: Goldstein G, Bach J-F and Wigzell H, (Eds). Immune regulation by characterized polypeptides. UCLA Symposia on Molecular and Cellular Biology, Vol 41. Alan R Liss, N.Y. in press.

Hirano T, Kumagai Y, Okumura K, and Ovary Z (1983) Regulation of murine IgE production: Importance of a not-yet-described T cell for IgE secretion demonstrated in SJA9 mice. Proc Natl Acad Sci USA 80:3435-3439.

Isakson PC, Pure E, Vitetta ES, and Krammer PH (1982) T cell-derived B cell differentiation factor(s): Effect on the isotype switch of murine B cells. J Exp Med 155:734-748.

Ishizaka K (1976) Cellular events in the IgE antibody response. Advances in Immunology 23:1-75.

Ishizaka K (1984) Regulation of IgE synthesis. Ann Rev Immunol 2:159-182

Itaya T and Ovary Z (1979) Suppression of IgE antibody production in SJL mice. IV. Interaction of primed and unprimed T cells. J Exp Med 150:507-516.

Katz DH (1980) Recent studies on the regulation of IgE antibody synthesis in experimental animals and man. Immunology 41:1-24.

Kumagai Y, Hirano T, Watanabe N, Okumura K, and Ovary Z (1983) Studies on IgE production in mice. I. Spontaneous suppression of IgE production in SJA/9 mice. Immunogenetics 18:147-153.

Lee F, Yakota T, Otsuka T, Meyerson P, Villaret D, Coffman R, Mosmann T, Rennick D, Roehm N, Smith C, Zlotnik A, and Arai K (1986) Isolation and characterization of a mouse interleukin cDNA clone that expresses BSF-1 activities and T cell and mast cell stimulating activities. Proc Natl Acad Sci USA: in press.

Mond JJ, Finkelman FD, Sarma C, Ohara J, Serrate S (1985) Recombinant interferon-γ inhibits the B cell proliferative response stimulated by soluble but not by sepharose-bound anti-immunoglobulin antibody. J Immunol 135:2513-2517.

Mosmann TR, Cherwinski H, Bond MW, Giedlin MA, Coffman RL (1986) Two types of murine helper T cell clones: 1. Definition according to profiles of lymphokine activities and secreted proteins. J Immunol in press.

Noelle R, Krammer PH, Ohara J, Uhr JW, and Vitteta ES (1984) Increased expression of Ia antigens on resting B cells: an additional role for B-cell growth factor. Proc Natl Acad Sci USA 81:6149-6153.
Ohara J, Lahet S, Inman J, and Paul WE (1985) Partial purification of murine B cell stimulatory factor (BSF)-1. J Immunol 135:2518-2523.
Rabin EM, Ohara J, and Paul WE (1985) B-cell stimulatory factor (BSF)-1 activates resting B cells. Proc Natl Acad Sci USA 82:2935-2939.
Suemura M, Shiho O, Deguchi H, Yamamura Y, Bottcher I, and Kishimoto T (1981) Characterization and isolation of IgE class-specific suppressor factor (IgE-TsF) 1. The presence of binding site(s) for IgE and of the H-2 gene products in IgE-Tsf. J Immunol 127:465-471.
Vitetta ES, Ohara J, Myers C, Layton J, Krammer PH, and Paul WE (1985) Serological, biochemical and functional identity of B cell stimulatory factor-1 and B cell differentiation factor for IgG1. J Exp Med 162:1726-1731.
Young M, Leung DYM, and Geha, RS (1984) Production of IgE-potentiating factor in man by T cell lines bearing Fc receptors for IgE. Eur J Immunol 14:871-876.

Interleukin-4 (B Cell Growth Factor-II/Eosinophil Differentiation Factor) is a Mitogen and Differentiation Factor for Preactivated Murine B Lymphocytes

Anne O'Garra, David J. Warren, Colin J. Sanderson,
Anthony I. Magee and Gerry G.B. Klaus
National Institute for Medical Research, London

1 Introduction

Type II B cell growth factor (BCGF II) was originally detected by its capacity to induce proliferation of the murine B cell lymphoma BCL_1 in vitro (Swain & Dutton, 1982: Swain et al, 1983). Its effects on normal B cells have not been well defined, since it has proved difficult to separate BCGF II from other potentially relevant factors. We have recently described a novel source of BCGF II which is free of any other lymphokine believed to act on B cells. This activity is produced by a murine T cell hybrid NIMP-TH1, which was selected for its capacity to secrete the eosinophil differentiation factor (EDF) (Warren & Sanderson, 1985: Sanderson et al, 1986). The BCGF II and EDF co-purify in every fractionation procedure employed (Fig. 1) : both activities migrate with an approximate Mr of 44,000 (Fig. 2) and a pI of approximately 5.0 (unpublished data). These findings, together with earlier evidence that BCGF II and EDF are co-ordinately produced by a large panel of T cell clones (Sanderson et al, 1985) strongly suggested that the two activities are due to the same molecule, which has therefore been named interleukin 4 (IL-4) (Sanderson et al, 1986). We have examined the effects of this factor on normal murine B cells.

Current Topics in Microbiology and Immunology, Vol. 132

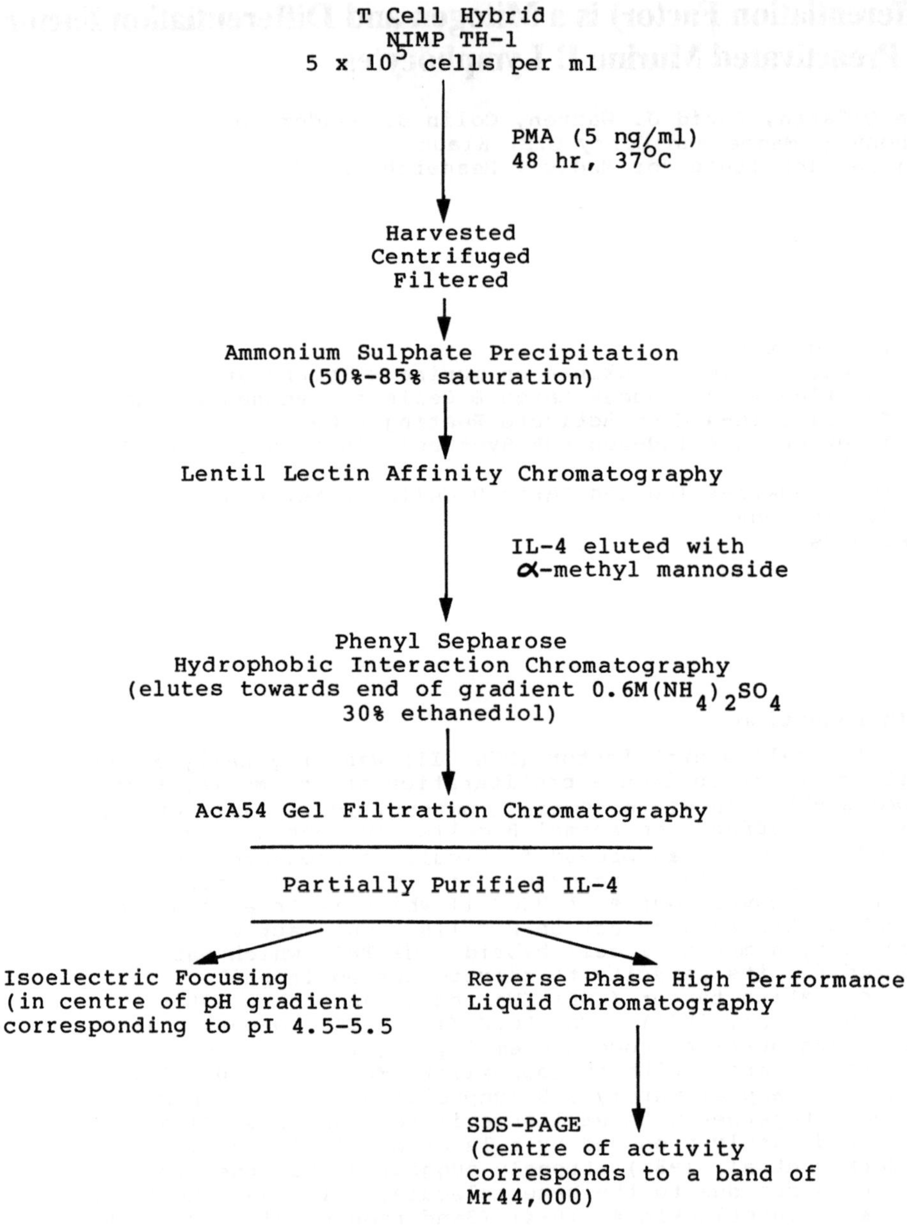

Fig. 1. Purification of IL-4

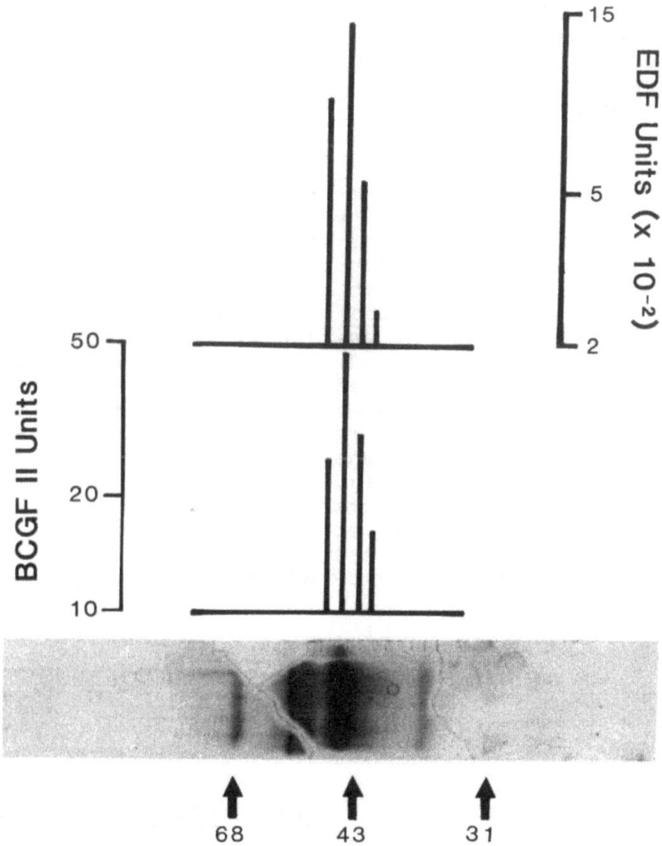

Fig. 2. Polyacrylamide gel electrophoresis of IL-4. Pooled active fractions from reverse phase HPLC were separated by $NaDodSO_4$-PAGE under non-reducing conditions. Panel (A) is a silver-stained portion of the gel, with positions of molecular weight weight markers (Mr x 10^{-3} Da) indicated. In panel (B), eluted material from each gel slice was assayed for EDF and for BCGF II.

2 Effects of IL-4 on normal murine B cells.

2.1 IL-4 induces large B cells to synthesize DNA.

Partially purified IL-4 was tested for its capacity to induce proliferation in B cells of different densities, obtained by Percoll density gradient centrifugation (Fig. 3) (O'Garra et al, 1986). The factor did not induce DNA synthesis in small dense B cells. As expected, these cells did respond to costimulation with anti-Ig plus conditioned medium from an alloreactive T cell clone (CM-T2) which contains both BSF-1 and IL-4. However, IL-4 stimulated marked DNA synthesis in large (low density) B cells, obtained from the 65%/50%

interface of the gradient, inducing a response which was comparable to that elicited by CM-T2 plus anti-Ig. These results suggested (but did not prove) that IL-4 acts on B cells that have been preactivated in vivo, but does not induce proliferation in resting B cells.

2.2 IL-4 does not activate resting B cells

It is now clear that BSF-1 alone markedly increases the levels of Ia antigens on murine B cells, which is an early indicator of B cell activation (Roehm et al, 1984; Noelle et al, 1984). In contrast, IL-4 had no effect on the levels of Ia antigens on small dense B cells (O'Garra et al, 1986).

A more direct way to demonstrate that resting B cells have entered cycle is by use of priming cultures (Klaus et al, 1984): cells are activated (primed) for 24-48 hr with various stimuli, washed and then recultured with a mitogen in readout cultures. Cells which have entered cycle will commence DNA synthesis earlier in response to restimulation. Fig. 4 shows that IL-4 did not prime small, dense B cells to respond to a mitogenic concentration of anti-Ig. In contrast, and as expected, anti-Ig or CM-T2 (presumably because it contains BSF-1, data not shown, see Rabin et al, 1985) induced significant activation. These results therefore indicate that resting B cells can be activated by BSF-1, but not by IL-4.

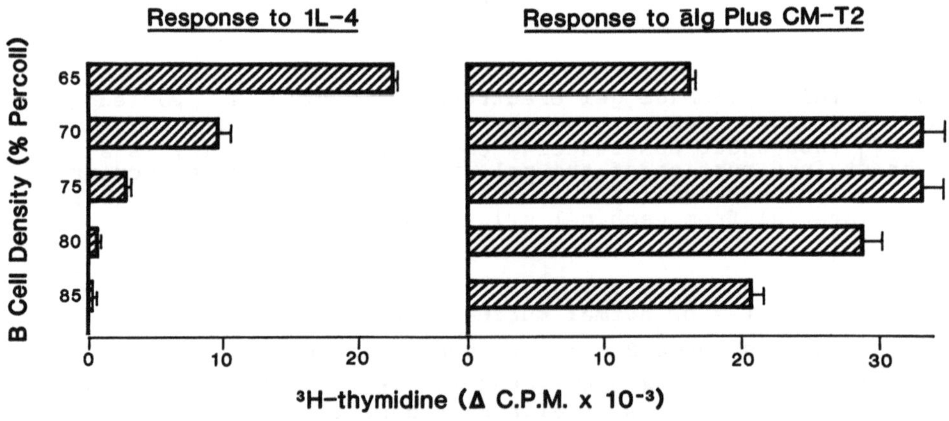

Fig. 3. IL-4 induces large but not small B cells to synthesize DNA. B cells separated on a discontinuous gradient of Percoll were cultured with partially purified IL-4 or with a submitogenic dose of anti-Ig and CM-T2 (which contains BSF-1). ^{3}H-thymidine uptakes were measured on day 3.

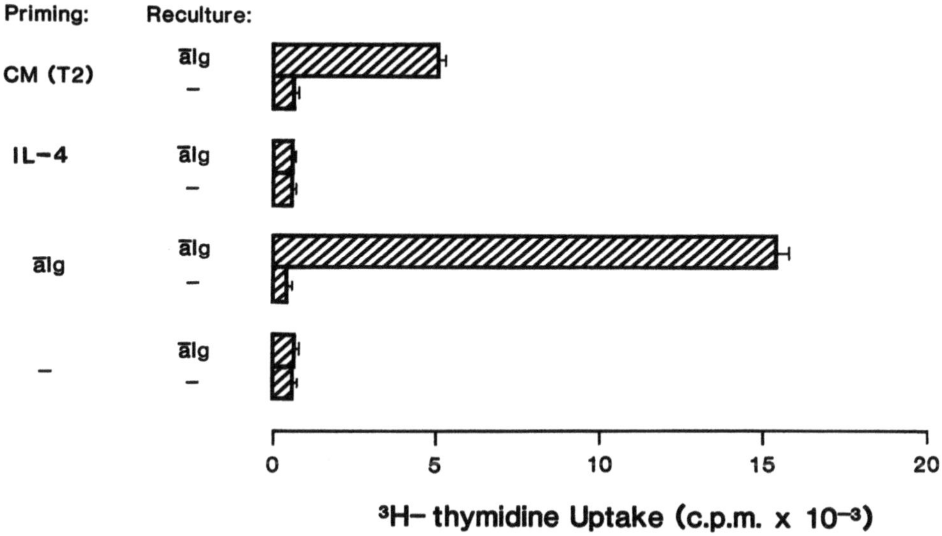

Fig. 4. Activation of B cells with growth factors for responsivenes to anti-Ig. Small dense B cells obtained as previously described were cultured (primed) for 24 hr with partially purified IL-4, CM-T2, anti-Ig, or medium alone. Cells were then washed, counted and recultured with medium alone or with a mitogenic dose of anti-Ig. ^{3}H-thymidine incorporation in these second cultures was assayed after 24 hr.

2.3 IL-4 induces DNA synthesis in preactivated B cells

We then tested the proliferative responses of B cells activated by anti-Ig to restimulation with IL-4 (Fig. 5). B cells primed with 2 or 10 ug/ml anti-Ig for 24 hr did not respond to IL-4 in the readout cultures, but responded well to anti-Ig. However, cells primed for 40 hr with 10 ug/ml anti-Ig (but not with 2 ug/ml) became responsive to IL-4. Anti-Ig causes dose-dependent cell cycle progression of B cells (DeFranco et al, 1985; Klaus et al, 1985). Ten ug/ml anti-Ig stimulates a substantial proportion of B cells to progress through G_1, whilst 1-2 ug/ml induces the cells to leave G_0 but not to progress substantially through G_1 (Klaus et al, 1985). The observation that resting B cells only become responsive to IL-4 after >30 hr priming with 10 ug/ml (and not 2 ug/ml) anti-Ig therefore strongly suggests that IL-4 acts as a mitogen on cells in late G_1. This, however, needs to be confirmed by cell cycle analysis.

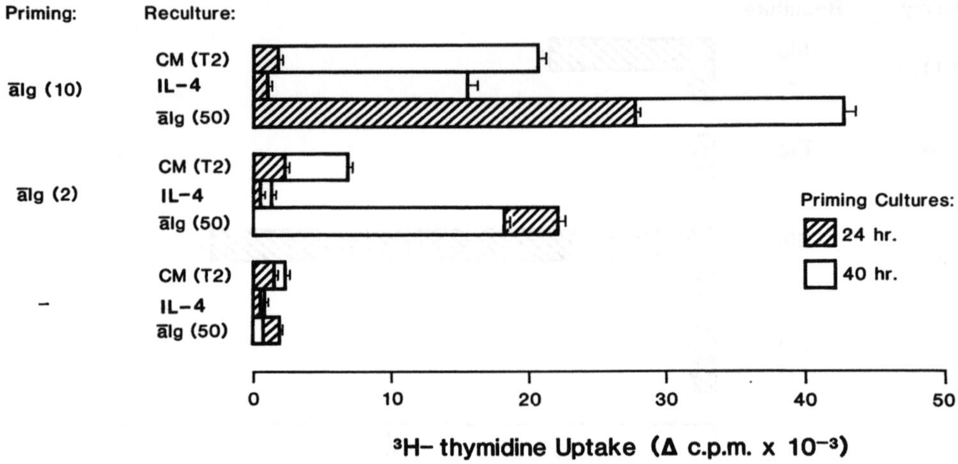

Fig. 5. Activation of B cells by anti-Ig for responsiveness to IL-4. Small dense B cells were cultured for 24 hr (hatched bars), or 40 hr (open bars) with 10 or 2 ug/ml anti-Ig, or medium alone. Cells were then washed, counted and recultured with medium alone, CM-T2, partially purified IL-4, or a mitogenic dose of anti-Ig. ^{3}H-thymidine incorporation in these readout cultures was assessed after 24 hr.

Recently, Muller et al, 1985, found that a factor with a Mr of 40-50 Kd produced by the EL4 cell line induced proliferation and IgM secretion in B cells activated by anti-Ig for 48 hr. This appeared to be distinct from IL-2 and BSF-1, but has not been extensively purified. They did not test its effects on naturally occurring large B cells. However, Layton et al, 1985, have reported that crude supernatants from various T cell sources stimulated such B cells to both DNA synthesis and Ig secretion. In our experience, complete separation of BCGF II and BSF-1 (from EL4 cells or CM-T2) by physicochemical means is extremely difficult. Our source of BCGF II is free of any other lymphokines believed to act on B cells, which therefore obviates this problem.

2.4 IL-4 induces large B cells to secrete IgM and IgG

In the light of the above findings it became important to establish if preactivated B cells could also be induced to secrete antibody by IL-4. Large (low density) B cells (O'Garra et al, 1986) were therefore cultured with IL-4, CM-T2, or LPS, and the cultures were then assayed for IgM and IgG secreting cells (Dresser & Popham, 1980; Carter & Dresser, 1985). Such cultures contained small numbers of IgM PFC on day 0, which increased markedly after culture with LPS or factors, and reached a plateau on days 5 to 7 (unpublished data). After 7 days culture with IL-4, CM-T2 or LPS the cultures produced large numbers of IgM PFC and significant levels of IgG PFC (Table 1). In contrast, small dense B cells responded to LPS, but not to IL-4 (not shown). Earlier studies had suggested that proliferation and maturation to antibody secretion in B lymphocytes are controlled by different lymphokines (Swain and Dutton, 1982). Recent evidence however indicates that the proliferative and differentiation activities cannot be separated by a variety of biochemical techniques (Muller et al, 1985; Harada et al, 1985). In agreement with this, IL-4 not only stimulates proliferation of large B cells recovered from Percoll gradients (Fig 3) but also evokes the maturation of IgM secreting and lesser numbers of IgG secreting cells (Table 1). Both BCGF and differentiation activities of the lymphokine are not separable by a series of biochemical techniques, including reverse phase HPLC and $NaDodSo_4$-PAGE (see O'Garra et al, 1986).

Table 1.

Additions	PFC/Culture	
	IgM	IgG
-	1,134 (39)	0
IL-4 (2 units/ml)	10,835 (374)	635 (55)
CM-T2 (5%)	25,333 (785)	2,323 (4)
LPS (10 ug/ml)	26,900 (393)	2,040 (52)

Large B cells (from the 65%/50% interface of Percoll gradients) were cultured with the indicated concentrations of partially purified IL-4, CM-T2, LPS, or medium. IgM and IgG PFC were assayed on day 7.

3. Conclusions

Our results clearly demonstrate that IL-4 does not affect resting B cells but induces both DNA synthesis and Ig secretion in naturally occurring large B cells (presumably preactivated), and stimulates DNA synthesis in B cells appropriately activated by anti-Ig. Furthermore, all the bioactivities of IL-4 are associated with a protein band with a Mr of 44,000 on $NaDodSo_4$-PAGE (Fig. 2 and O'Garra et al, 1986). It now remains to be shown if this factor exerts distinct signals for growth and differentiation in B cell blasts, since it is possible that it merely prolongs proliferation sufficiently to allow the cells to secrete Ig. Furthermore, although it seems likely that IL-4 acts directly on preactivated B cells, we cannot at present exclude the possibility that it may synergize with other factors produced by residual cells contaminating our culture system. Clearly, much further work is required to establish the precise physiological role of this lymphokine in B cell growth and maturation.

Acknowledgements. We are grateful to Mary Holman and Angela Popham for technical help. Anne O'Garra was supported by a fellowship from Glaxo Group Research.

References

Carter J, and DW Dresser (1985) Fetal stimulation of maternal immunoglobulin production in mice. J Reprod and Fertil 74:535-542

DeFranco AL, Raveche ES, and Paul WE (1985) Separate control of B lymphocyte early activation and proliferation in response to anti-IgM antibodies. J Immunol 135:87-94

Dresser DW, and Popham AM (1980) Plaque assay for rheumatoid factors. Immunology 41:569-577

Harada N, Kikuchi Y, Tominaga A, Takaki S, Takatsu K (1985) BCGF II activity on activated B cells of a purified murine T cell replacing factor (TRF) from a T cell hybridoma (B151K12). J Immunol 134:3944-3951

Klaus, GGM, Hawrylowicz CM, Holman M, Keeler KD (1984) Activation and proliferation signals in mouse B cells. III Intact (IgG) anti-Ig antibodies activate B cells but inhibit induction of DNA synthesis Immunology 53:693-701

Klaus, GGB, Hawrylowicz CM, Carter CJ (1985) Activation and proliferation signals in mouse B cells. VI Anti-Ig antibodies induce dose-dependent cell cycle progression in B cells Immunology 55:411-418

Layton JE, Krammer PH, Hamaoka T, Uhr JW, Vitetta ES (1985) Small and large B cells respond differently to T cell-derived B cell growth and differentiation factors. J Mol Cell Immunol 2:155-167

Muller W, Kuhn R, Goldman W, Tesch H, Smith FI, Radbruch A, Rajewsky K (1985) Signal requirements for growth and differentiation of activated murine B lymphocytes J Immunol 135:1213-1219

Noelle R, Krammer PH, Ohara J, Uhr JW, Vitetta ES (1984) Increased expression of Ia antigens on resting B cells: An additional role for B-cell growth factor Proc Natl Acad Sci USA 81:6149-6153

O'Garra A, Warren DJ, Holman M, Popham AM, Sanderson CJ, Klaus GGB (1986) Interleukin-4 (B cell growth factor-II/eosinophil differentiation factor) is a mitogen and differentiation factor for preactivated murine B lymphocytes Proc Natl Acad Sci USA In press

Sanderson CJ, O'Garra A, Warren DJ, Klaus GGB (1986) Eosinophil differentiation factor also has B cell growth factor activity Proposed name Interleukin-4 Proc Natl Acad Sci USA 83:437-440

Sanderson CJ, Strath M, Warren DJ, O'Garra A, Kirkwood TBL (1985) The production of lymphokines by primary alloreactive T-cell clones: a co-ordinate analysis of 233 clones in seven lymphokine assays. Immunology 56:575-583

Swain SL, Dutton RW (1982) Production of a B cell growth-promoting activity, (DL) BCGF, from a cloned T cell line and its assay on the BCL_1 B cell tumour J Exp Med 156:1821-1834

Swain SL, Howard M, Kappler J, Marrack P, Watson J, Booth R, Wetzel GD, Dutton RW (1983) Evidence for two distinct classes of murine B cell growth factors with activities in different functional assays J Exp Med 158:822-835
Warren DJ, Sanderson CJ (1985) Production of a T cell hybrid producing a lymphokine-stimulating eosinophil differentiation 54:615-623

Note Added in Proof:
In previous publications, (Sanderson et al. 1986. PNAS. 83: 437; O'Garra et al. PNAS. In Press) we have referred to EDF/BCGF II as Interleukin-4 (IL-4). This name has also been coined for BSF-1 (Noma et al. 1986. Nature 319: 640).

Role of the LFA-1 Molecule in B Cell Differentiation

Gail Abendroth Bishop and Geoffrey Haughton

Department of Microbiology and Immunology and The Lineberger Cancer Research Center, The University of North Carolina at Chapel Hill, Chapel Hill, NC 27514

INTRODUCTION

The lymphocyte function-associated antigen-1 (LFA-1) was first identified as a T cell surface antigen, and antibodies to LFA-1 have been shown to inhibit responses of T cells to antigen and/or major histocompatibility complex (MHC) molecules (Springer 1982, Krensky 1983, Ware 1983, Collins 1984, Krensky 1984, Golde 1985, Naquet 1985). However, LFA-1 molecules are also present on the surface of B cells (Davignon 1981), and the possible functional role played by B cell LFA-1 has received little attention.

The murine B cell lymphoma CH12 has surface IgM with specificity for the phosphatidyl choline moiety of sheep erythrocyte (SRBC) membranes (Arnold 1983, Mercolino 1986) and can be induced to differentiate to immunoglobulin (Ig) secretion by antigen-specific, MHC-restricted signals, as well as by mitogens (LoCascio 1984). A tissue culture-adapted subclone of CH12, CH12.LX, now provides a valuable model with which to study regulation of B cell differentiation, free from possible contamination by host cells.[1] In this report, CH12.LX cells and monoclonal antibodies (Mabs) to the LFA-1 molecule were used to examine the role of LFA-1 in B cell differentiation.

MATERIALS AND METHODS

B Cells.

The surface IgM+ B cell clone CH12.LX was derived by single-cell cloning of the B cell lymphoma CH12, which arose in a B10.H-2^aH-4^b p/Wts mouse, and has been described previously (Arnold 1983). CH12.LX cells were maintained in suspension culture, in RPMI 1640 medium supplemented with 10% fetal calf serum, 300μg/ml glutamine, 10^{-5} M 2-mercaptoethanol, and antibiotics (complete medium, CM).

T Cells.

E2.21, the I-E^k-specific alloreactive T helper (Th) cell hybridoma used in these studies, was provided by Dr. A. Augustin, who has previously described its derivation (Augustin 1984).

Antibodies.

The Mabs used in these studies were 14-4-4S (anti-I-E^k; Ozato 1980), 30C7 (anti-Lgp 100, Ledbetter 1981), M17 (anti-LFA-1 α chain; Sanchez-Madrid 1983), and M18 (anti-LFA-1 β chain; ibid). Mabs were used as tissue culture supernatants

---

[1] Bishop, GA, Haughton, G. Induced differentiation of clonal Ly-1+ B cells by T cells and antigen. Submitted.

Current Topics in Microbiology and Immunology, Vol. 132

from hybridomas provided by the American Type Culture Collection, Rockville, MD. 14-4-4S is a mouse monoclonal alloantibody; 30C7, M17, and M18 are IgG rat anti-mouse monoclonal Mabs.

Assay for B cell Differentiation.

To measure induced differentiation, 2 x 10^5 CH12.LX cells were cultured in 2 ml of CM in 24-well plates as described (LoCascio 1984). Th cells (Fig 1A) were exposed to 1500R of gamma irradiation prior to addition to cultures; 5 x 10^4 Th cells were added/culture. When SRBC were added as a source of antigen (Fig. 1A & B), 10^6 were included/culture. Mitogen-stimulated cultures (Fig. 1C) contained 50 µg/ml of LPS. Phorbol myristate acetate (TPA)-treated cultures (Fig. 1D) contained 50 ng/ml of TPA. Incubation of CH12.LX cells with the DNA synthesis inhibitor mitomycin C (MC, Table 1) was performed for 30 minutes at 37°C, after which cells were washed three times prior to culture. All cultures were performed in duplicate. Direct hemolytic plaque-forming cells (pfc) in cultures of CH12.LX cells were determined by the method of Cunningham (1968).

Aggregation Assay.

To measure the relationship between pfc formation and aggregation by CH12.LX cells, cultures were performed in quadruplicate. Two cultures were assesed for pfc as described above, and two were resuspended gently, centrifuged in a 12 x 75mm round-bottom tube for 5 minutes at 700 rpm, and gently resuspended in 0.25ml of RPMI 1640. The percentage of aggregated cells (2-10 cells/aggregate) was determined by counting > 500 cells/sample in a hemacytometer.

Assay for Cell Proliferation.

Cultures were performed as above, in 0.2ml/culture in a 96-well microtitration plate. Four hours prior to the end of culture, each well was pulsed with 1 µCi of ^{3}H-thymidine. Cells were harvested and uptake of ^{3}H-thymidine measured as described (Bradley 1980).

RESULTS

Anti-LFA-1 Mediated Inhibition of Antigen-Specific, MHC-Restricted B cell Differentiation.

CH12.LX cells are induced to differentiate to IgM secretion in the simultaneous presence of an antigen which binds their surface Ig (SRBC) and Th cells which bind to their I-E molecules[1]. Since antibodies to the LFA-1 molecule have been shown to block antigen presentation to T cells by B cell hybridomas (Golde 1985, Naquet 1985), we wished to determine whether such antibodies block antigen-specific, Th cell-mediated induction of CH12.LX differentiation. Fig. 1A demonstrates that Mabs to both the α and β chains of the LFA-1 molecule blocked B cell differentiation induced by I-E^k-specific Th cells and SRBC. This inhibition was dependent on the dose of Mab, and Mab to the LFA-1 α chain (M17) was somewhat more inhibitory than Mab to the β chain (M18), although both Mabs were successful in inhibiting B cell differentiation.

Both CH12.LX B cells and E2.21 T cells bind M17 and M18 Mabs (data not presented). Thus, the inhibition of B cell differentiation seen in Fig. 1A could be mediated through binding of either B or T cell LFA-1 molecules, or both. Since we have recently found that monoclonal antibodies to I-E^k can substitute for I-E^k-specific Th cells in delivering a differentiative signal to CH12. LX cells[1], we next examined whether anti-LFA-1 Mabs can block B cell differentiation in the absence of T cells. Fig. 1B shows that a 1:1 mixture of M17 and M18 hybridoma supernatants was effective in blocking spontaneous differentiation of CH12.LX cells, as well as that induced in the simultaneous presence of SRBC and 14-4-4S Mab (previous studies have shown that neither antigen, T cells, nor anti-I-E^k antibody alone stimulate CH12.LX cells to differentiate.[1]) Finally, a control rat Mab to Lgp 100, 30C7, had no effect upon the induced differentiation of CH12.LX cells.

Anti-LFA-1-mediated Inhibition of Nonspecific Induction of B Cell Differentiation.

Data presented in Fig. 1B demonstrated that anti-LFA-1 Mabs could inhibit B cell differentiation directly, via the B cell LFA-1 molecule. We next examined whether this inhibition also extended to differentiation induced by mechanisms other than antigen or MHC-specific signals. It was found that anti-LFA-1 Mabs also inhibited, in a dose-dependent manner, differentiation of CH12.LX cells induced by the B cell mitogen LPS (Fig. 1C).

We have found that drugs which inhibit DNA synthesis in CH12.LX cells stimulate their differentiation[2]. We thus considered the possibility that anti-LFA-1 Mabs exert their inhibitory effect upon the differentiation of CH12.LX cells by increasing their proliferation. However, as Fig. 1C demonstrates, M17/M18 antibodies did not alter the ^{3}H-thymidine uptake of CH12.LX cells at any Mab dose tested. In addition, anti-LFA-1 antibodies used at the highest concentration tested in Fig. 1A-C (a 1/5 dilution) had no effect on the differentiation of CH12.LX cells induced by treatment with the DNA synthesis inhibitor MC (Table 1).

Correlation Between Anti-LFA-1-mediated Inhibition of B Cell Differentiation and Aggregation.

Prior studies present evidence supporting a role for the LFA-1 molecule in mediating or enhancing cell-cell adhesion (Pattaroyo 1985). To determine whether Mab to LFA-1 inhibited contact between B cells as a mechanism for its inhibitory effects upon B cell differentiation, the ability of M17/M18 to inhibit spontaneous and TPA-induced aggregation was tested. Fig. 1D shows that anti-LFA-1 Mabs (1/5 dilution) inhibited both aggregation and differentiation of CH12.LX cells, both spontaneous and induced by TPA. A control rat Mab (30C7) had no effect on aggregation or differentiation.

Table 1. Effect of anti-LFA-1 upon MC-induced B cell Differentiation.[a]

	[MC], µg/ml[b]				
Treatment	0	6.25	12.5	25	50
MC alone	4921	6850	12,888	11,333	51,000
MC + M17/M18[c]	3076	6598	10,444	10,000	49,333

[a]pfc/10^6 cells determined as described in Material and Methods.

[b]Treatment with MC performed as described in Materials and Methods.

[c]anti-LFA-1 monoclonal antibodies, used at a 1/5 dilution.

[2]Bishop GA, Haughton G. Role of the interleukin 2 receptor in differentiation of a clone of Ly-1^+ B cells. Manuscript in preparation.

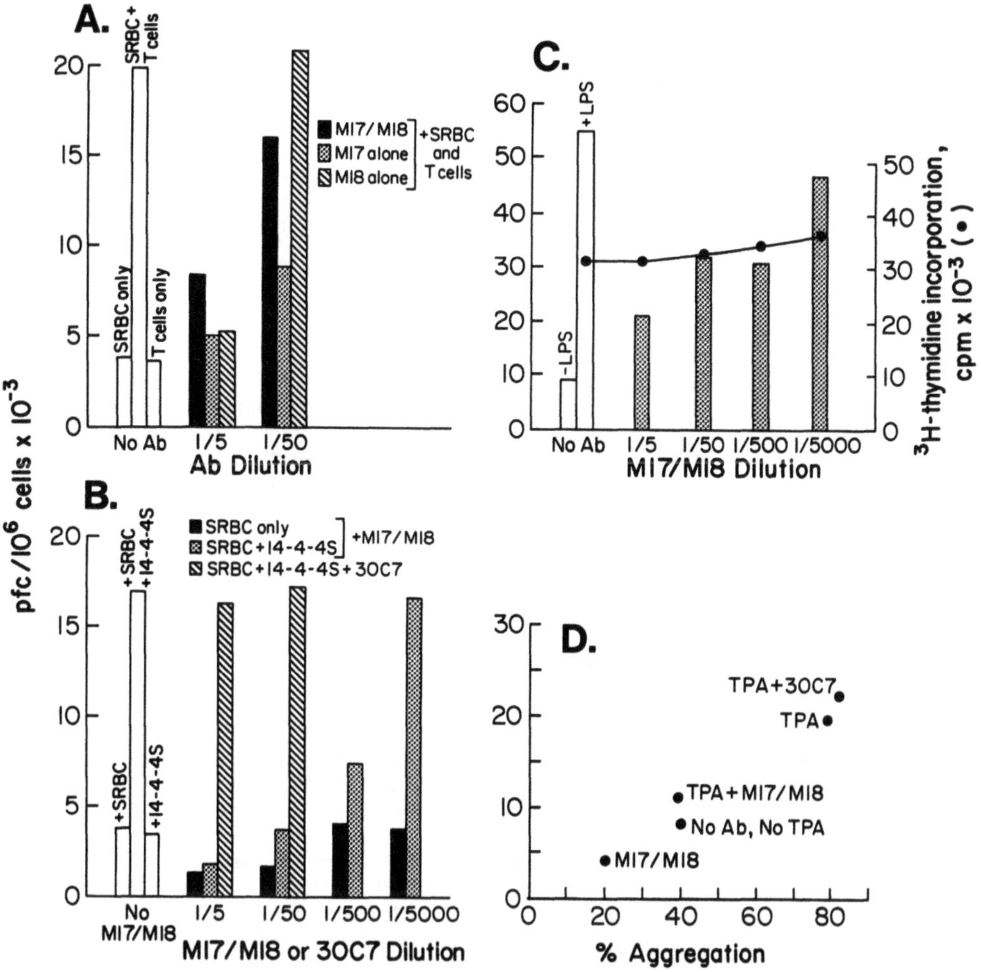

Fig. 1. Effects of antibodies to LFA-1 on B cell differentiation. CH12.LX clonal B cells were cultured and assayed for pfc formation as described in Materials and Methods. M17 and M18 are rat Mabs to the LFA-1 α(M17) and β(M18) chains, 30C7 is a control rat Mab to Lgp100 (not present on CH12.LX), and 14-4-4S is a mouse Mab to I-E^k. All antibodies were used as hybridoma tissue culture supernatants, at the indicated dilutions. A)Differentiation of CH12.LX induced by SRBC plus I-E^k-alloreactive T hybridoma cells. B) Differentiation of CH12.LX induced by SRBC plus anti-I-E^k Mab (14-4-4S, used at a 1/100 dilution). C) Differentiation of CH12.LX induced by mitogen. All cultures except those labeled "-LPS" contained 50 μg/ml of LPS. Uptake of ^{3}H-thymidine by CH12.LX cells was also measured in this experiment (O----O). D) Differentiation and aggregation of CH12.LX induced by TPA. Mabs (M17/M18 or 30C7) were used at a 1/5 dilution.

Studies on Transferrin Receptor Expression in Mouse Plasmacytoma Cells

L.M. Neckers, R. Nordan, S. Bauer and M. Potter

Laboratory of Pathology and Laboratory of Genetics, NCI, NIH, Bethesda, MD

INTRODUCTION

Transferrin receptor (TfR) expression in lymphoid cells is normally regulated by interaction of tissue-specific growth factors with their receptors (Neckers and Cossman 1983, Neckers et al. 1984). Malignant transformation of T and B lymphocytes generally leads to constitutive expression of TfR (Neckers 1985). Mouse plasmacytomas are an example of terminally differentiated B cells which continue to proliferate in an uncontrolled manner and constitutively express TfR *in vivo* . However, *in vitro* growth of most plasmacytomas requires the presence of a macrophage-derived growth factor (plasmacytoma growth factor, PCT-GF) described elsewhere in this volume (Nordan et al.; see also Nordan and Potter 1986). In this report we characterize the relationship between PCT-GF and TfR in plasmacytoma cell lines and describe a TfR mRNA species uniquely found in mouse plasmacytomas.

ROLE OF TfR IN PLASMACYTOMA GROWTH *IN VITRO*

The plasmacytoma cell line 1165 grows in culture but is dependent on added PCT-GF (Nordan et al., this volume). When rat anti-mouse TfR antibody is added to cultures containing PCT-GF, growth of 1165 cells is completely inhibited, although cell viability is not affected (Fig. 1). Thus TfR expression is required for the growth of these cells even in the presence of PCT-GF.

TfR expression itself is dependent on the presence of PCT-GF, as can be seen in Fig. 2. Removal of PCT-GF from the cultures of three different dependent cell lines results in rapid loss of surface TfR and a concomitant synchronization of the cells in the G1 phase of the cell cycle. Removal of PCT-GF from a growth factor independent cell line does not result in either a loss of surface TfR (Fig. 2, top curve), or G1 synchronization.

The relative specificity of this phenomenon is supported by the observation that surface expression of two other antigens (H2 and PC-1) does not decay following removal of PCT-GF (data not shown). Finally, the reduction in surface expression of TfR is representative of an overall reduction in TfR number, since total TfR (surface and cytoplasmic receptors) are reduced by a similar degree following removal of PCT-GF (data not shown).

MOUSE PLASMACYTOMA CELLS POSSESS A UNIQUE SPECIES OF TfR mRNA

Our studies on TfR expression in these cells led us to examine plasmacytoma TfR mRNA expression. In these studies we utilized a full-length human TfR cDNA - pTFR1 (generously supplied by A. McClelland and F. Ruddle, Yale University) - and two mouse cDNA probes - mTFR2 and mTFR1 - which we cloned and which hybridize respectively to coding and non-coding regions of the TfR mRNA.

Current Topics in Microbiology and Immunology, Vol. 132

REFERENCES

Arnold LW, LoCascio NJ, Lutz PM, Pennell CA, Klapper DG, Haughton G (1983) Antigen-induced lymphomagenesis: Identification of a murine B cell lymphoma with known antigen specificity. J. Immunol. 131:2064-2068
Augustin AA, Sim GK (1984) T-cell receptors generated via mutations are specific for various MHC antigens. Cell 39:5-12
Bradley LM (1980) Mitogen-induced responses. In Mishell BB, Shiigi SM (eds) Selected methods in cellular immunology. WH Freeman & Co., San Francisco, p 156
Collins T, Krensky AM, Clayberger C, Fiers W, Gimbrone MA, Burakoff SJ, Pober JS (1984) Human cytolytic T lymphocyte interactions with vascular endothelium and fibroblasts: role of effector and target cell molecules. J. Immunol. 133:1878-1884
Cunningham AJ, Szenberg A (1968) Further improvements in the plaque technique for detecting single antibody-forming cells. Immunology 14:599-601
Davignon D, Martz E, Reynolds T, Kurzinger K, Springer TA (1981) Monoclonal antibody to a novel lymphocyte function-associated antigen (LFA-1): Mechanism of blockade of T lymphocyte-mediated killing and effects on other T and B lymphocyte functions. J. Immunol. 127:590-595
Golde WT, Kappler JW, Greenstein J, Malissen B, Hood L, Marrack PM (1985) MHC-restricted antigen receptor on T cells. VIII. Role of the LFA-1 molecule. J. Exp. Med. 161:635-640
Krensky AM, Sanchez-Madrid F, Robbins E, Nagy JA, Springer TA, Burakoff SJ (1983) The functional significance, distribution, and structure of LFA-1, LFA-2, and LFA-3: Cell surface antigens associated with CTL-target interactions. J. Immunol. 131:611-616
Krensky AM, Robbins E, Springer TA, Burakoff SJ (1984) LFA-1, LFA-2, and LFA-3 antigens are involved in CTL-target conjugation. J. Immunol. 132:2180-2182
Lanier LL, Arnold LW, Raybourne RB, Russell S, Lynes MA, Warner NL, Haughton G (1982) Transplantable B-cell lymphomas in B10.H-2^{a}H-4^{b} p/Wts mice. Immunogenetics 16:367-371
Ledbetter JA, Herzenberg LA (1981) Xenogeneic monoclonal antibodies to mouse lymphoid differentiation antigens. Immunol. Rev. 47:63-90
LoCascio NJ, Arnold LW, Corley RB, Haughton G (1984) Induced differentiation of a B cell lymphoma with known antigen specificity. J. Mol. Cell. Immunol. 1:177-187.
Mercolino, TJ, Arnold LW, Haughton G (1986) Phosphatidyl choline is recognized by a series of Ly-1^{+} murine B cell lymphomas specific for erythrocyte membranes. J.Exp.Med. 163:155-165.
Naquet P, Malissen B, Bekkhoucha F, Pont S, Pierres A, Hood L, Pierres M (1985) L3T4 but not LFA-1 participates in antigen presentation by A^{k}-positive L cell transformants. Immunogenetics 22:247-256
Ozato K, Mayer N, Sachs DH (1980) Hybridoma cell lines secreting monoclonal antibodies to mouse H-2 and Ia antigens. J. Immunol. 124:533-540
Pattarroyo M, Beatty PG, Fabre JW, Gahmberg CG (1985) Identification of a cell surface protein complex mediating TPA-induced adhesion among human mononuclear leukocytes. Scand. J. Immunol. 22:171-182
Sanchez-Madrid F, Simon P, Thompson S, Springer TA (1983) Mapping of antigenic and functional epitopes on the α and β subunits of two related mouse glycoproteins involved in cell interactions, LFA-1 and Mac-1. J. Exp. Med. 158:586-602
Springer TA, Davignon D, Ho M, Kurzinger K, Martz E, Sanchez-Madrid F (1982) LFA-1 and Lyt 2,3 molecules associated with T lymphocyte-mediated killing; and Mac-1, an LFA-1 homologue associated with complement receptor function. Immunol. Rev. 68:171-196
Ware CF, Sanchez-Madrid F, Krensky AM, Burakoff SJ, Strominger JL, Springer TA (1983) Human LFA-1: Identification of multiple antigenic epitopes and their relationship to CTL-mediated cytotoxicity. J. Immunol. 131:1182-1188
Zubler RH, Lowenthal JW, Erard F, Hashimoto N, Devos R, MacDonald HR (1984) Activated B cells express receptors for, and proliferate in response to, pure interleukin 2. J. Exp. Med. 160:1170-1183

Studies on Transferrin Receptor Expression in Mouse Plasmacytoma Cells

L.M. Neckers, R. Nordan, S. Bauer and M. Potter

Laboratory of Pathology and Laboratory of Genetics, NCI, NIH, Bethesda, MD

INTRODUCTION

Transferrin receptor (TfR) expression in lymphoid cells is normally regulated by interaction of tissue-specific growth factors with their receptors (Neckers and Cossman 1983, Neckers et al. 1984). Malignant transformation of T and B lymphocytes generally leads to constitutive expression of TfR (Neckers 1985). Mouse plasmacytomas are an example of terminally differentiated B cells which continue to proliferate in an uncontrolled manner and constitutively express TfR *in vivo* . However, *in vitro* growth of most plasmacytomas requires the presence of a macrophage-derived growth factor (plasmacytoma growth factor, PCT-GF) described elsewhere in this volume (Nordan et al.; see also Nordan and Potter 1986). In this report we characterize the relationship between PCT-GF and TfR in plasmacytoma cell lines and describe a TfR mRNA species uniquely found in mouse plasmacytomas.

ROLE OF TfR IN PLASMACYTOMA GROWTH *IN VITRO*

The plasmacytoma cell line 1165 grows in culture but is dependent on added PCT-GF (Nordan et al., this volume). When rat anti-mouse TfR antibody is added to cultures containing PCT-GF, growth of 1165 cells is completely inhibited, although cell viability is not affected (Fig. 1). Thus TfR expression is required for the growth of these cells even in the presence of PCT-GF.

TfR expression itself is dependent on the presence of PCT-GF, as can be seen in Fig. 2. Removal of PCT-GF from the cultures of three different dependent cell lines results in rapid loss of surface TfR and a concomitant synchronization of the cells in the G1 phase of the cell cycle. Removal of PCT-GF from a growth factor independent cell line does not result in either a loss of surface TfR (Fig. 2, top curve), or G1 synchronization.

The relative specificity of this phenomenon is supported by the observation that surface expression of two other antigens (H2 and PC-1) does not decay following removal of PCT-GF (data not shown). Finally, the reduction in surface expression of TfR is representative of an overall reduction in TfR number, since total TfR (surface and cytoplasmic receptors) are reduced by a similar degree following removal of PCT-GF (data not shown).

MOUSE PLASMACYTOMA CELLS POSSESS A UNIQUE SPECIES OF TfR mRNA

Our studies on TfR expression in these cells led us to examine plasmacytoma TfR mRNA expression. In these studies we utilized a full-length human TfR cDNA - pTFR1 (generously supplied by A. McClelland and F. Ruddle, Yale University) - and two mouse cDNA probes - mTFR2 and mTFR1 - which we cloned and which hybridize respectively to coding and non-coding regions of the TfR mRNA.

Current Topics in Microbiology and Immunology, Vol. 132

The TfR gene is comprised of at least 19 exons extending over 33 kb of DNA (McClelland et al. 1984). The gene transcribes an unusually long (4.9 kb) mRNA, less than half of which codes for the TfR protein. The function of the remaining 3' untranslated portion of the mRNA is not known but has been postulated to relate to regulation of receptor expression (Kuhn et al. 1984).

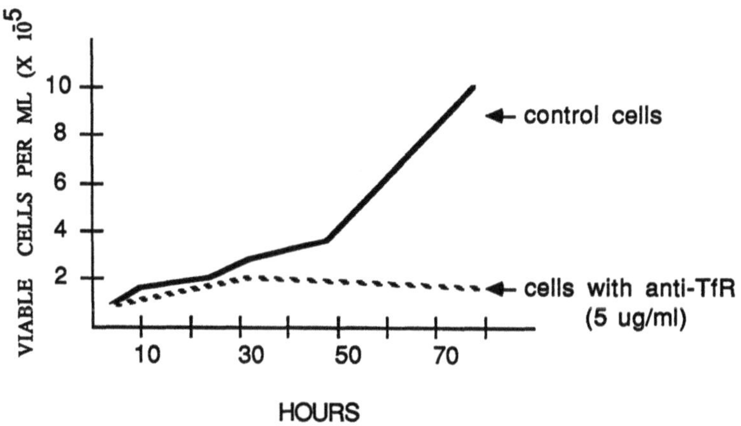

Fig. 1. Plasmacytoma cell growth is inhibited by anti-TfR antibodies in the presence of PCT-GF. Cell number is expressed as viable cells/ml x 100,000. Anti-TfR antibodies were added at start of culture.

In all mouse and human cells examined to date only a 4.9 kb TfR mRNA has been observed. This includes the LPS-stimulated mouse splenic B cell - presumably the progenitor of the plasmacytoma cell. However, when mRNA isolated from mouse plasmacytoma cells is examined, a second smaller TfR specific mRNA species is observed (Fig. 3). This 2.7 kb transcript appears in all mouse plasmacytomas examined to date, whether derived from pristane primed mice, pristane/Abelson virus treated mice, or pristane/J3 virus treated mice. In the first two instances, resultant tumors possess a translocated and activated endogenous c-myc gene (Potter and Boyce 1962; Anderson and Potter 1969; Potter et al. 1973). In the latter case, the mice have been injected with a hybrid v-myc construct and the resultant tumors express high levels of v-myc mRNA (Rapp et al. 1985).

The 2.7 kb TfR transcript appears to contain the TfR coding sequences but lacks most of the non-coding region of the full length TfR mRNA. This was deduced by hybridizing plasmacytoma mRNA - size fractionated on formaldehyde-agarose gels - with various parts of the full length human cDNA and both mouse cDNA's. The data is depicted in Fig. 4. Briefly, three fragments representing parts of the coding region of the full length message all hybridize to both the 4.9 kb and 2.7 kb transcripts, as does the coding region specific mouse cDNA mTFR2. However, two fragments representing the untranslated portion of the full length message hybridize only to the 4.9 kb message but not to the 2.7 kb transcript. This is also true for the mouse cDNA mTFR1 - specific for the non-coding region of the full length mRNA.

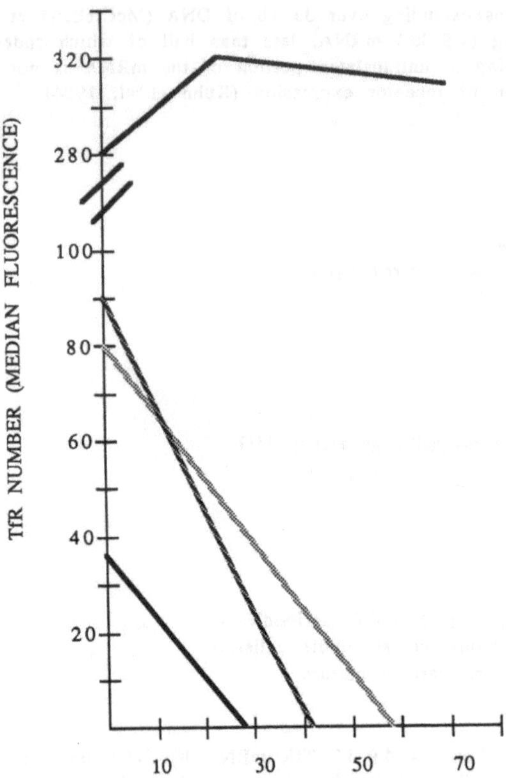

Fig. 2. Surface TfR number declines following removal of PCT-GF. Units on the y-axis represent median fluorescence intensity as measured by flow cytometric analysis. The x-axis refers to hours following removal of PCT-GF. The uppermost curve represents surface TfR on a PCT-GF independent cell line following removal of PCT-GF. The three declining curves represent surface TfR expression on three different PCT-GF dependent cell lines.

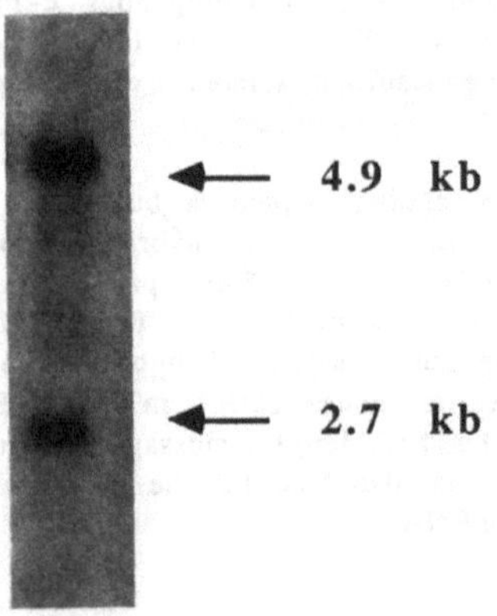

Fig. 3. TfR mRNA in mouse plasmacytomas. A unique 2.7 kb transcript is observed

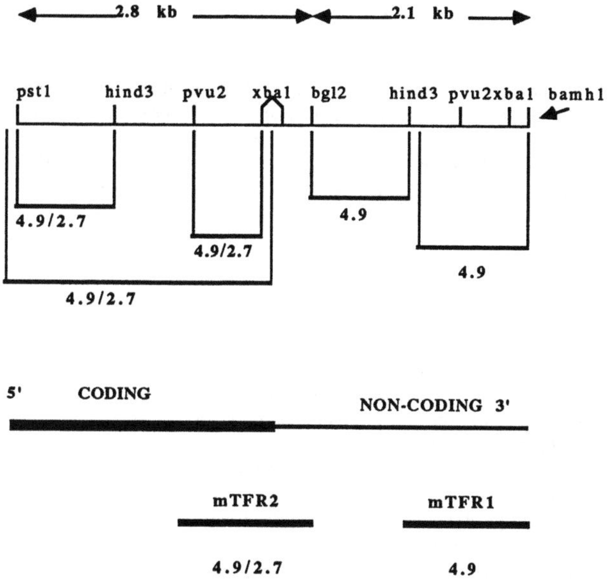

Fig. 4. Hybridization of several fragments of human TfR cDNA and two mouse cDNA's to the 4.9 kb and 2.7 kb TfR transcripts seen in plasmacytoma cells. Only those cDNA's which recognize the coding region hybridize to the 2.7 kb transcript.

The appearance of this novel transcript is not due to rearrangement of the TfR gene in plasmacytomas, since restriction enzyme analysis of cellular DNA does not reveal any alteration in gene structure (data not shown).

CONCLUSIONS

We have demonstrated that mouse plasmacytoma cell growth depends on TfR expression, which in turn is regulated by PCT-GF. In these cells, a novel TfR transcript appears, comprising the coding region of the full length TfR mRNA, but lacking most of the untranslated part of the 4.9 kb message. The unique transcript does not arise via gene rearrangement but may be an example of alternative processing of the 4.9 kb mRNA species.

It should be emphasized that all mouse plasmacytomas examined possess this unique TfR transcript. While not all these tumors possess a translocated endogenous c-myc gene, all demonstrate high levels of either c-myc or v-myc expression. Neither human multiple myeloma (end stage human B cells) nor Burkitt's lymphoma cells (more immature human B cells possessing c-myc translocations) express a 2.7 kb TfR mRNA. We speculate that its occurence depends on the presence of high myc levels in a terminally differentiated B cell. To test this hypothesis we are currently examining TfR transcripts in one human plasma cell leukemia which carries a c-myc translocation (Hollis and Kirsch, this volume). At the same time, we have infected another human plasma cell leukemia lacking c-myc rearrangement with a viral construct in which mouse c-myc is under the control of viral long terminal repeat elements (Wolff et al., this volume). In this way we hope to artificially induce high myc expression in this tumor and study the resultant size of the TfR transcripts. These studies are currently in progress.

Although the function of the 2.7 kb mRNA is currently under study, it is known that the presence of the long untranslated portion of the full length message is not necessary for expression of the human TfR cDNA in mouse L cells (Kuhn et al. 1984, Kuhn 1985). Since a regulatory role has been proposed for the 3' untranslated part of the full length transcript, one might speculate that the appearance of the 2.7 kb mRNA in all mouse plasmacytomas, and its absence in normal proliferating B cells, is etiologically significant.

REFERENCES

Neckers LM, Cossman J (1983) Transferrin receptor induction in mitogen-stimulated human T lymphocytes is required for DNA synthesis and cell division and is regulated by interleukin 2. Proc Natl. Acad. Sci. USA 80: 3494-3498

Neckers LM, Yenokida G, James SP (1984) The role of the transferrin receptor in human B lymphocyte activation. J Immunol 133: 2437-2441

Neckers LM (1985) Transferrin receptor regulation of proliferation in normal and neoplastic B cells. Curr Top Microbiol Immunol 113: 62-68

Nordan R, Potter M (to be published) A macrophage-derived factor required by plasmacytoma cells for survival and proliferation *in vitro* . Science

McClelland A, Kuhn LC, Ruddle FH (1984) The human transferrin receptor gene: Genomic organization, and the complete primary structure of the receptor deduced from a cDNA sequence. Cell 39:267-274

Kuhn LC, McClelland A, Ruddle FH (1984) Gene transfer, expression, and molecular cloning of the human transferrin receptor gene. Cell 37:95-103

Anderson PN and Potter M (1969) Induction of plasma cell tumors in BALB/c mice with 2,6,10,14-tetramethylpentadecane (pristane). Nature 222: 994-995

Potter M and Boyce C (1962) Induction of plasma cell neoplasms in strain BALB/c mice with mineral oil and mineral oil adjuvants. Nature 193:1086-1087

Potter M, Sklar MD and Rowe WP (1973) Rapid viral induction of plasmacytomas in pristane primed BALB/c mice. Science 182: 592-594

Kuhn LC (1985) Human transferrin receptor expressed from a transfected cDNA is functional in murine cells. In: Spik G, Montreuil J, Crichton RR, and Mazurier J. (eds.) Proteins of Iron Storage and Transport, Elsevier Science Publishers, New York, p.369

Rapp UR, Cleveland JL, Fredrickson TN, Holmes KL, Morse III HC, Jansen HW, Patschinsky T and Bister K (1985) Rapid induction of hemopoietic neoplasms in newborn mice by a *raf(mil)/myc* recombinant murine retrovirus. J Virol 55: 23-33

Structure and Expression of c-*myb* Protooncogene mRNA in Murine B-Cells

T.P. Bender and W.M. Kuehl

NCI-Navy Medical Oncology Branch, National Cancer Institute, National Institutes of Health, Naval Hospital, Bethesda, Maryland 20814

INTRODUCTION

The c-myb proto-oncogene, which encodes a nuclear DNA binding protein (Boyle 1984, Kempnauer 1984) has been reported to be expressed predominantly in normal tissue and tumor cells of hematopoietic origin (Westin 1982; Gonda 1982). Moreover, for each hematopoietic lineage examined, the steady state levels of c-myb mRNA expression are highest in immature cells. These properties of the c-myb gene and its products are consistent with the idea that c-myb regulates hematopoietic maturation by controlling the expression of other genes. We have begun to examine this hypothesis using B-cell tumor lines.

EXPRESSION OF c-myb mRNA IN MURINE B-LYMPHOID TUMOR CELL LINES

Using a panel of murine B-lymphoid tumor cell lines which represent various stages of B-cell development, we have analyzed c-myb mRNA expression by Northern blot analyses of total RNA and total poly A-positive RNA. We examined four pre-B cell lines, 8 intermediate B-cell lines (which include immature B-cell lines such as WEHI-231 and very mature B-cell lines such as A20.2J), and four plasmacytoma lines. The pre-B cell lines include the LS8.T2 and 1881.B4 Abelson virus transformed cell lines, as well as the carcinogen induced 70Z/3.12 cell line. The fourth pre-B cell line, HAFTL-1 was derived by virus transformation of fetal liver cells, and may actually represent a pre-B cell progenitor as it expresses the B220 cell surface marker and its H-chain genes are in a germline configuration although they spontaneously rearrange at a high frequency upon subcloning (J. Pierce, personal communication). The intermediate B-cell lines include WEHI-279, BAL.17, BFO.3, X16.8C, 2PK3, and M12, in addition to the two lines mentioned above. The four plasmacytoma lines include S107, 45.6TG, MOPC-21, and CBOHC. CBOHC is a variant derived from the C1 cell line which was adapted to culture from a spontaneous plasmacytoma in a C3H strain mouse.

All cell lines express detectable levels of a predominant 3.8 kb c-myb mRNA species, although in many instances minor species at 4.0 and 4.2 kb were detected as well. All four pre-B cell lines contain similar amounts of c-myb mRNA, while the intermediate B-cell and plasmacytoma lines contain 0.05 to less than 0.005 units of c-myb mRNA as the pre-B cell lines. It should be noted that Mushinski (1983) has reported that Abelson virus induced pre-B cell lymphosarcomas express high levels of c-myb mRNA, whereas Abelson virus/pristane induced plasmacytomas expressed no detectable c-myb mRNA using an avian v-myb probe. Our results suggest that maturation from the pre-B cell to the immature B cell includes a marked down-regulation of c-*myb* mRNA expression. This maturation appears to involve more than expression of surface IgM since a subclone (IH6A) of the 1881 cell line which has functionally rearranged a kappa light chain gene and expresses surface IgM continues to express the same high levels of c-*myb* mRNA as the parental 1881 line and other pre-B cell lines. In most studies correlating c-*myb* mRNA expression with hematopoietic maturation, it has not been possible to conclude whether the higher level of c-*myb* mRNA expression in immature cells is due to the state of differentiation or the rate of proliferation. However, since we isolated RNA from exponentially growing cell lines, our results indicate that the marked down-regulation of c-*myb* mRNA is not due to changes in the growth properties of the cells, but rather correlates with maturation beyond the pre-B cell stage of development.

CORRELATION OF c-*myb* mRNA LEVELS WITH PHENOTYPE IN HYBRID CELL LINES

To further examine the regulation of c-*myb* mRNA expression and to correlate it with phenotype, we have constructed two types of hybrid cell lines by somatic cell fusion. First, a group of pre-B cell lymphoma x plasmacytoma hybrids (PBP) was made by fusing the plasmacytoma 45.6TG ($HPRT^-$) with the pre-B cell lymphoma 70Z/3B (TK^-). Second, a group of pre-B cell lymphoma x B-cell lymphoma hybrids (PBB) was made by fusing 70Z/3B to the mature B-cell lymphoma A20.2J ($HPRT^-$).

Pre-B cell lymphoma x plasmacytoma hybrids have previously been characterized and used to analyze various aspects of immunoglobulin biosynthesis (Riley 1981). These studies have concluded that hybrid cell lines of this type phenotypically resemble the terminally differentiated plasmacytoma parent in terms of the level of immunoglobulin expression, immunoglobulin secretion and J-chain production. All five PBP hybrid lines examined secrete immunoglobulin bearing the H-chain isotype of each parental line, and also express very low levels of c-*myb* mRNA, indistinguishable from the plasmacytoma parent. Thus, these hybrid cell lines phenotypically resemble the parental 45.6TG plasmacytoma line including low levels of c-*myb* mRNA expression.

Detailed analysis of pre-B cell x B-cell hybrids will be reported elsewhere. Southern blotting data showed that the rearranged H- and L-chain genes from the 70Z/3B and A20.2J parental lines were present in each of the hybrids examined. The IgG_{2a} expressed by A20.2J includes both membrane and secreted forms, with the latter being quantitatively secreted. In contrast, 70Z/3B cells express cytoplasmic mu H-chain but no L-chain, and do not secrete immunoglobulin. Although the H-chain protein of each parental isotype and kappa L-chains encoded by each parent is expressed in each hybrid line, no secretion of immunoglobulin bearing either isotype was detected by immunoprecipitation and SDS-polyacrylamide gel electrophoresis. We have not yet determined whether the immunoglobulin produced is retained in the cytoplasm or inserted in the cell membrane. In contrast to A20.2J, which makes abundant J-chain mRNA and is Ia^+ by FACS analysis, the hybrids -- like the 70Z/3B pre-B cell lymphoma parent -- do not make detectable levels of J-chain mRNA and are Ia^-. Northern blot analysis shows that the high levels of c-*myb* mRNA in the hybrid lines is indistinguishable from the 70Z/3B pre-B cell lymphoma parent. Thus, the phenotype of these cells closely resemble that of the 70Z.3B pre-B cell parent.

These studies of hybrid cell lines show that in contrast to the terminally differentiated plasma cell phenotype, which is consistently dominant in cell fusion experiments between B-lymphoid tumors (Riley 1981), the mature A20.2J B-cell phenotype is reversible when fused to the 70Z/3B pre-B cell tumor line. This includes the low steady state level of c-myb mRNA expression associated with mature B-cell lymphomas. These experiments clearly correlate high levels of c-myb mRNA expression with the pre-B cell stage of differentiation, regardless of whether or not light chain is expressed.

STEADY STATE LEVELS OF c-myb mRNA DECREASE DURING LPS INDUCTION OF A PRE-B CELL LYMPHOMA LINE

The 70Z/3.12 cell line is a carcinogen induced pre-B cell lymphoma (Paige 1978). Though it has productive rearrangements of both H- and Kappa L-chain genes only the H-chain gene is transcribed and expressed as cytoplasmic mu H-chain. Treatment of 70Z/3.12 with LPS reversibly induces transcription of the kappa locus resulting in mIgM expression on >90% of the cells and thus a phenotype similar to an immature B-cell. We have utilized this cell line to more carefully examine events at the pre-B/B-cell junction.

Parallel cultures of 70Z/3.12 were established by seeding $5x10^5$ cells/ml in RPMI 1640 with 10% FCS and 10uM 2-mercaptoethanol. One set of cultures was treated with LPS at a final concentration of 10 ug/ml. Induced and uninduced cultures were harvested and total cellular RNA was prepared, fractionated electrophoretically, transferred to nitrocellulose and sequentially hybridized to nick translated probes specific for murine c-myb, c-myc and kappa L-chain. Over this time course there was no difference in the growth rates of LPS induced and uninduced cultures.

Hybridization of Northern blots to a 3.8 kb Xbal/BamH1 murine kappa L-chain constant region probe shows that upon induction with LPS kappa L-chain mRNA expression rapidly and markedly increases within 6 hours. After 12 hours post-induction this expression does not change. No kappa mRNA was detected in uninduced cultures. By contrast, c-myb mRNA levels gradually decrease approximately 12 fold during LPS induction while no change in c-myb message expression was seen in uninduced cultures. It is noted that the down-regulation of c-myb mRNA levels takes place later in the time course than the rapid increase in kappa mRNA expression. Over the same time course c-myb mRNA expression did not change. Thus, as the 70Z/3.12 cell line is induced to progress from a pre-B cell to a state phenotypically resembling an immature B-cell the steady state level of c-myb mRNA decreases to a level nearly within the range seen in B-cell lymphomas.

STRUCTURE OF c-myb mRNA AND EVIDENCE FOR EXTREME 5' HETEROGENEITY

To begin analysis of c-myb mRNA regulation during B-cell development we have recently published the structure of two overlapping c-myb cDNA clones obtained from a murine pre-B cell lymphoma (70Z/3B) cDNA library (Bender and Kuehl, in press). The composite c-myb mRNA sequence derived from these clones includes 3413 nucleotides not including a poly A tail. There is a single long open reading frame which begins at the first base of the sequence and extends to a TGA termination codon at position 2173. The first Met codon of the long open reading frame is at position 265 and is contained in a consensus eukaryotic translation initiation start sequence. If this is the correct start site, the primary translation product would contain 636 amino acids and have a size of about 71 kD. This is in good agreement with the 75 kD size reported for the avian c-myb protein (Klempnauer 1983). In addition, we have used a rabbit anti-v-myb serum (kindly provided by K. Moelling) which precipitates a protein of approximately 73 kD from the 70Z/3B pre-B cell lymphoma cell line. Twenty-six nucleotides upstream from the vestigial poly A tail is an AATAAA consensus polyadenylation signal. Three other cDNA clones examined terminated at this same position. A second AATAAA sequence is also present at position 2468 though at present we have no evidence that it is used. The c-myb mRNA includes 1241 nucleotides of 3' untranslated region.

To further characterize the 5' end of the c-myb transcription unit we have cloned and sequenced a 1136 bp BamH1 murine genomic clone which includes 799 bp 5' and 50 bp of intron 3' of a sequence identical to nucleotides 1-287 of our composite c-myb mRNA. Thus, in addition to the putative 7 amino terminal codons this fragment includes nearly one kilobase of 5' flanking/untranslated sequence. When this fragment was used as a probe in S1-nuclease protection studies with 70Z/3B total cellular RNA at least 13 protected products were detected with approximate sizes ranging from 184-970 nucleotides. Using other probes derived from our cDNA clones we have shown that all of the heterogeneity takes place 5' of the translation initiation codon. The largest protected product when combined with the appropriate region of our c-myb mRNA sequence is sufficient to account for a 4.2 kb message. The other protected species would predict mRNA species of about 3.4-4.0 kb. Thus, the major 3.8 kb message seen on RNA blots may represent an average of multiple species.

We have examined independent preparations of 70Z/3B total cellular RNA as well as total poly A positive mRNA, and found identical patterns of heterogeneity. In addition, similar patterns of heterogeneity were seen in RNA derived from two other pre-B cell lymphoma lines (1881.B4 and LS8.T2) as well as three B-cell lymphomas (BFO.3, BAL.17 and A20.2J) and a plasmacytoma (45.6TG). Therefore, we do not find significant differences in this heterogeneity between tumors of different developmental phenotypes. Also, when cytoplasmic and nuclear RNA were examined similar patterns of protection were seen making post-transcriptional modification an unlikely explanation for this finding. Although the mechanism and biological relevance of this heterogeneity are not presently understood we are analyzing this region for promoter/regulatory sequences.

STRUCTURAL HOMOLOGIES BETWEEN THE PREDICTED MURINE AND AVIAN c-myb PROTEINS

The primary translation product of the murine c-myb gene derived from our composite mRNA sequence would initiate translation at the first Met codon of the long open reading frame and contain 636 amino acids. Fig. 1 shows a diagrammatic comparison of the murine c-myb protein to that predicted for the avian protein (Rosson 1986). We have arbitrarily divided the c-myb protein into subregions based on amino acid sequence homology. Subregion II contains the three tandem repeats of approximately 50 amino acids each reported for the murine, avian and Drosphila c-myb proteins (Gonda 1985; Rosson 1986; Katzen 1985). As shown this region is very highly conserved between chicken and mouse (98%). In addition, the remarkable homology of subregions, I, IV, VI, and VIII (86, 99, 94, and 90% respectively) suggests that there may be multiple non-contiguous regions in the c-myb protein which are important for its function. As shown by the dashed box in Fig. 1, the predicted avian protein is reported to have 58 additional

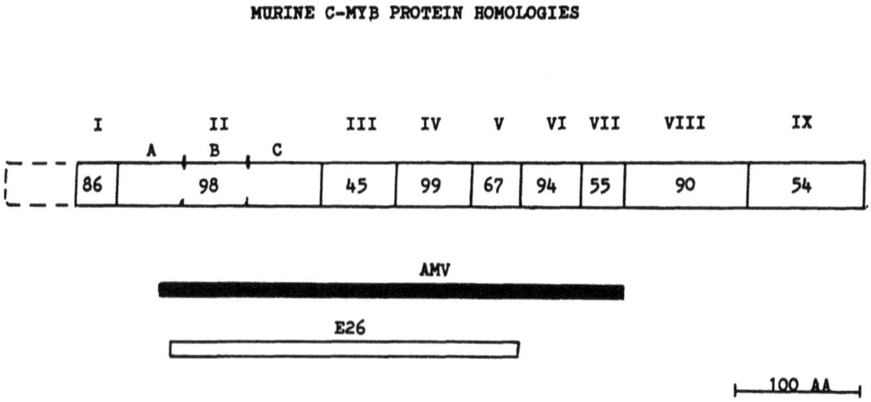

Fig. 1. Schematic representation of amino acid homologies between the predicted sequences of the murine and avian c-*myb* proteins. Subregions are marked by Roman numerals. Arabic numbers represent percent amino acid homology within subregions. The dashed box at the amino terminus repesents 58 extra amino acids reported for the avian c-*myb*. Regions of homology with AMV and the E26 virus are marked below the c-*myb* protein with solid and open bars respectively.

amino acids at the amino terminus relative to the murine protein. In this regard we have recently obtained human c-*myb* genomic clones homologous to the 5' end of the murine c-*myb* gene. Sequence analysis of these clones predicts that in contrast to the avian c-*myb* translation of the human c-*myb* mRNA would initiate at the same point as in the mouse. Also, this sequence shows that nucleotide homology with the mouse of >80% continues for at least 400 bp into the 5' flanking/ untranslated region. We note that the v-*myb* proteins coded for by AMV (Klempnauer 1982) and the E26 virus (Nunn 1984) are truncated forms of the c-*myb* protein with deletions in highly conserved regions at both the amino and carboxy terminal ends of the protein. In addition, Shen-Ong (1986) has shown that the c-*myb* locus can be activated by retrovirus insertion at either the 5' or 3' ends which disrupt protein coding sequences in highly conserved regions and potentially result in truncated c-*myb* proteins.

SUMMARY

The results presented here demonstrate that levels of c-*myb* mRNA expression dramatically decrease during B-cell development and that events at the pre-B cell/B-cell junction down-regulate this expression. Furthermore, since this down-regulation has been demonstrated in exponentially growing cells these results indicate that it is not due to changes in growth properties but rather due to maturation beyond the pre-B cell stage. At present, we have made a series of vectors for expression of c-*myb* protein after transfection into eukaryotic cells. These vectors will be used to examine the regulation of c-*myb* mRNA expression as well as its potential role in B-cell development.

REFERENCES

Bender TP, Kuehl WM (in press) Murine *myb* protoconcogene messenger RNA:

cDNA sequence and evidence for 5' heterogeneity. Proc Natl Acad Sci

Boyle WJ, Lampert MA, Lipsick JS, Baluda MA (1984) Avian myeloblastosis virus and E26 virus oncogene products are nuclear proteins. Proc Natl Acad Sci 81:4265-4269

Gonda TJ, Sheiness DK, Bishop JM (1982) Transcripts from the cellular homologs of retroviral oncogenes: distribution among chicken tissues. Mol Cell Biol 2:617-624

Katzen AL, Kornberg TB, Bishop JM (1985) Isolation of the proto-oncogene c-myb from D. Melanogaster. Cell 41:449-456

Klempnauer K, Gonda TJ, Bishop JM (1982) Nucleotide sequence of the retroviral leukemia gene v-myb and its cellular progenitor c-myb: the architecture of a transduced oncogene. Cell 31:453-463

Klempnauer H, Ramsey G, Bishop JM, Moscovici MG, Moscovici C, McGrath JP, Levinson AD (1983) The product of the retroviral transforming gene v-myb is a truncated version of the protein encoded by the cellular oncogene c-myb. Cell 33:345-355

Klempnauer K, Symonds J, Evan GI, Bishop JM (1984) Subcellular localization of proteins encoded by oncogenes of avian myeloblastosis virus and avian leukemia virus E26 and by the chicken c-myb gene. Cell 37:537-547

Mushinski JF, Potter M, Bauer SR, Reddy EP (1983) DNA rearrangement and altered RNA expression of the c-myb oncogene in mouse plasmacytoid lymphosarcomas. Science 220:795

Nunn M, Weiher H, Bullock P, Duesberg P (1984) Avian erythroblastosis virus E26: nucleotide sequence of the tripartite onc gene and of the LTR, and analysis of the cellular prototype of the viral ets sequence. Virology 139:330-339

Paige CJ, Kincade PW, Ralph P (1978) Murine B cell leukemia line with inducible surface immunoglobulin expression. J Immunol 121:641-647

Riley SC, Brock EJ, Keuhl WM (1981) Induction of light chain expression in a pre-B cell line by fusion to myeloma cells. Nature 289:804-806

Rosson D, Reddy EP (1986) Nucleotide sequence of chicken c-myb complementary DNA and implications for myb oncogene activation. Nature 319:604-606

Shen-Ong GLC, Morse HC, Potter M, Mushinski JF (1986) Two modes of c-myb activation in virus induced mouse myeloid tumors. Molecular and Cell Biol 6:380-392

Westin EH, Gallo RC, Arya SK, Eva A, Sauza LM, Baluda MA, Aaronson SA, Wong-Staal F (1982) Differential expression of the amv gene in human hematopoietic cells. Proc Natl Acad Sci 79:2194-2198

Genomic Activity and Translocation in Lymphocytes

I.R. Kirsch, C.T. Denny, and G.F. Hollis

NCI-Navy Medical Oncology Branch, National Cancer Institute National Institutes of Health, Bethesda, Maryland 20892

Analyses of chromosomal aberrations associated with specific cancers are providing insight into fundamental issues of cellular development and differentiation as well as oncogenesis. We have previously reported our findings in support of the concept that chromosomal aberrations often reflect the particular differentiated state of the cells and cell types in which they occur (Kirsch 1985). This concept developed not just from data dealing with the involvement of immunoglobulin genes in the chromosomal aberrations seen in Burkitt's and other B cell tumors, but also from observations we reported on the involvement of the globin encoding regions in translocations seen in erythroleukemias. It was with this as a foundation that we speculated that chromosomal aberrations associated with T cell disorders might involve chromosomal regions to which T cell specific functions would be localized. This prediction has now been fulfilled as we (Caccia 1985) and others (Croce 1985, Isobe 1985, LeBeau 1985, Morton 1985, Murre 1985) have localized the alpha, beta, and gamma chains of the T cell antigen receptor to three of the four most common and consistent hotspots of chromosomal breakage in malignant and non-malignant (or pre-malignant) T cells (Kaiser-McCaw 1975, Aurias 1980, Scheres 1980, Wake 1982, Taylor 1982, Williams 1984, Zech 1984, Smith 1986) The fact that these breakpoints can be seen in non-cancerous states brings up the question of whether each and every one of the specific cancer associated chromosomal aberrations is directly causal or contributory to malignant transformation. We have completed an analysis of a T cell line derived from the tumor cells of a patient with T cell lymphoma which may begin to provide a perspective on this question. This work has been fully reported in a separate article (Denny 1986). This T cell line contained a distinctive inversion of one of its chromosomes 14. Sequencing the breakpoint of this inversion reveals that is has been caused by a site-specific recombination event between a T cell receptor alpha chain joining (J) segment and an immunoglobulin heavy chain variable (V) segment (Fig. 1). The recombination event occurred in-frame and a potentially functional hybrid (part T cell receptor, part immunoglobulin) transcript is expressed by the tumor cells.

This finding implies that the same recombination system can catalyze site specific recombination in both the T cell receptor and immunoglobulin gene loci and, in fact, unify them. This postulate is supported by recent work of Yancopoulos (1986). This also suggests that at some point in the development of this particular lymphocyte both the T cell receptor and immunoglobulin loci, heretofore heretofore felt to be disparately activated during development, were simultaneously accessible to this V-J recombination system.

The relationship of this inversion to the development of the lymphoma remains uncertain. The inversion may not be directly contributory

Current Topics in Microbiology and Immunology, Vol. 132

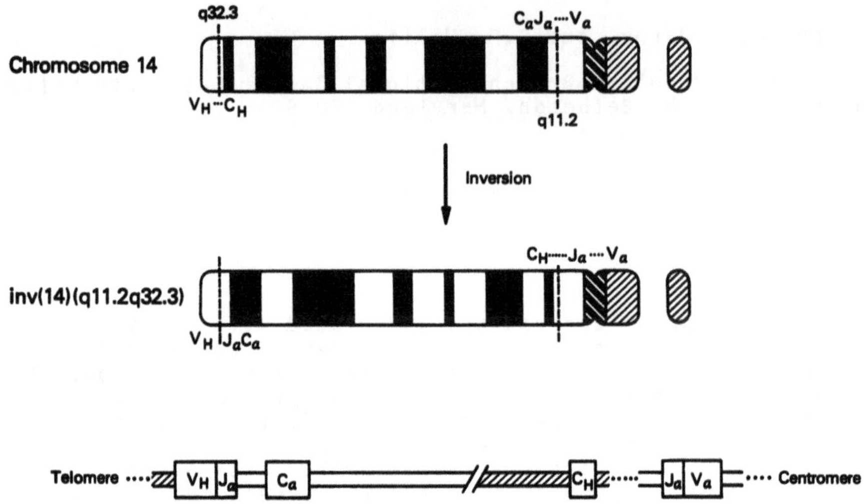

Fig. 1. A model of how site-specific recombination between a T cell receptor J segment and immunoglobulin V segment causes an inversion of chromosome 14. Reprinted from Nature (Denny 1986).

to the malignant event; perhaps it is only a reflection (though a very interesting one) of the differentiated state of the cell. It is possible that a yet to be identified oncogene resides near the heavy chain V region and the recombination with the T cell receptor locus somehow activates or deregulates it akin to c-myc deregulation in Burkitt's lymphoma. Another possibility is that the hybrid gene itself possibly translated into a hybrid protein causes an abnormal mitogenic stimulus and contributes to the development of this lymphoma.

The inversion of chromosome 14 is not the only abnormality in this cell line. A translocation between the beta chain of the T cell receptor (J. Sklar, pers. commun.) and a genomic region on chromosome 9 also is present in this cell. Furthermore, we have recently characterized a rearrangement of the c-myc locus in this tumor cell line (Kirsch submitted). Any, all, or none of these aberrations may be crucial to the development of cancer in the six year old male from whom this cell line was derived, but by carrying out detailed analyses on this line and others we may begin to discern the necessary, sufficient, and unifying features of cell type specific chromosomal abnormalities.

We are pursuing many of the questions raised here by searching for a hybrid protein product made by this cell line, further assessing c-myc gene function in similar T cell lymphomas, and critically analyzing an early B cell tumor which appears to carry the same morphological inversion of chromosome 14.

REFERENCES

Aurias A, Dutrillaux B, Buriot D, Lejeune J (1980) High frequencies of inversions and translocations of chromosomes 7 and 14 in ataxia telangiectasia. Mutation Research 69:369-374

Caccia N, Bruns GAP, Kirsch IR, Hollis GF, Bertness V, Mak TW (1985) T cell receptor alpha chain genes are located on chromosome 14 at 14q11-14q12 in humans. J Exp Med 161:1255-1260

Croce CM, Isobe M, Palumbo A, Puck J, Ming J, Tweardy D, Erikson J, Davis M, Rovera G (1985) Gene for alpha-chain of human T-cell receptor: Location on chromosome 14 region involved in T-cell neoplasms. Science 277:1044-1047.

Denny CT, Yoshikai Y, Mak TW, Smith SD, Hollis GF, Kirsch IR (1986) A chromosome 14 inversion in a T cell lymphoma is caused by site-specific recombination between immunoglobulin and T cell receptor loci. Nature 320:549-551

Isobe M, Erikson J, Emanuel BS, Nowell PC, Croce CM (1985) Location of gene for beta subunit of human T-cell receptor at band 7q35 a region prone to rearrangement in T cells. Science 228:580-582

Kaiser-McCaw B, Hecht F, Harnden DG, Teplitz RL (1975) Somatic rearrangement of chromosome 14 in human lymphocytes. Proc Natl Acad Sci USA 72:2071-1075.

Kirsch IR, Brown JA, Lawrence J, Korsmeyer S, Morton CC (1985) Translocations that highlight chromosomal regions of differentiated activity. Cancer Genet Cytogenet 18:159-171.

Kirsch IR, Denny CT, Bertness V, Smith SD, Hollis GF (submitted) Disruption of the c-myc protooncogene in a human T cell lymphoma cell line

LeBeau MM, Diaz MO, Rowley JD, Mak TW (1985) Chromosomal localization of the human T cell receptor beta-chain genes. Cell 41:335

Morton CC, Duby AD, Eddy RL, Shows TB, Seidman JG (1985) Genes for beta chain of human T cell antigen receptor map to regions of chromosomal rearrangements in T cells. Science 228:582-585

Murre C, Waldmann RA, Morton CC, Bongiovanni KF, Waldman TA, Shaws TB, Seidman JG (1985) Human gamma-chain genes are rearranged in leukemic T cells and map to the short arm of chromosome 7. Nature 316:549-552

Scheres JMJC, Hustinx TWJ, Weemaes CMR (1980) Chromosome 7 in ataxia-telangictaxia. J Pediatr 97:440-441

Smith SD, Morgan R, Link MP, McFall P, Hecht F (1986) Cytogenetic and immunophenotypic analysis of cell lines established from patients with T cell leukemia/lymphoma. Blood 67:650-656

Taylor AMR (1982) Cytogenetics of ataxia-telangictasia. In: Bridges BA and Harndern DG (eds) Ataxia-telangiectasia: A cellular link between cancer, neuropathology, and immunodeficiency. John Wiley and Sons, New York, pp 53-81

Wake N, Minowada J, Park B, Sandberg AA (1982) Chromosomes and causation of human cancer and leukemia. XLVII. T-cell acute leukemia in ataxia-telangiectasia. Cancer Genet Cytogenet 6:345-357.

Williams DL, Look AT, Melvin SL, Roberson PK, Dahl G, Flake T, Stass S (1984) New chromosomal translocations correlate with specific immunophenotypes of childhood acute lymphoblastic leukemia. Cell 36:101-109

Yancopoulos GD, Blackwell TK, Suh H, Hood L, Alt FW (1986) Introduced T cell receptor variable region gene segments recombine in pre-B cells: Evidence that B and T cells use a common recombinase. Cell 44:251-259

Zech L, Gahrton G, Hammarstrom L, Juliusson G, Mellstedt H, Robert KH, Smith CIE (1984) Inversion of chromosome 14 marks human T-cell chronic lymphocytic leukemia. Nature 308:858-860

Possible Role of Immunoglobulin Recombination Sequences in the Genesis of Variant t(2;8) Translocations of Burkitt Lymphoma

M. Lipp and P. Hartl

Institut für Biochemie, Ludwigs-Maximilians-Universität, Karlstrasse 23, D-8000 München 5, FRG

INTRODUCTION

Various chromosomal abberations have been regularly found in cytogenetic investigations and can be associated with specific human neoplasia (Rowley 1980; Yunis 1983). However, few of them are accessible to molecular analysis providing the necessary information for understanding the mechanisms and functional consequences of such drastic changes in the otherwise higly conserved structural order of genetic material. Some of the best analyzed examples are human Burkitt lymphomas and murine plasmacytomas carrying consistently a reciprocal translocation (t(8,14), t(2;8), and t(8;22) in man, and t(12;15) and t(6;15) in mice) which always involves one of the immunoglobulin heavy or light chain genes and the locus of the c-myc oncogene on human chromosome 8 and on mouse chromosome 15 (for review see Klein 1983, 1985)). Although a lot of new information has accumulated recently, the available data do not allow one to propose an unifying hypothesis explaining the mechanisms responsible for the genesis of translocations and for the activation of the c-myc gene.

We have molecularly analysed the reciprocal chromosomal breakpoints of the Burkitt lymphoma (BL) line BL64 carrying a variant t(2;8) translocation which appears in about 10% of all patients and involves the kappa light chain genes. In contrast to the common t(8;14) translocations observed in BL, the breakpoint of these variant translocations is usually far downstream of the c-myc gene, thus leaving the c-myc transcription unit intact. One important finding of this characterization is the detection of recognition sequences that apparently mediate site-specific recombination in the vicinity of both breakpoints. Thus it is probable that this translocation and other related chromosomal rearrangements have been catalyzed by the same enzymes normally involved in the V-J recombination process.

MOLECULAR ANALYSIS OF THE t(2;8) TRANSLOCATION OF BL64

In the variant t(2;8) translocations of Burkitt lymphoma determination of the breakpoint, based so far mainly on data obtained by in situ hybridization on metaphase chromosomes, revealed that the c-myc gene was retained on the $8q^+$ chromosome, and that a region 5' of the constant (C_k), within the joining (J_k), or the variable (V_k) region could be affected (Erikson 1983; Rappold 1984; Emanuel 1984; Taub 1984).

Current Topics in Microbiology and Immunology, Vol. 132

Localization of the Chromosomal Breakpoints within the J_k-Region

In order to narrow down the location of the chromosomal breakpoint within the kappa light chain locus we performed Southern blot analysis of genomic BL64 DNA. As shown in Fig. 1 (insert), hybridization of a ^{32}P-labeled J_k specific probe to nitrocellulose blots containing separated BamHI fragments revealed three bands of 9.5 kb, 8.0 kb, and 7.0 kb. Only the two largest of these BamHI fragments also hybridized to a C_k probe (data not shown) indicating that one or the other could contain either the breakpoint on chromosome $8q^+$ or the functional rearranged kappa light chain gene. The 7.0 kb BamHI fragment whould then be expected to carry the reciprocal breakpoint on chromosome $2p^-$.

Isolation of the Reciprocal Breakpoints of Chromosomes $8q^+$ and $2p^-$

To analyse in more detail the structural changes caused by the translocation, we screened a genomic library of BL64 with a J_k probe to isolate recombinant lambda phages containing one of these three BamHI fragments. Figure 1 summarizes the results of detailed mapping

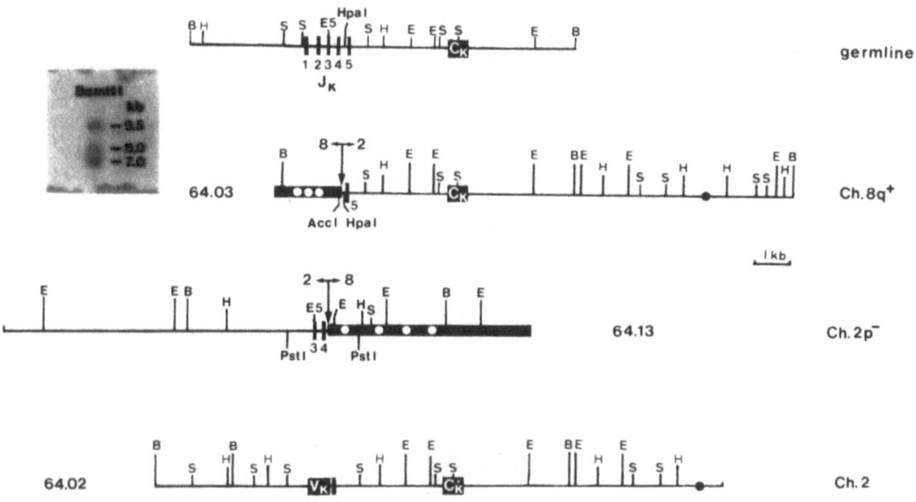

Fig. 1. Restrictionenzyme map of recombinant phage clones isolated from a genomic library of BL64 cells. Each clone contains one of the three particular BamHI fragments visualized with a J_k-specific probe in a Southern blot analysis of BL64 DNA (see insert). The structure of the germline BamHI fragment of the human kappa light chain is included for comparison. Clone 64.03 represents the breakpoint (arrow) on chromosome $8q^+$, clone 64.13 the reciprocal breakpoint on chromosome $2p^-$. Clone 64.02 contains the functional rearranged kappa light chain gene located on Chromosome 2. White and black dots indicate repetitive Alu-type sequences. Methods: BL64 cells were established from invaded bone marrow from a 4-year old Algerian boy in relapse from BL (Mark-Vendel 1983). Hybridization conditions, and origin and cloning of the J_k (1.8 kb SacI fragment), and C_k (2.5 kb EcoR1 fragment) specific probes were described previously (Rappold 1984). Preparation of the genomic library of the BL64 cell line was performed by insertion of a partial, size selected Sau3A digest of high-molecular-weight DNA into a BamHI-digested EMBL3A vector (Frischauf 1983). Abbreviations of the restriction enzymes: B, BamHI; E, EcoRI; E5, EcoRV; H, HindIII; S, SstI.

and rehybridization experiments with kappa-specific probes. The insert of clone 64.02 including the 9.5 kb BamHI fragment, hybridized with the V_k as well as with the C_k probe and represented the functional rearranged kappa light chain gene. Since clone 64.03 contained the 8.0 kb BamHI fragment, which could be shown to be positive for C_k, we supposed it was carrying the breakpoint located on chromosome $8q^+$. Consequently, clone 64.13, which included the 7.0 kb BamHI fragment and hybridized only with the J_k probe, had to represent the reciprocal breakpoint located on chromosome $2p^-$.

Detailed restriction enzyme analysis of the 2.3 kb BamHI-SstI fragment of clone 64.03 revealed that compared to the germline configuration of the J_k-region, only the HpaI-site located 5' of the J_5-segment was still conserved (Fig. 1). From these results the breakpoint concerning chromosome 2 could be narrowed down to a region between the J-segments four and five. As shown in Fig. 1 the EcoRV-site, which lies within the coding region of J_3, was still present in the 7.0 kb BamHI fragment of phage 64.13. However, the pattern of restriction sites further upstream differed from the germline configuration completely implying that nonfunctional V-J recombination has taken place in this allele. It is noteworthy that nearly all fragments located 3' of the EcoRV-site contain repetitive sequences (Fig. 1). Thus, with respect to chromosome 8 the translocation has occurred within a cluster of highly repetitive Alu-type sequences.

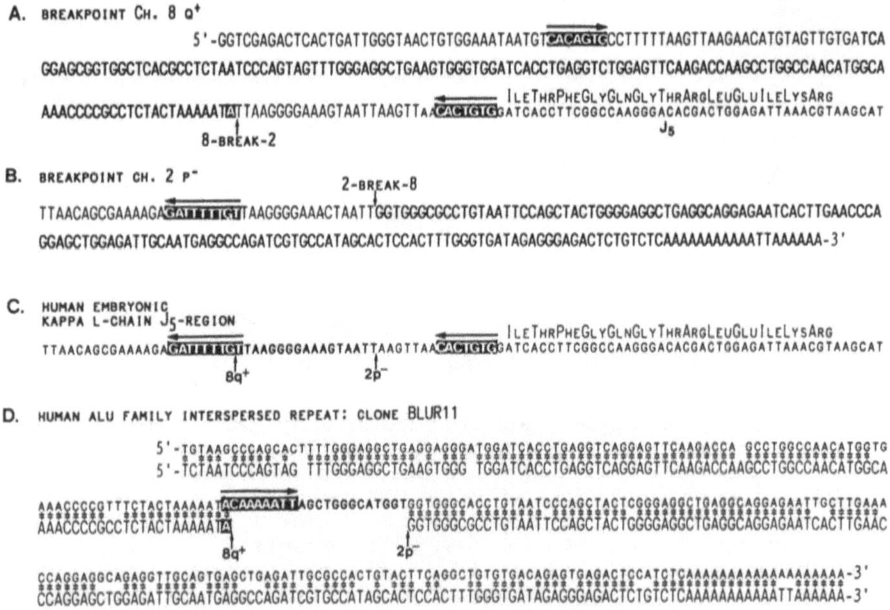

Fig. 2. DNA sequence spanning the breakpoint on chromosome $8q^+$ (A), and on chromosome $2p^-$ (B). The corresponding sequence of the human embryonic J_5-region is shown for comparison (C; Hieter et al., 1982). The sequence of clone BLUR11 of the human Alu family (Deininger et al., 1981) is compared with the Alu-repeat sequence spanning the breakpoints (D). This sequence is shown in boldface in A and B. Boxed regions and horizontal arrows indicate the conserved heptamer and nonamer recombination sequences. Dideoxy sequencing (Sanger 1977) was performed using double-stranded superhelical plasmid DNA as described by Chen (1985).

Presence of the V-J Recombination Signal Sequences Adjacent to the Chromosomal Breakpoints

To get further information about the possible mechanisms which may be involved in the genesis of translocations, we determined the nucleotide sequences spanning the breakpoints of both marker chromosomes. From the 2.3 kb BamHI-SstI fragment of phage 64.03 the 230 bp AccI-HpaI fragment was subcloned and sequenced, and from phage 64.13 the 1.8 kb PstI fragment (for location of the fragments see Fig. 1). The evaluation of the sequence data, shown in Fig. 2, revealed the following results: With respect to chromosome 2 the break occured exactly between the nonamer and heptamer nucleotide boxes 5' of J_5. A short sequence of 17 bp originating from chromosome 2 is present in both marker chromosomes (Fig. 2A and 2B; in Fig. 2C the corresponding portion of the human embryonic kappa light-chain J_5-region is shown for comparison). With respect to chromosome 8 the breakpoint lies right in the middle of a repetitive Alu-type sequence. Comparison of the Alu-repeat with published sequences revealed the best homology of 89% to clone Blur 11 of the Alu-family, but also revealed a 21 bp deletion ranging from position -22 to -42 of the Alu family consensus sequence (Deininger 1981; Fig. 2D).

Our finding that one of the chromosomal breaks has occurred between the putative V-J recombination signal caused us to look for similar target sequences, usually found 3' of non-rearranged V_k-genes, in the vicinity of the breakpoint of chromosome 8. Both signal boxes could be found as inverted repeats of the J-sequences. The nonamer 5'-A/CAAAAATT-3' corresponds to 5'-GATTTTTG/T-3' of J_k and includes the breakpoint (/) observed in chromosome $8q^+$. The eight nucleotides 3' of the break are part of the 21 bp deletion within the Alu-repeat. The heptamer 5'-CACAGTG-3' corresponds to 5'-CACTGTG-3' of J_k and is located at a distance of 155 bp upstream of the nonamer box, within the unique sequences of chromosome 8. These data strongly suggest that enzymes normally catalyzing V-J rearrangement could be involved in the genesis of the t(2;8) translocation in the Burkitt lymphoma described here.

CONCLUSIONS

Our detailed molecular analysis of the reciprocal breakpoints of a Burkitt lymphoma carrying a variant t(2;8) translocation provides new insights in the genesis of chromosomal rearrangements. The presence on both chromosomal partners of a complete signal structure consisting of a heptamer and an A/T-rich nonamer, which appear to be highly conserved between all immunoglobulin and T-cell receptor gene segments (for review see Tonegawa 1983; Hood 1985), led us to propose a secondary structure for the alignment of chromosome 2 and 8 (Fig. 3) based on the suggestions for V-J- or V-D-J-joining (Tonegawa 1983). Although the length of the spacer between the heptamer and the nonamer, which is normally 12 bases long and seems to be responsible for the direction of the recombination, is considerably longer on chromosome 8 (155 bases), we suggest that the putative recombinases can still recognize both sequences and stabilize the whole interchromosomal recombination structure. Consistent with this suggestion, it should be noted that the intrachromosomal V-J recombination is also an imprecise process, which was well documented by analysis of naturally occurring aberrant rearrangements (Kelley

1985; Seidman 1980; Höchtl 1983) and in vitro introduced immunoglobulin gene segments (Lewis 1984).

This interpretation of our results is further strengthened by a recently reported nuclear endonucleolytic activity that cleaves immunoglobulin recombination sequences (Hope 1986). This activity introduces a double-strand cut, and the cleavage occurs predominantly at the dinucleotide pair $\begin{smallmatrix}\mathrm{TG}\\ \mathrm{AC}\end{smallmatrix}$. The generation of the breakpoint on chromosome $8q^{+}$ could be easily explained by the action of such an enzyme introducing a double-strand cut (/) in the stem structure of the paired nonamers $\begin{smallmatrix}\mathrm{GATTTTTG/T}\\ \mathrm{TTAAAAAC/A}\end{smallmatrix}$ followed by ligation of the nucleotides 5'-A-T-3'(Fig. 3). It seems to us that this physical linkage of chromosome 8 to 2 could have been the crucial step for the initiation of the translocation. For all subsequent events common mechanisms suggested for homologous and non-homologous recombination could be responsible, including single-strand nicks, exonuclease activity, repair synthesis primed from free 3'-termini or by terminal homologies of a few nucleotides, and direct ligation of blunt ends (Szostak 1983; Roth 1985).

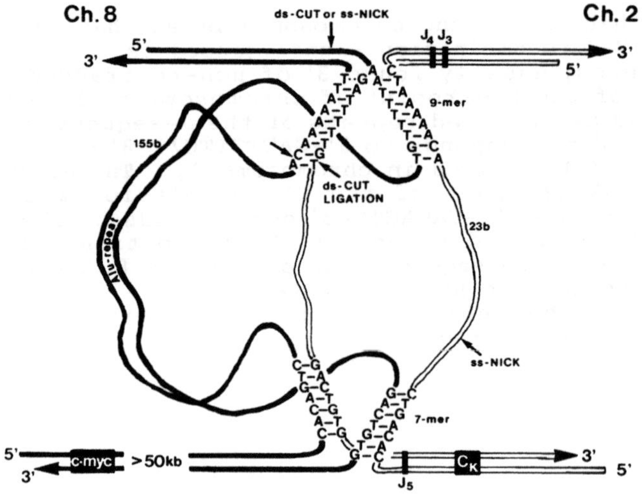

Fig. 3. Possible secondary structure for the alignment of chromosome 2 and 8 via the heptamer and nonamer recognition sequences. Arrows indicate the locations of the reciprocal breakpoints, and possible target sites for the putative recombinase system (for explanation see discussion). The c-myc gene is located at least 50 kb upstream of the breakpoint in the J_k-region. This result will be reported in detail elsewhere (P.H. and M.L., in preparation).

Additional evidence for an involvement of the immunoglobulin recombinase in the genesis of chromosomal rearrangements was recently found in a t(11;14) translocation of chronic lymphocytic leukeamia, where a weak homology to the J_H recombination sequences could be detected (Tsujimoto 1985). However, in cases of the common t(8;14) translocations of BL, where the breakpoint is often localized within the Sµ region of the heavy chain, no such homology could be found.

Possibly this is a special feature of the variant t(2;8) translocations. In fact, we and others have recently found a rearrangement in the J_k region in some additional cases (M.L., unpublished observation, and G.W. Bornkamm, personal communication), which will now be analyzed in detail. However, the perfect homology of the recombination target structures observed in the BL64 cell line could be an exception. Possibly, a weaker homology between a transcriptionally active site in the chromatin and the immunoglobulin loci could be sufficient to transiently stabilize an interchromosomal complex and to activate some of the components of the immunoglobulin recombination system leading to the initiation and an irreversible manifestation of a particular translocation.

ACKNOWLEDGEMENTS

We thank Gilbert M. Lenoir for providing us with the cell line BL64. The work was supported by the Deutsche Forschungsgemeinschaft (Li 374/1-1).

REFERENCES

Chen EJ, Seeburg PH (1985) Supercoil sequencing: a fast and simple method for sequencing plasmid DNA. DNA 4:165-170

Deininger PL, Jolly DJ, Rubin CM, Friedmann T, Schmid CW (1981) Base sequence studies of 300 nucleotide renatured repeated human DNA clones. J Mol Biol 151:17-33

Emanuel BS, Selden JR, Chaganti RSK, Jhanwar S, Nowell PC, Croce CM (1984) The 2p breakpoint of a 2;8 translocation in Burkitt lymphoma interrupts the V_k locus. Proc Natl Acad Sci USA 81:2444-2446

Erikson J, Nishikura K, Ar-Rushdi A, Finan J, Emanuel B, Lenoir G, Nowell PC, Croce CM (1983) Translocation of an immunoglobulin kappa-locus to a region 3'of an unrearranged c-myc oncogene enhances c-myc transcription. Proc Natl Acad Sci USA 80:7581-7585

Frischauf A-M, Lehrach H, Poustka A, Murray N (1983) Lamda replacement vectors carrying polylinker sequences. J Mol Biol 170:827-842

Hieter PA, Maizel JV, Leder P (1982) Evolution of human immunoglobulin kappa J region genes. J Biol Chem 257:1516-1522

Höchtl J, Zachau HG (1983) A novel type of aberrant recombination in Ig genes and its implications for V-J joining mechanism. Nature 302:260-263

Hood L, Kronenberg M, Hunkapiller T (1985) T cell antigen receptor and the immunoglobulin supergene family. Cell 40:225-229

Hope TJ, Aguilera RJ, Minie ME, Sakano H (1986) Endonucleolytic activity that cleaves immunoglobulin recombination sequences. Science 231:1141-1145

Kelley DE, Wiedemann LM, Pittet A-C, Strauss S, Nelson KJ, Davis J, Van Ness B, Perry RP (1985) Nonproductive kappa immunoglobulin genes: Recombinational abnormalities and other lesions affecting transcription, RNA processing, turnover, and translation. Mol Cell Biol 5:1660-1675

Klein G (1983) Specific chromosomal translocations and the genesis of B-cell-derived tumors in mice and men. Cell 32:311-315

Klein G, Klein E (1985) Evolution of tumours and the impact of molecular oncology. Nature 315:190-195

Mark-Vendel E, Philip T, Ladjaj Y, Aboulola M, Lenoir GM (1983)

Chromosomal translocation in algerian Burkitt's lymphoma. The Lancet ii:788
Lewis S, Gifford A, Baltimore D (1984) Joining of V-kappa to J-kappa gene segments in a retroviral vector introduced into lymphoid cells. Nature 308:425-428
Rappold GA, Hameister H, Cremer T, Adolph S, Henglein B, Freese U-K, Lenoir GM, Bornkamm GW (1984) c-myc and immunoglobulin kappa light chain constant genes are on the $8q^+$ chromosome of three Burkitt lymphoma lines with t(2;8) translocation. EMBO J 3:2951-2955
Roth DB, Porter TN, Wilson JH (1985) Mechanisms of nonhomologous recombination in mammalian cells. Mol Cell Biol 5:2599-2607
Rowley JD (1980) Chromosome abnormalities in Cancer. Cancer Genetics and Cytogenetics 2:175-198
Sanger F, Micklen S, Coulson AR (1977) DNA sequencing with chain-terminating inhibitors. Proc Natl Acad Sci USA 74:5463-5467
Seidman JG, Leder P (1980) A mutant immunoglobulin light chains is formed by aberrant DNA and RNA splicing events. Nature 286:779-783
Szostak JW, Orr-Weaver TL, Rothstein RJ (1983) The double-strand-break repair model for recombination. Cell 33:25-35
Taub R, Kelly K, Battey J, Latt S, Lenoir GM, Tantravahi U, Tu Z, Leder P (1984) A novel alteration in the structure of an activated c-myc gene in a variant t(2;8) Burkitt lymphoma. Cell 37:511-520
Tonegawa S (1983) Somatic generation of antibody diversity. Nature 302:575-581
Tsujimoto Y, Jaffe E, Cossman J, Gorham J, Nowell PC, Croce CM (1985) Clustering of breakpoints on chromosome 11 in human B-cell neoplasms with the t(11;14) chromosome translocation. Nature 315:340-343
Yunis JJ (1983) The chromosomal basis of human neoplasia. Science 221:227-236

C-Myc Activation in Spontaneous Rat Immunocytomas Containing a 6;7 Chromosomal Translocation

Warren S. Pear, Gunilla Wahlström, Stanley F. Nelson, Sigurdur Ingvarsson, Hervé Bazin[1], George Klein, and Janos Sumegi

Dep't of Tumor Biology, Karolinska Institute, S-104 01 Stockholm, Sweden
[1]Experimental Immunology Unit, Faculty of Medicine, University of Louvain, Brussels, Belgium

The Lou/Wsl rat immunocytoma (RIC) is a plasma cell tumor (Bazin et al, 1972; for review, see Bazin, 1986), and histologically resembles the mouse plasmacytoma. Tumors arise spontaneously in the ileocecal lymph nodes in approximately 28% of rats of the Lou/Wsl strain, and are detectable at about one year of age. The tumors kill the animals approximately one month after becoming palpable. Although the most frequently secreted myeloma protein is IgE, all isotypes and Bence-Jones proteins are secreted. In addition to the genetic predisposition of the Lou/Wsl strain, both parasites and sex have been postulated as factors in immunocytoma development (Bazin, 1985).

Similar to the non-random chromosomal translocations identified in Burkitt's lymphoma (BL) and mouse plasmacytoma (MPC) (reviewed in Klein and Klein, 1985), it has been shown that the RIC contains a consistent chromosomal translocation between chromosomes 6 and 7 (Wiener et al, 1982). The 6;7 translocation has been identified in all 15 RICs examined cytogenetically (Table 1) (Wiener et al, 1982; Szeles and Wiener, unpublished results). In their paper describing the cytogenetics of the RIC, Wiener et al (1982) noted that the RIC translocation resembles the MPC, and hypothesized that the translocation in the RIC would involve the same loci as in the 12;15 MPC translocation.

By utilizing rat/mouse somatic cell hybrids (Szpirer et al, 1984), we have shown that the same genes involved in the 12;15 MPC translocation, c-myc and IgH, are located on the chromosomes involved in the RIC translocation (Table 2). The c-myc gene has been localized to chromosome 7 (Sumegi et al, 1983) and the immunoglobulin heavy chain cluster (IgH) to chromosome 6 (Pear et al, 1986). Cytogenetic studies of 15 RICs have not identified any tumors which display a translocation between the chromosomes containing the c-myc (7) and Ig kappa locus (4) (Szeles and Wiener, personal communication). We are in the process of localizing the rat Ig lambda locus.

Cleavage of rat genomic DNA with EcoR1 generates a 17 kb c-myc-specific fragment which contains all 3 exons and 5' and 3' flanking sequences. Hybridization of the human c-myc 3rd exon probe, pMC41-3RC (Dalla-Favera et al, 1982) to EcoR1 digested DNA from 15 RICs showed that the c-myc-carrying fragment is

Current Topics in Microbiology and Immunology, Vol. 132

Table 1: Summary of Lou/Wsl rat immunocytomas

TUMOR	TRANSLOC TYPE	COPIES t6;7	IG SECR	SIZE OF ECORI REARR C-MYC	IG COMIG
IR9	t(6;7)	1	BJ	None	*
IR27	t(6;7)	1	gamma1/K	>23	*
IR33	t(6;7)	1	gamma2a/K	>23	*
IR49	t(6;7)	1	BJ-K	>23	*
IR50	ND	ND	epsilon/K	>23	*
IR72	t(6;7)	1	epsilon/K	>23	*
IR74	t(6;7)	1	none	>23	*
IR75	t(6;7)	1	epsilon/K	12	S_u
IR88	t(6;7)	1	epsilon/K	>23	*
IR89	t(6;7)	1	epsilon	>23	ND
IR209	t(6;7)	1	gamma2a/K	12	*
IR222	t(6;7)	1	epsilon	18	*
IR223	t(6;7)	2	BJ	20	epsilon
IR241	ND	ND	gamma1/K	>23	*
IR304	ND	ND	gamma2a/K	None	*

Notes: ND-Not Determined; *-No Co-migration detected; TRANSLOC-Translocation; Ig SECR- Secreted Immunoglobulin; K-Kappa; BJ-Bence-Jones; Ig COMIG-Immunoglobulin Co-migration

rearranged in 13 of these tumors (Table 1 and Figure 1). As shown in Table 1, the rearranged c-myc-containing EcoR1 fragment is greater than 23 kb in the majority of these tumors. In two tumors, IR75 and IR209, the rearranged c-myc carrying EcoR1 fragment is approximately 12 kb. The rearranged c-myc-carrying EcoR1 fragments from both of these tumors have been cloned into EMBL4.

Analysis of the c-myc breakpoints in the IR75 and IR209 has shown that the breakpoints occur upstreams of the proximal c-myc promoter, approximately 800 bps in the IR75 and 600 bps in the IR209. This is upstreams of the most frequent c-myc breakpoints in both MPC and BL (reviewed in Cory, 1986). Sequence analysis has demonstrated that the IR75 has undergone multiple rearrangements which juxtapose part of the switch mu region with the c-myc gene in opposite transcriptional orientations. Upstreams of the juxtaposed switch mu sequences are sequences derived from upstreams of the switch gamma1 region. Thus, like both BL and MPC, the translocation in the IR75 has juxtaposed c-myc and an Ig loci. Since the chromosome 6 breakpoint is located at 6q3.2, this is most likely the location of the rat IgH locus. Likewise, the c-myc gene is located at 7q3.

Table 2: Chromosomal Location of C-Myc, IgH,and Ig Kappa Loci

LOCUS	RAT CHROMOSOME	
C-MYC	7	(Sumegi et al, 1983)
IgH	6	(Pear et al, 1986)
IgKappa	4	(Perlmann et al, 1985)

We have utilized genomic hybridization to determine the c-myc breakpoint in 13 other RICs (Figure 2). Two RICs, IR9 and IR304, do not show rearrangement with EcoR1. Further chromosome walking has demonstrated that these two tumors are not rearranged within at least 23 kb of the proximal c-myc promoter. As shown in Figure 2, the c-myc-associated breakpoints are clustered within a 900 bp BamH1 fragment which contains the proximal c-myc promoter and approximately 700 bps of 5' flanking sequence. This is the same region in which viral insertion occurs in murine T-cell lymphomas (Corcoran et al, 1984; Li et al, 1984; Selten et al, 1984) and in Moloney virus-induced rat thymomas (Steffen, 1984). The breakpoint in IR49 occurs in the intron between exons 1 and 2; similar to the most common breakpoint in Balb/c MPCs.The breakpoints in IR74 and IR241 occur at least 700 bps upstreams of the proximal promoter. As in BL and MPC, no breakpoints have been identified which interrupt the c-myc coding exons.

Co-migration experiments between the rearranged c-myc-carrying fragment and Ig switch and constant region probes have shown that the translocation in the IR223 has juxtaposed the c-epsilon locus with the c-myc gene. Suprisingly, none of the other 13 analyzed tumors has shown co-migration between the rearranged c-myc and Ig switch and constant region probes. As with the IR75, however, it is possible that rearrangement takes place within other regions of the IgH cluster. Analysis of other cloned RICs should elucidate which Ig regions are involved in the translocation event.

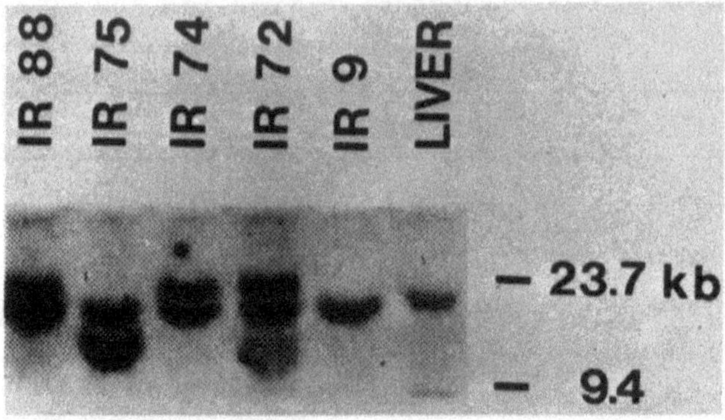

Figure 1: C-myc rearrangement in the RIC. DNA was digested with EcoR1 and transferred to nitrocellulose. The filter was hybridized to the ^{32}P-labeled human c-myc 3rd exon probe, pMC41-3RC (Dalla-Favera et al, 1982). High stringency washings were done in 0,2 X SSC, 0,2% SDS for 1 hr at 65 degrees.

In summary, our studies of the RIC show that in 3 different tumors (BL, MPC, RIC) in 3 different species (human, mouse, rat), nearly identical genetic loci (c-myc, Ig) are juxtaposed via chromosomal translocation. These 3 tumors represent at least two different stages of B cell maturation, and the natural histories and modes of induction of the tumors are very different. The finding that c-myc/Ig juxtapositon occurs in these three tumors suggests that this configuration plays a central role in the genesis of these B cell tumors.

Figure 2: Identification of translocation breakpoints within the 17 kb EcoR1 c-myc-carrying fragment in 15 RICs

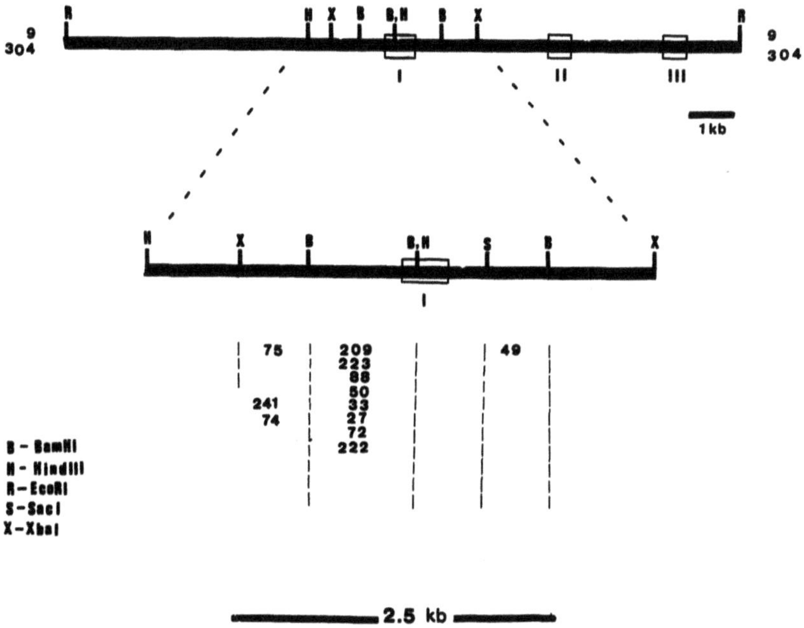

Acknowledgements: This work was supported by PHS grant number 3R01CA14054 awarded by the National Cancer Institute, DHHS and by the Swedish Cancer Society. W.S.P, S.I., and J.S. are recipients of fellowships from the Cancer Research Institute and the Concern Foundation.

References:

Bazin, H, Deckers, C, Beckers, A, and Heremans, JF (1972) Transplantable Ig-secreting tumors in rats. Int. J. Cancer 10: 568-580.

Bazin, H (1985). In: Mechanisms of B Cell Neoplasia. Editiones Roche, Basil, p. 208.

Bazin, H (1986) Louvain rat immunocytomas. Adv. Cancer Res.: in press.

Corcoran, LM, Adams, JM, Dunn, AR, and Cory, S (1984)

Transposition of the immunoglobulin heavy chain enhancer to the myc oncogene in a murine plasmacytoma. Cell 40: 71-79.

Cory, S (1986) Activation of cellular oncogenes in hemopoietic cells by chromosomal translocation. Adv Cancer Res: in press.

Dalla-Favera, R, Gelmann, EP, Martinotti, S, Franchini, G, Papas, T, Gallo, R, and Wong-Staal, F (1982) Cloning and characterization of different human sequences related to the onc gene (v-myc) of avian myelocytomatosis virus (MC29). Proc. Natl. Acad. Sci. USA 79: 6497-6501.

Klein, G and Klein, E (1985) Myc/Ig juxtaposition by chromosomal translocation: some new insights, puzzles, and paradoxes. Immunology Today 6: 208-215.

Li, Y, Holland, CA, Hartley, JW, and Hopkins, N (1984) Viral integration near c-myc in 10-20% of MCF 247-induced AKR lymphomas. Proc. Natl. Acad. Sci. USA 81: 6808-6811.

Pear, WS, Wahlström, G, Szpirer, J, Levan, G, Klein,G, and Sumegi, J (1986) Localization of the rat immunoglobulin heavy chain locus to chromosome 6. Immunogenetics: in press.

Perlmann, C, Sumegi, J, Szpirer, C, Levan, G, and Klein, G (1985) The rat immunoglobuliln kappa light chain locus is on chromosome 4. Immunogenetics 22: 97-100.

Selton, G, Cuypers, HT, Zijlstra, M, Melief, C, and Berns, A (1984) Involvement of c-myc in MULV-induced T cell lymphomas in mice: frequency and mechanisms of activation. EMBO J. 3:3215-3222.

Steffen, D (1984) Proviruses are adjacent to c-myc in some murine leukemia virus-induced lymphomas. Proc. Natl. Acad. Sci. USA 81: 2097-2101.

Szpirer, J, Levan G, Thorn, M, and Szpirer, C (1984) Gene mapping in the rat by mouse-rat somatic cell hybridization: synteny of the albumin and alpha-fetoprotein genes and assignment to chromosome 14. Cytogenet. Cell Genet. 38: 142-149.

Sumegi, J, Spira, J, Bazin, H, Szpirer, J, Levan, G, and Klein, G (1983) Rat c-myc is located on chromosome 7 and rearranges in immunocytomas with t(6;7) chromosomal translocation. Nature 306: 497-498.

Wiener, F, Babonits, M, Spira, J, Klein, G, and H Bazin (1982) Non-random chromosomal changes involving chromosomes 6 and 7 in spontaneous rat immunocytomas. Int. J. Cancer 29: 431-437.

The Molecular Genetics of Human T Cell Leukemias and Lymphomas

Jan Erikson[1] and Carlo M. Croce

The Wistar Institute of Anatomy and Biology, 36th Street at Spruce, Philadelphia, Pennsylvania 19104

Specific chromosomal translocations are consistently associated with particular malignancies suggesting they play a role in neoplastic development (Klein 1981; Yunis 1983). Studies on the translocations present in Burkitt's lymphoma have shown they result in the association of the c-myc oncogene with the 5' end of either the IgH locus on chromosome 14, or the C_κ or C_λ loci on chromosome 2 and 22 respectively. A consequence of this juxtaposition is the deregulation of the participating c-myc oncogene (Croce and Nowell 1985). In addition the IgH locus has been implicated in the translocations present in other B cell leukemias and lymphoma (Tsujimoto et al. 1984a, 1984b). The Ig loci's unique feature of B cell restricted DNA rearrangement prior to functional expression may be responsible for targeting the Ig loci for B cell associated translocations. Similarly, the alpha and beta chain genes which compose the serologically defined T cell receptor are rearranged and expressed specifically in T cells (Davis et al. 1984). The experiments presented in this paper demonstrate the participation of the T cell receptor α chain gene in the t(11;14) and the t(8;14) translocations in T cell malignancies and show that in the later case this participation may be responsible for the deregulation of the c-myc oncogene.

The locus for the α-chain of the T cell receptor has been mapped to band q11.2 on chromosome 14 (Croce et al. 1985), a chromosome region that is involved in inversions and translocations in T cell neoplasms (Hecht et al. 1984). One of the most common alterations in acute lymphocytic leukemia (ALL) of the T cell type is a t(11;14) (p13;q11) chromosome translocation (Williams et al. 1984). By analyzing a panel of human-mouse somatic cell hybrids generated from two clinical isolates harboring this translocation, we have been able to show that the α-chain gene is split by this translocation event and that the α-chain gene is split by this translocation event and that the Vα segments are proximal to the Cα segment within band 14q11.2 (Fig. 1) (Erikson et al. 1985). The α-chain locus may be involved in the activation of a putative oncogene at band p13 on chromosome 11 in a manner similar to the involvement of the Ig loci in Burkitt's lymphoma.

Recently a t(8;14) translocation has been described in several T cell neoplasms (Caubet 1985) with breakpoints at 8q24, where the c-

[1]Department of Medical Microbiology, Stanford University School of Medicine, Stanford, California 94305

Current Topics in Microbiology and Immunology, Vol. 132

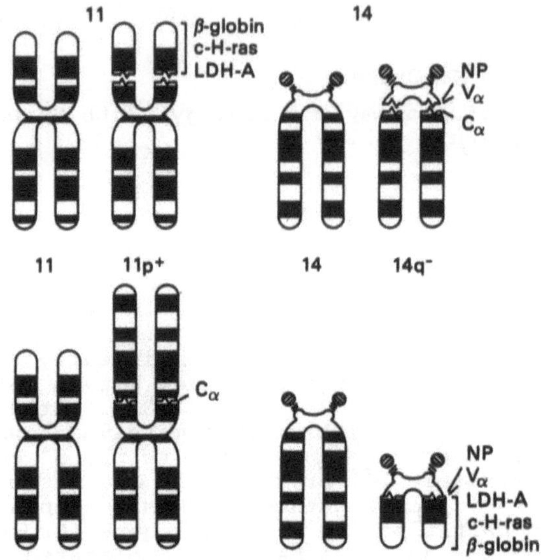

Fig. 1. The t(11;14) (p13;q11) translocation in T-ALL. The translocation breakpoint on chromosome 14 splits the locus for the α-chain of the T-cell receptor. The Vα genes remain on the $14q^-$ chromosome, while the Cα translocates to the involved chromosome 11 ($11p^+$). The gene for human nucleoside phosphorylase remains on the involved chromosome 14 ($14q^-$). The genes LDH-A, β-globin, and c-H-ras translocate to the involved chromosome 14 ($14q^-$).

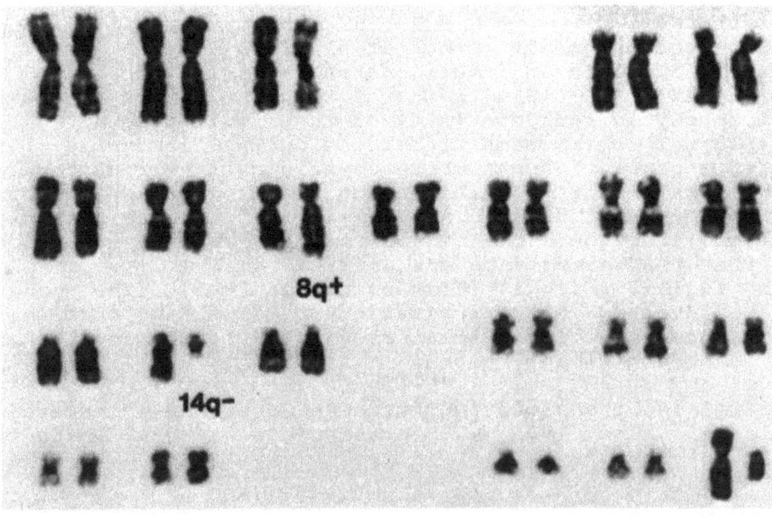

Fig. 2a. Representative karyotype of leukemic cells from patient DeF with t(8;14) translocation and pericentric inversion of chromosome 9 as the only abnormalities (the latter was shown to be a constitutional variant in normal T cells during clinical remission).

The breakpoint on chromosome 14 is at band q11, and the segment translocated to chromosome 8 reflects loss, and possible rearrangement, of chromosome 14 material. The molecular data (see text) indicate that the breakpoint on chromosome 8 is distal to the c-myc locus at 8q24.

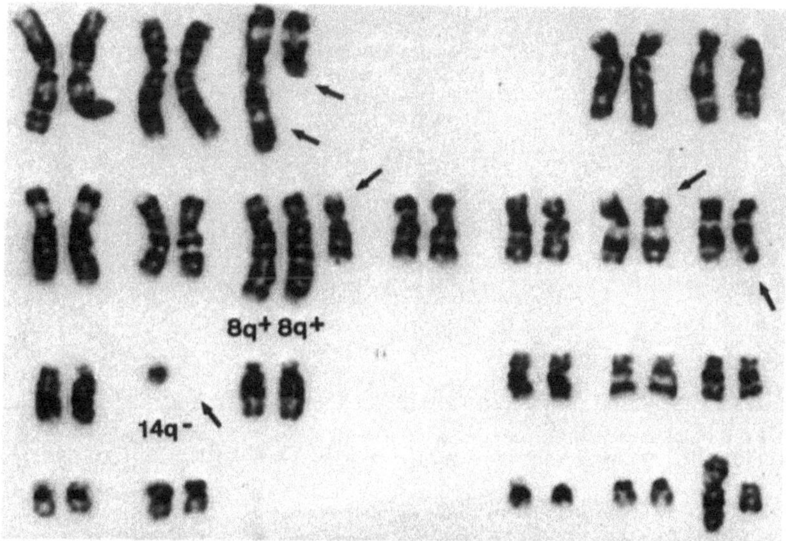

Fig. 2b. Representative karyotype of T cell leukemia cell line SKW-3 with t(8;14) (q24;q11) translocation. In addition to two copies of the $8q^+$ chromosome and a $14q^-$, resulting from the translocation, other abnormalities (arrows) include: a t(3q;3q) translocation, a t(8p;11p) translocation, a $12q^+$, and absence of the other chromosome 14. These results are consistent with the previous cytogenetic analysis of SKW-3 cells (Shima 1985).

myc oncogene resides (Dalla Favera et al. 1982), and 14q11, where the alpha chain locus resides (Croce et al. 1985). We examined two such cases to determine if the alpha chain locus may be involved in c-myc deregulation in these T cell malignancies. Figure 2a shows the karyotype of leukemic cells from the bone marrow of a patient (DeF), with T-ALL where the t(8;14) translocation and a constitutional inversion of chromosome 9 are the only alterations. Figure 2b shows the karyotype of a cell line, SkW-3, derived from a 55 year-old female with T cell chronic lymphocytic leukemia (CLL). This cell line carries two copies of the $8q^+$ chromosome derived from a t(8;14) translocation as well as other chromosomal abnormalities.

The relative positions of the c-myc and α-chain genes as a result of the translocation were determined by analyzing a series of somatic cell hybrids derived from the leukemic cells of patient DeF and

Table 1. Human genes in DeF-BW5147 cell hybrids

Cell lines	mos	myc	IgH	Cα	Vα	NP	Human chromosomes[a]				Human c-myc transcripts
							8	$8q^+$	14	$14q^-$	
DeF	+	+	+	+	+	+	++	++	++	++	+++
BW5147	-	-	-	-	-	-	-	-	-	-	-
563 BC5	+	+	+	+	+	+	+	-	++	++	-
563 BB4	+	+	+	+	+	+	±	-	++	+	ND
563 BD3	+	+	-	-	+	+	+	-	-	++	-
563 AA1	+	+	-	-	+	+	+	-	-	+	ND
563 BB2	+	+	+	+	-	-	-	+	-	-	ND
563 BD2	-	-	-	-	+	+	-	-	-	++	ND
563 BA5-BC10	+	+	+	+	-	-	-	++	-	-	++
563 BA5-BB3	+	+	+	+	-	-	ND[b]	ND	ND	ND	ND
563 BA5-DE7	+	+	+	+	+	+	±	+	+	++	ND
563 AC3	+	+	+	+	+	+	-	+	-	++	+

[a] Percentages of metaphases containing the relevant human chromosome. A minimum of 18 metaphases of each hybrid were examined. - = none; ± = 1-10%; + = 10-30%; ++ = >30%.

[b] ND = Not done.

the mouse thymoma fusion partner, BW5147. Hybrids were tested for the presence of human chromosomes, for the c-mos oncogene located at band 8q11 (Caubet et al. 1985), for the c-myc oncogene, for the variable (Vα) and constant (Cα) regions of the alpha chain gene and for nucleoside phosphorylase (NP) which we have previously mapped proximal to the Vα genes at 14q11 (Table 1) (Erikson et al. 1985). We can conclude from these results that the chromosome breakpoint on chromosome 14 is between Vα and Cα genes and that the c-myc oncogene remains on the $8q^+$ chromosome with Cα sequences translocating to a region 3' to the involved c-myc oncogene (Fig. 3) (Erikson et al. 1986). Using probes spanning 38 kb 3' of c-myc (Fig. 4a) we did not detect rearrangement in DeF cells. We did detect, however, rearrangements 3' of the c-myc gene in the other t(8;14) case we examined (SkW-3) (Fig. 4b). The breakpoint in these cells is between the first EcoR1 and the first HindIII site 3' of the c-myc gene. These results illustrate that the 5' end of the α-chain gene is associated with the c-myc gene. As was the case in the Burkitt lymphoma variant t(2;8) and t(8;22) translocations where the Ig loci on 2 and 22 are oriented centromere 5'-3', as is the α-chain locus on chromosome 14, this association is

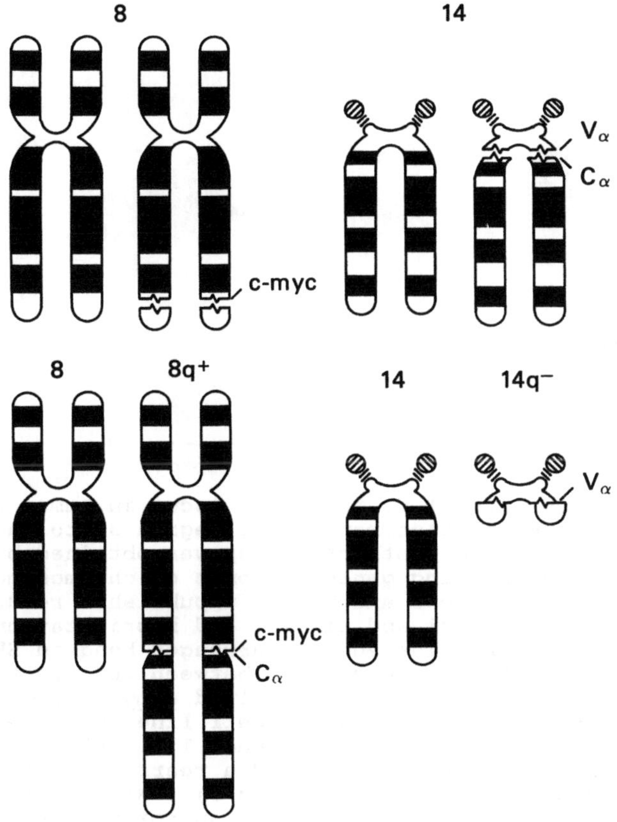

Fig. 3. Diagram of the t(8;14) (24, q11) chromosome translocation in T cell leukemias. The breakpoint on chromosome 8 is distal to the involved c-myc oncogene, while the breakpoint on chromosome 14 involves directly the locus for the α chain of the T cell receptor.

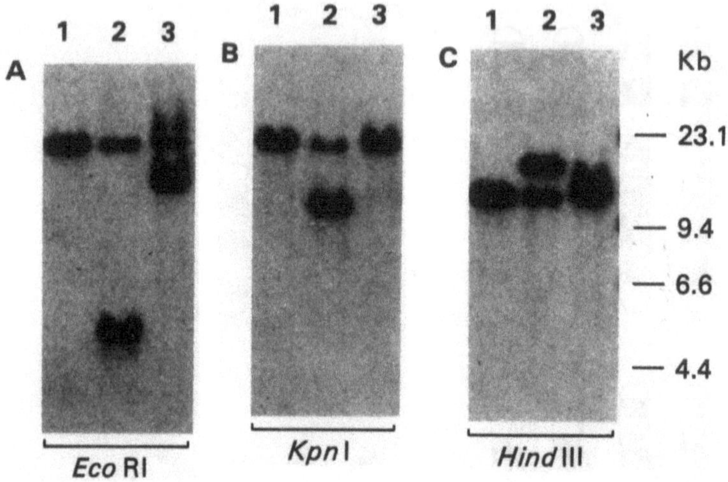

Fig. 4. Rearrangement distal to the c-myc locus in human T cell leukemia cells: a) restriction map of the region 3' to the c-myc locus on chromosome 8. The restriction map was obtained by chromosome walking using overlapping genomic clones of chromosome 8 of human PA 682 cells (Lee, Showe and Croce, unpublished results). b) Digestion with EcoR1, Kpn1 and HindIII and hybridization with pCA 1.7S DNA showed a germ line and a rearranged band in SKW-3 cells (lanes 2). Thus the breakpoint is between the first EcoR1 and the first HindIII site 3' to the involved c-myc oncogene (Fig. 2a). Molt 4 is a human T cell leukemia cell line that does not carry a rearrangement of chromosome 8 (lanes 1). BL2 is a Burkitt lymphoma with a t(8;22) translocation and a rearrangement distal (3') to the involved c-myc oncogene (lanes 3). We have cloned the breakpoint of BL2 cells and found it to be approximately 10 kb 3' to the involved c-myc oncogene (Erikson and Croce, unpublished results). The band representing the rearranged c-myc locus is more intense than the germ line band because SKW-3 cells contain two copies of the $8q^+$ chromosome (Fig. 2b).

achieved by translocation to the 3' of the c-myc gene. In addition there is heterogeneity in breakpoints on chromosome 8 in the T associated t(8;14) as there was in the Burkitt t(2;8) and t(8;22) translocations (Croce and Wunell 1985).

To determine what effect this translocation had on c-myc expression we compared transcription from the translocation-associated gene on the $8q^+$ chromosome to that of the normal c-myc gene on chromosome 8 in somatic cell hybrids between BW5.47 mouse cells and human DeF leukemia cells protection using a S1 nuclease assay (Erikson et al. 1986). As shown in Fig. 5, hybrids containing the 8q$^+$ chromosome express human c-myc transcripts while hybrids containing the normal 8 do not have detectable levels of steady-state mRNA. These results indicate that the translocation of the Cα locus to a region 3' of the c-myc gene results in c-myc deregulation thus implicating this oncogene in T cell malignancies.

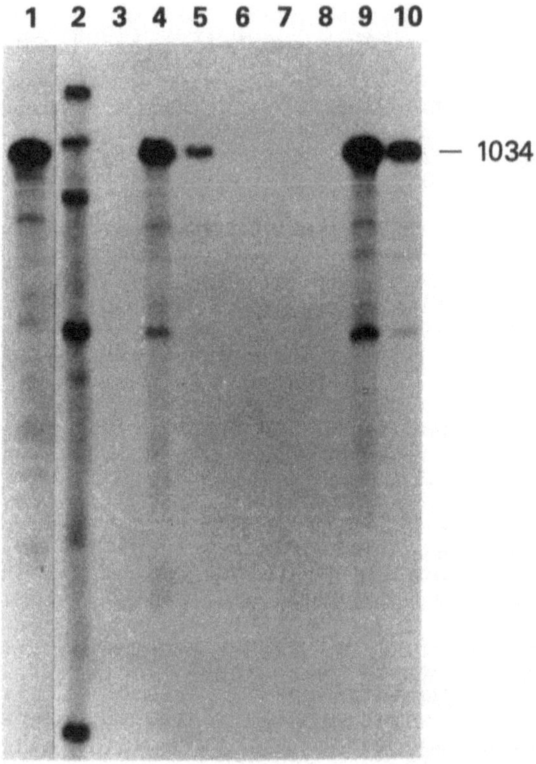

Fig. 5. S1 nuclease protection analysis of RNA expressed in parental and hybrid cells. The S1 probe was pRyc 7.4, a human c-myc cDNA clone that carries 1.2 kb insert of the human c-myc cDNA in pBR322. The pRyc 7.4 plasmid DNA was digested by BclI, 5'-^{32}P end labeled and used as a probe as described previously (Croce and Nowell 1985). The expected fragment protected by human c-myc mRNA (1,034 nucleotides) encompasses most of the protein coding sequence. We detected the expression of human c-myc transcripts in DeF human leukemia cells (lane 1), in Jurkat human T cell lymphoma cells (lane 9), in SKW-3 T cell leukemia cells (lane 4) and in GM1500-6TG-OUB tumorigenic human lymphoblastoid cells, in which the expression of c-myc transcripts is very elevated (lane 10) (18). The mouse BW5147 leukemic cells express mouse c-myc transcripts (data not shown) that are not detectable by using the human c-myc probe (lane 8). Size markers are in lane 2. No RNA is in lane 3.

We detected human c-myc transcripts in hybrid 563 BA5-BC10 that carries the $8q^+$ chromosome but not the normal 8 (Table 1) (lane 5). We did not detect, however the expression of human c-myc transcripts in hybrids 563 BD3 and 563 BC5 that have retained the normal chromosome 8, but have lost the $8q^+$ (Table 1) (lanes 6 and 7). We also detected human c-myc transcripts in hybrid 563 AC3 that carries the $8q^+$ chromosome in 10% of its cells, but has lost the normal chromosome 8 (data not shown) (Table 1).

REFERENCES

Caubet JF, Bernheim A, Larsen CJ, Berger R (1985) Human proto oncogene c-mos maps to 8q11. EMBO J 4:2245-2248

Croce CM, Isobe M, Palumbo A, Puck J, Ming J, Tweardy D, Erikson J, Davis M, Rovera G (1985) Gene for α-chain of human T-cell receptor: Location on chromosome 14 region involved in T-cell neoplasms. Science 227:1044-1047

Croce CM, Nowell PC (1985) Molecular basis of human B cell neoplasia. Blood 65:1-7

Dalla Favera R, Bregni M, Erikson J, Patterson D, Gallo RC, Croce CM (1982) Human c-myc oncogene is located in the region of chromosome 8 that is translocated in Burkitt lymphoma cells. Proc Natl Acad Sci USA 79:7824-7826

Davis MM, Chien Y-h, Gascoigne NRJ, Hedrick SM (1984) Murine T cell receptor gene complex: Isolation, structure and rearrangement. Immunol Rev 4:235-258

Erikson J, Finger L, San L, ar-Rushdi A, Nishikura K, Minowada J, Finan J, Emanual B, Nowell PC, Croce CM (1986) c-myc deregulation by translocation of the alpha-locus of T cell receptor in T cell leukemias. Science, in press

Erikson J, Williams DL, Finan J, Nowell PC, Croce CM (1985) Locus of the α-chain of the T-cell receptor is split by chromosome translocation in T-cell leukemias. Science 229:784-786

Hecht F, Morgan R, Hecht BKM, Smith STD (1984) Common region on chromosome 14 in T-cell leukemia and lymphoma. Science 226:1445-1447

Klein G (1981) The role of gene dosage and genetic transposition in carcinogenesis. Nature 294:313-315

Tsujimoto Y, Yunis J, Onorato-Showe C, Erikson J, Nowell PC, Croce CM (1984a) Molecular cloning of the chromosomal breakpoint of B-cell lymphomas and leukemias with the t(11;14) chromosome translocation. Science 224:1403-1407

Tsujimoto Y, Finger L, Yunis J, Nowell PC, Croce CM (1984b) Molecular genetics of follicular lymphoma: Cloning of the chromosome breakpoint of neoplastic B-cells with the t(14;18) chromosome translocation. Science 226:1097-1100

Williams D, Look AT, Melvin SL, Roberson PK, Dahl G, Flake T, Strass S (1984) New chromosomal translocations correlate with specific immunophenotypes of childhood acute lymphoblastic leukemia. Cell 36:101-109

Yunis J (1983) The chromosomal basis of human neoplasia. Science 221:227-232

Molecular Genetics of Human B-cell Neoplasia

Y. Tsujimoto and C. M. Croce

The Wistar Institute, 3601 Spruce Street, Philadelphia, PA 19104

INTRODUCTION

Specific chromosome rearrangements, predominantly translocations and inversions, are observed in the great majority of human hematopoietic malignancies (Van Den Berghe, et. al. 1978, Yunis et. al. 1982, 1984). In Burkitt lymphoma the specific chromosomal translocations involve directly one of the human immunoglobulin loci and the c-myc oncogene (Dalla Favera, et. al. 1982, Croce, et. al. 1983, Erikson et. al. 1983). The consequence of the juxtaposition of the immunoglobulin loci and of the c-myc oncogene is a deregulation of the transcription of the involved c-myc oncogene that is transcribed constitutively at elevated levels (Croce, et. al. 1983, Erikson, et. al. 1983, Nishikura, et. al. 1983). Other specific chromosomal translocations involving band 14q32, where the immunoglobulin heavy chain locus resides (Croce et. al. 1979, Erikson et. al. 1982), are observed in B cell neoplasms. A t(11;14) (q13;q32) chromosome translocation has been observed in chronic lymphocytic leukemia of the B cell type (Nowell et. al. 1981), in diffuse B cell lymphoma (Yunis et. al. 1982, 1984) and in multiple myeloma (Van Den Berghe et. al. 1984). This translocation juxtaposes the bcl-1 locus to the heavy chain locus (Tsujimoto et. al. 1984, 1985a, b). In most cases of follicular lymphoma, one of the most common human hematopoietic maligancies, a t(14;18) (q32;q21) chromosome translocation has been observed (Yunis et. al. 1982, 1984).

The t(11;14) and t(14;18) Chromosome Translocations Are Due to Mistakes in VDJ Joining

By taking advantage of the involvement of immunoglobulin heavy chain locus (IgH) in the t(11;14) and t(14;18) chromosome translocations, we have molecularly cloned the breakpoints of these translocations by using IgH DNA as probe (Tsujimoto et. al. 1984, 1985b). From the structural and DNA sequencing analysis of the breakpoints from two cases of chronic lymphocytic leukemia (CLL) with the t(11;14) and from four cases of follicular lymphoma with the t(14;18) translocation, we have shown that these chromosome translocations are mediated by the VDJ joining recombinase (Tsujimoto et. al. 1985a, c). This is based on the fact that (1) the breakpoints occur at the 5' region of J segment, (2) 7mer-9mer signal sequences for VDJ joining are present at the breakpoint regions, and (3) extranucleotides (N region-like sequences) are present at the joining sites (Fig. 1).

Current Topics in Microbiology and Immunology, Vol. 132

Figure 1 summarizes the DNA sequences of the breakpoints of the t(14;18) chromosome translocation. The breakpoinats of the t(14;18) chromosome translocation in four cases of follicular lymphoma are tightly clustered within about 100 bp region.

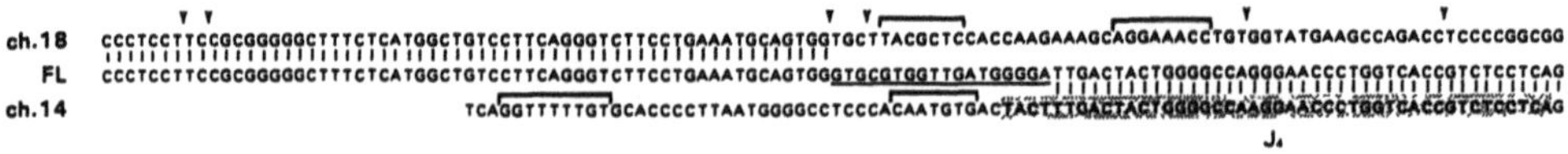

Fig. 1. DNA sequences of the breakpoint of the t(14;18) chromosome translocation. The top line represents normal chromosome 18 sequences. The open triangles indicate the breakpoints on chromosome 18 from 14q+ chromosome in 6 cases of follicular lymphoma so far analyzed (Tsujimoto et. al., 1985C; Bakhshi et. al., 1985; Cleary and Sklar, 1985). The middle and bottom line represents a representative t(14;18) breakpoint sequence and J4 segment sequence t(14;18) respectively. N region-like sequence is underlined.

The t(14;18) Chromosome Translocation Directly Involves the bcl-2 Gene at Chromosome 18 Band q21

The chromosome 18 probe flanking the breakpoint region (probe A in Fig. 2) has been shown to detect transcripts (Tsujimoto et. al., 1985d). These transcripts are expressed in many different kinds of hematopoietic cells including B, T and myeloid cells. The gene defined by these probes, for which we propose the name bcl-2 is transcribed into at least three messages, 8.5 kb, 5.5 kb and 3.5 kb (Tsujimoto et. al., 1986). The 8.5 kb mRNA seems to utilize another polyadenylation site further downstream from the one which is used for the 5.5 kb mRNA. As described below, the bcl-2 gene is interrupted by chromosome translocation in most cases of follicular lymphoma with the t(14;18) translocation. The Northern blot hybridization shows that follicular lymphoma cell lines with the t(14;18) produce aberrant transcripts (Tsujimoto et al. 1986).

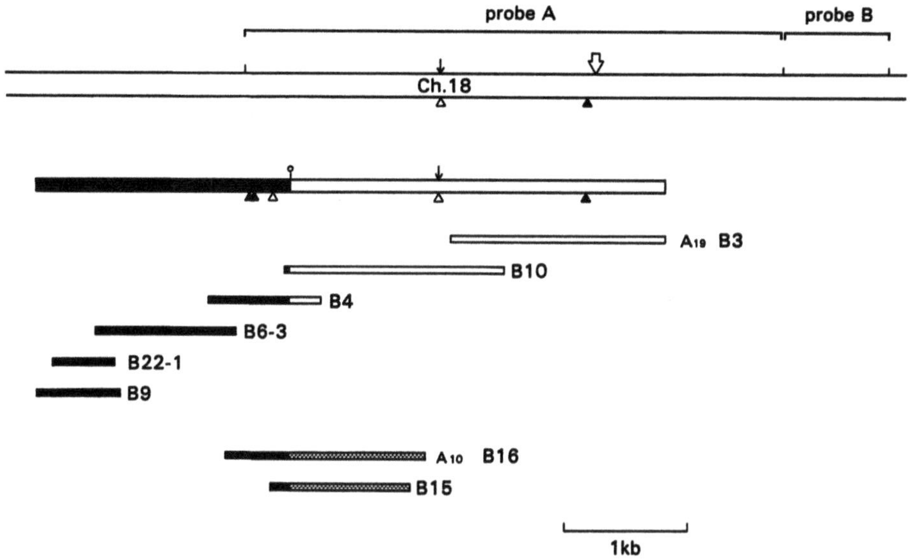

Fig. 2. bcl-2 cDNA clones.

Top double lines represent genomic restriction map corresponding to 3' part of cDNA (2nd exon). The restriction map of genomic DNA was deduced by analysis of the several overlapping genomic clones which were previously described (Tsujimoto et. al. 1985b, d). The hot spot of the breakpoint of the t(14;18) chromosome translocation is shown by ⇩

Structure of cDNA clones are shown below the genomic restriction map. The clones B3, 4, 10, 15 and 16 were obtained from 380 cDNA library made by using oligo(dT) as primer. The other clones, 22-1, 6-3, and 9 were obtained from the primer extension library. The open box represents the second exon and the filled and dotted boxes represent the first exon. The restriction sites are shown by ∇ SstI, ▼SstII, | HindIII ⚲, BamHI, and ↓ EcoRI.

Molecular Cloning of bcl-2 cDNA

To analyze the bcl-2 gene we have constructed a cDNA library in λgt11 vector from polyA$^+$ mRNA of the pre B cell leukemia cell line 380. By screening aproximately 2 x 10^5 recombinants with chromosome 18 probe (A) (Fig. 2), we have obtained three independent cDNA clones which are overlapping each other (B3, 4, 10). As shown in Fig. 2, clone B3 contains 19 A residues at the end, indicating that this clone represents the 3' end of mRNA. The restriction maps of cDNA clones and genomic sequences are colinear from the 3' end of the cDNA clone B3 until just before the BamHI site of the cDNA sequence. The cDNA sequence beyond this point diverges from genomic sequences (data not shown). Thus cDNA sequences consist of at least two genomic regions.

The 5' part of cDNA clone B4 (5' end to BamHI site) detects another set of cDNA clones, B15 and B16 (Fig. 2). These two cDNA clones share the same sequences at the 5' region with B4 but totally different at the 3' part from B3, 4 and 10 (see Fig. 2).

In order to obtain cDNA sequences further upstream, we also constructed a cDNA library by primer extension and obtained a series of overlapping clones, 6-3, 22-1 and 9. The cDNA sequences clone B9 to B3 represents 5.5 kb transcript and those from B9 to B16 represent 3.5 kb bcl-2 transcript. From the orientation of bcl-2 gene transcription and the location of the t(14;18) translocation breakpoint, it is concluded that the 5' end of the bcl-2 gene is more distal than its 3' end out bound 18q21 and that, after translocation, the transcription of bcl-2 gene and of the IgH locus occurs in the same direction.

<u>Nucleotide Sequence of the bcl-2 Gene</u>

Nucleotide sequence derived from 5.5 kb bcl-2 mRNA is shown in Fig. 3A. The DNA sequence of 5105 bp reveals one possible open reading frame consisting of 239 amino acid residues (bcl-2 protein). The nucleotide sequence corresponding to the 3.5 kb bcl-2 mRNA is shown in Fig. 3B. As shown in Fig. 3B, 3.5 kb mRNA codes for another protein consisting of 205 amino acid residues (bcl-2β protein) which is identical to bcl-2 protein except at the carboxyl terminus. Thus bcl-2 gene seems to code for two different protein products.

In order to determine whether the open reading frame observed on the basis of the cDNA sequences is biologically active, the strategy shown in Fig. 4A was used. The cDNA sequence with the open reading frame for bcl-2 protein was cloned under the promoter of the C. coli phage T7 and trascribed by T7 RNA polymerase <u>in vitro</u>. The RNA transcripts made <u>in vitro</u> were assayed in an <u>in vitro</u> translation system and the protein products, labelled with ^{35}S-methionine, were analyzed by SDS-PAGE. As shown in Fig. 4B antisense RNA transcribed RNA transcribed from DNA constructs in which the cDNA sequence is inserted in wrong orientation with respect to the T7 promoter, did not produce any protein. On the other hand, sense RNA produced two major protein products of approximately 28-30 kd molecular weight, which are close to the size expected for the bcl-2 protein products from the DNA sequence analysis. The two proteins are presumably initiated from the two ATG codons at +1 and at +46. The small size differences could be due to the high proline content of the bcl-2 gene products. To confirm that these 28 kd proteins are derived from the open reading frame of bcl-2, sense RNA was made from a DNA construct in which the open reading frame was truncated by cleavage with the restriction enyzyme BamHI (at +563 in Fig. 3A). As shown in Fig. 4B this truncated sense RNA produced smaller size proteins instead of the 28-30 kd proteins, confirming that the 28-30 kd proteins are derived from the bcl-2 open reading frame shown in Fig. 3A. Computer search did not show any homology of bcl-2 alpha and beta products to any protein so far sequenced. Since the predicted amino acid sequences of the bcl-2 proteins do not show transmembrane domain or leader peptide, the bcl-2 proteins do not seem to be either a membrane or a secreted protein.

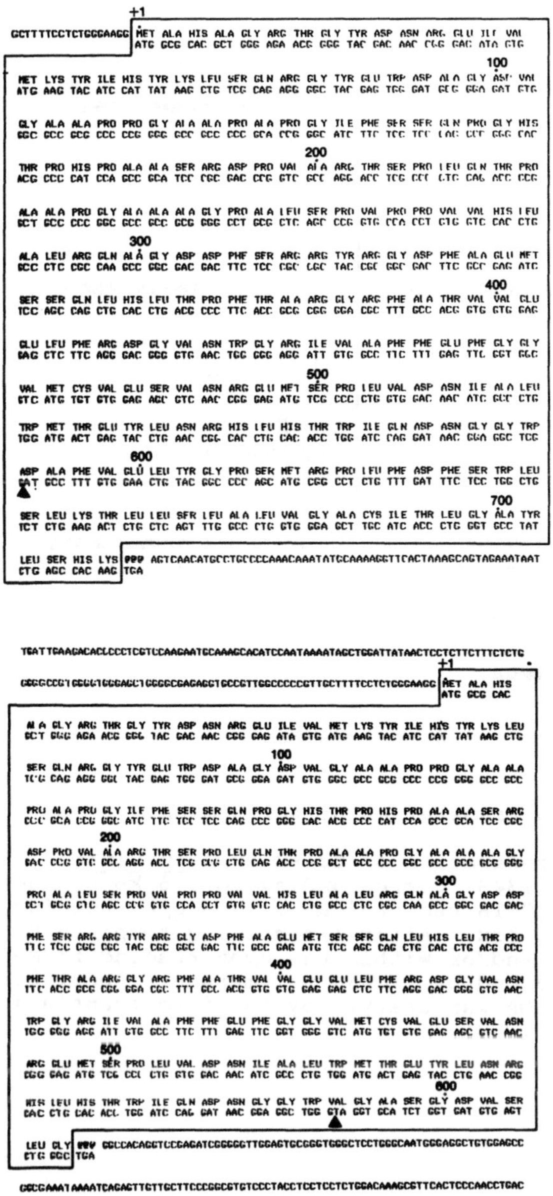

Fig. 3. Nucleotide sequence of bcl-2 cDNA. Nucleotide sequence of bcl-2 cDNA were determined from overlapping cDNA clones shown in Fig. 2. The open reading frames are shown by boxes. The splicing site is shown by ∇

(A) cDNA sequences corresponding to 5.5 kb bcl-2 transcript. Only open reading frame region is shown.

(B) cDNA sequences corresponding to 3.5 kb transcript. Only DNA sequences surrounding the open reading frame are shown. The possible initiation codon ATG is counted at +1. The breakpoints of the t(14;18) translocation in four cases of follicular lymphoma which were previously reported are shown by ∇ (Tsujimoto et. al., 1985c).

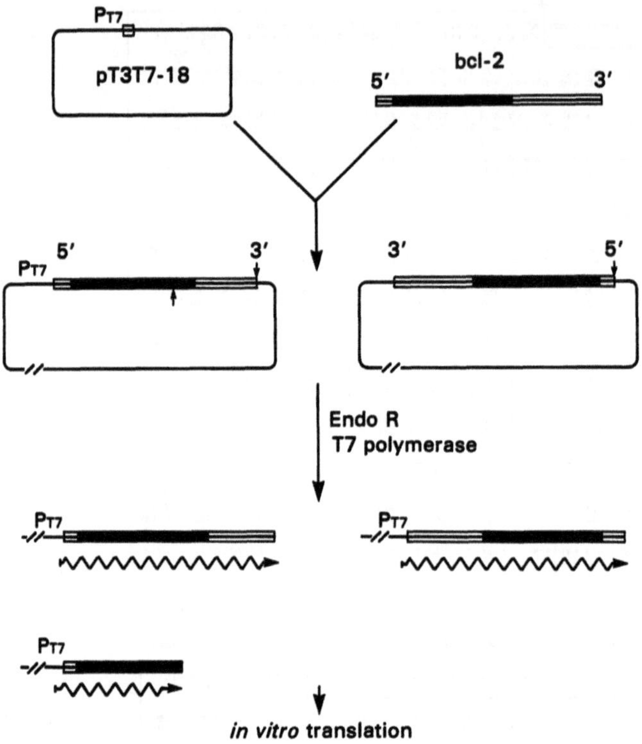

Figure 4. In vitro translation of bcl-2 mRNA.

(A) Strategy for preparation of bcl-2 mRNA in vitro. The cDNA sequences (-93 to +1348) corresponding to 5.5 kb transcript were subcloned into pT3T7-18 vector (BRL). The open reading frame is shown by the filled box. After linearizing template DNAs at the end of cDNA insert and/or within the open reading frame (at +563), bcl-2 mRNA was produced by T7 RNA polymerase. About 0.5 ug (shown by wavy lines) of RNA was assayed by in vitro translation system (Ricciardi et al., 1979).

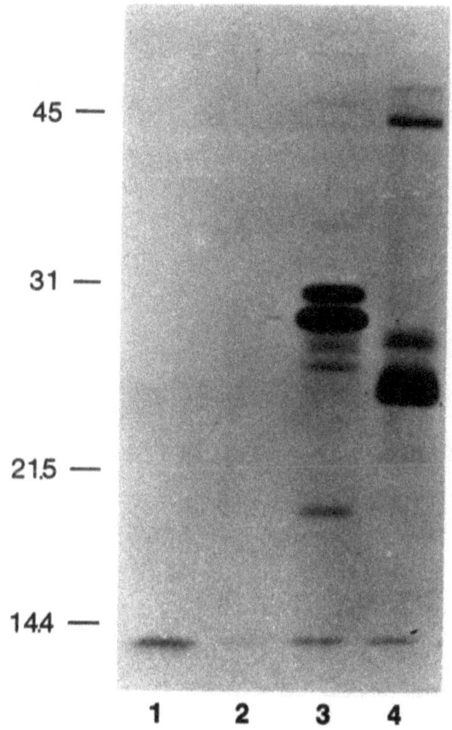

(B) Analysis of in vitro translation product by SDS 12.5% polyacrylamide gel electrophoresis. Lane 1, no RNA; lane 2, antisense bcl-2 RNA; lane 3, sense RNA; lane 4, sense RNA truncated within the open reading frame (at +563 in Fig. 3). The size is shown in kilo dalton.

Genomic Organization of bcl-2 Gene

As described above, cDNA sequences corresponding to 5.5 kb transcript consists of at least two exons. To identify the 5' exon(s), the genomic clone, 18-27 was obtained which hybridized with the 5' region of the B4 clone (5' end to BamHI site). The restriction map of 18-27 is shown in Fig. 5. The restriction mapping and DNA sequencing of the part of genomic clone indicate that 18-27 DNA has all cDNA sequences 5' to the splice site and also that the genomic DNA sequences are colinear to B16 and B15 cDNA sequences without any intervening sequence. Thus, 3.5 kb mRNA is transcribed from this 5' exon without any intron. On the other hand, 5.5 kb transcript is produced by splicing within the first exon and joining to the second (3') exon. The genomic clone 18-27 does not overlap with any genomic clones containing DNA sequences of or 5' to the second exon which has been described previously (Tsujimoto et. al. 1985d). This indicates that two exons are separated by more than 50 kb intervening sequence.

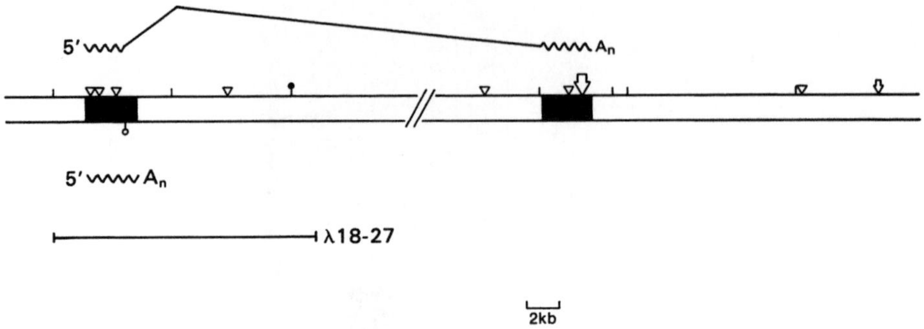

Fig. 5 Genomic organization of bcl-2 gene.

The filled boxes represent two exons of bcl-2 gene. Two difference mRNA, 5.5 kb and 3.5 kb are also shown by wavy lines. 18-27 genomic clone was obtained by screening 380 genomic DNA library with 5' region probe of B4 cDNA clone. The two breakpoint hot spots of the t(14;18) translocation are shown by arrows (⇩). The restriction sites are shown by ▽ for SstI ⫯ for HindIII, ⫰ for BamHI and ⌈ for SalI.

The bcl-2 gene represents a likely candidate for being involved directly in the pathogenesis of follicular lymphoma as a result of its transcriptional deregulation. To determine whether deregulation of the bcl-2 gene results in B cell neoplasia, we intend to introduce the bcl-2 open reading frames in retrovirus vectors and to assess their transforming activity.

REFERENCES:

Bakshi, A., Jensen, J. P., Goldman, P., Wright, J. J., McBride, O. W., Epstein, A. L. and Korsmeyer, S. J. (1985). Cloning the chromosomal breakpoint of t(14;18) human lymphomas: clustering around J_H on chromosome 14 and near a transcription unit on 18. Cell 41:899-906.

Cleary, ML, Sklar J (1985). Nucleotide sequence of a t(14;18) chromosomal breakpoint in follicular lymphoma and demonstration of a breakpoint-cluster region near a transcriptionally active locus on chromosome 18. Proc Natl Acad Sci USA 82:7439-7443.

Croce, CM, Shander M, Martinis J, Cicurel L, D'Ancoma GG, Dolby TW, Koprowski H (1979). Chromosomal location of the genes for human immunoglobulin heavy chains. Proc Natl Acad Sci USA 76:3416-3419.

Croce, Thierfelder W, Erikson J, Nishikura K, Finan J, Lenoir G, Nowell PC (1983). Transcriptional activation of an unrearranged and untranslocated c-myc oncogene by translocation of a Cλ locus in Burkitt lymphoma cells. Proc. Natl. Acad. Sci. USA 80:6922-6926.

Dalla Favera R, Bregni M, Erikson J, Patterson D, Gallo RC, Croce CM (1982). Human c-myc oncogene is located on the region of chromosome σ that is translocated in Burkitt lymphoma cells. Proc Natl Acad Sci USA 79:7824-7827.

Erikson J, Finan J, Nowell, PC, Croce CM (1982). Translocation of immunoglobulin V_H genes in Burkitt lymphoma. Proc Natl Acad Sci USA 79:5611-5615.

Erikson J, Nishikura K, ar-Rushdi A, Finan J, Emanuel BS, Lenoir G, Nowell PC, Croce CM (1983). Translocation of an immunoglobulin κ locus to a region 3' of an unrearranged c-myc oncogene enhances c-myc transcription. Proc Natl Acad Sci USA 80:7581-7585.

Nishikura K, ar-Rushdi A, Erikson J, Watt R, Rovera G, Croce CM (1983). Differential expression of the normal and of the translocated human c-myc oncogenes in B cells. Proc. Natl. Acad. Sci. USA 80:4822-4826.

Nowell PC, Shankey TV, Finan J, Guerry D, Besa E (1981). Proliferation, differentiation and cytogenetics of chronic leukemic B lymphocytes cultured with mitomycin-treated normal cells. Blood 57:444-451.

Ricciardi RP, Miller JS, Roberts BE (1979). Purification and mapping of specific nRNAs by hybridization - selection and cell-free translation. Proc Natl. Acad. Sci. USA 76:4927-4951.

Tsujimoto Y, Yunis J, Onorato-Showe L, Nowell PC, Croce CM (1984). Molecular cloning of the chromosomal breakpoint of B-cell lymphomas and leukemias with the t(11;14) chromosome translocation Science 224:1403-1406.

Tsujimoto Y, Jaffe E, Cossman J, Gorham J, Nowell PC, Croce CM (1985a). Clustering of breakpoints on chromosome 11 in human B-cell neoplasms with the t(11;14) chromosome translocation. Nature, 315:340-343.

Tsujimoto Y, Finger LR, Yunis J, Nowell PC, Croce CM (1985b). Cloning of the chromosome breakpoint of neoplastic B-cells with the t(14;18) chromosome translocation. Science 226:1097-1099.

Tsujimoto Y, Gorhma J, Cossman J, Jaffe E, Croce CM (1985c). The t(14;18) chromosome translocations involved in B-cell neoplasms result from mistakes in V-D-J joining. Science 229:1390-1393.

Tsujimoto Y, Cossman J, Jaffe E, Croce CM (1985d). Involvement of bcl-2 gene in human follicular lymphoma. Science 228:1440-1443.

Van den Berghe H, Parloir C, David G, Michaux JL, Sokal G (1979). A new characteristic karyotypic anomaly in lymphoproliferative disorders. Cancer 44:188-195.

Van den Berghe H, Vermaelen K, Louwagie A, Criel A, Mecucci C, Vaerman J-P (1984). High incidence of chromosome abnormalities in IgG3 myeloma. Cancer Genet. Cytogenet. 11:381-387.

Yunis JJ, Oken MM, Kaplan ME, Ensrud KM, Howe RB, Theologides A (1982). Distinctive chromosomal abnormalities in histologic subtypes of non-Hodgkin's lymphoma. N. Engl. J. Med. 307:1231-1236.

Yunis JJ, Oken MM, Theologides A, Howe RB, Kaplan ME (1984). Recurrent chromosomal defects are found in most patients with non-Hodgkin's-lymphoma. Cancer Genet. Cytogenet. 13:17-28.

c-*myc* and Functionally Related Oncogenes Induce Both High Rates of Sister Chromatid Exchange and Abnormal Karyotypes in Rat Fibroblasts

C. Cerni[+], E. Mougneau[*], M. Zerlin[°], M. Julius[°], K.B. Marcu[°], and F. Cuzin[*]

[+] Institute of Tumorbiology-Cancer Research, University of Vienna, A-1090 Vienna, Austria
[°] Department of Biochemistry, State University of New York, Stony Brook, N.Y. 11794, USA
[*] Centre de Biochimie, Université de Nice, Parc Valrose, 06034 Nice, France

INTRODUCTION

Activated myc genes are found in a broad variety of spontaneous malignancies in rodents and humans as well: Burkitt Lymphoma (Klein and Klein 1985; Croce et al. 1984; Dalla-Favera et al. 1985; this volume), neuroblastoma (Schwab 1985), small cell lung carcinoma (Nau et al. 1985), mouse plasmacytoma (Klein and Klein 1985; this volume) and rat immunocytoma (Pear, this volume).

On the cytogenetic level these malignant diseases have in common either specific chromosomal translocations or chromosomal alterations characteristic for gene amplification, both involving myc genes. This has led to the conclusions that 1. c-myc is overexpressed by specific rearrangements, and 2. activation of myc somehow causes malignant transformation. However, clonality of myc-induced neoplasia in transgenic mice (Stewart et al. 1984; Adams et al. 1985; this volume) points to the need for a rare second event in myc-expressing tissues to generate malignancy. Similarly, the tumorigenic conversion of cultured rat lines expressing high levels of myc is not a direct consequence of deregulated myc gene expression but also requires other genetic events (Zerlin et al., this volume).

Data are presented on a feature of c-myc and functionally related oncogenes by which they might contribute to this process of malignant transformation. Transfer of these genes into cultured rat fibroblast cells are associated with an increase in genetic recombination.

SISTER CHROMATID EXCHANGE

DNA rearrangements seem to play a crucial role in the oncogenic transformation pathway (Cairns 1981). Determination of SCE frequencies, the exchange of two DNA strands at apparently homologous loci, has proven to be a general measure of recombinational events induced by almost all mutagenic and/or carcinogenic agents (Wolff 1982). We have re-examined the question of their relationship with cell transformation by studying SCE rates in a collection of rat cell lines transformed by various oncogenes. For SCE determination, cells were exposed to 20µM bromodeoxyuridine (BrdU), a concentration within the range where the number of SCE does not depend on the dose of BrdU (Cerni 1984).

Current Topics in Microbiology and Immunology, Vol. 132

Studies of SCE in FR3T3 cells, a diploid, non-transformed, high-serum dependent rat cell line (Seif and Cuzin 1977), revealed a distribution centered around 0.27 SCE per chromosome (see Fig. 2), with less than 5% of the total above 0.40 ("high SCE fraction"). This was considered a suitable reference point for SCE comparison among various Fisher rat derived cell lines (Cerni and Mougneau 1984). Results obtained on cell lines derived from primary rat embryo fibroblast (REF) were always in good agreement with those obtained on FR3T3 derivatives.

SCE increase in FR3T3 cells expressing high levels of myc

We prepared clones of FR3T3 cells that express high levels of c-myc from one of two mouse expression vectors: SVc-myc1 (Land et al. 1983) and FVXMc-myc (Zerlin et al., this volume). Details on myc expression in these lines are presented elsewhere (Zerlin et al., this volume). Figure 1 shows characteristic metaphases of a control line and a line expressing high levels of c-myc.

A B

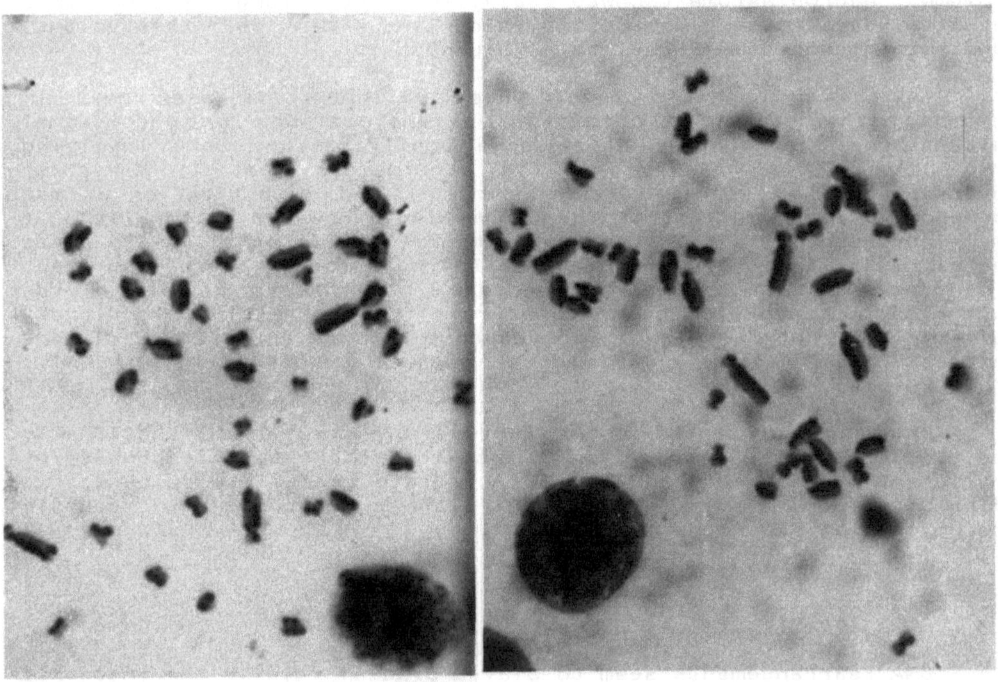

Fig. 1. Differentially stained metaphases of FR-pSVc-myc (A) and FR-pSVneo (B)

SCE distribution patterns of individual clones and of populations which comprise about 200 clones are shown in Fig. 2. FR3T3 samples denoted with an (e) or an (l) refer to lines that were maintained for less than 10 or more than 60 transfers in culture respectively (Zerlin et al., in preparation). The SCE rates in these cell lines revealed an increase of the high-SCE-fraction to 33%-55% of the metaphases, a 8 to 15 fold increase above the values observed in the parental FR3T3 or in a control line, FR-pSVneo (Fig. 1).

FR3T3 cells were also infected at early and late passages with the MMCV(neo) retrovirus that expresses the OK10 v-myc gene (Wagner et al. 1985). SCE inducibility was found to be high in both cases.

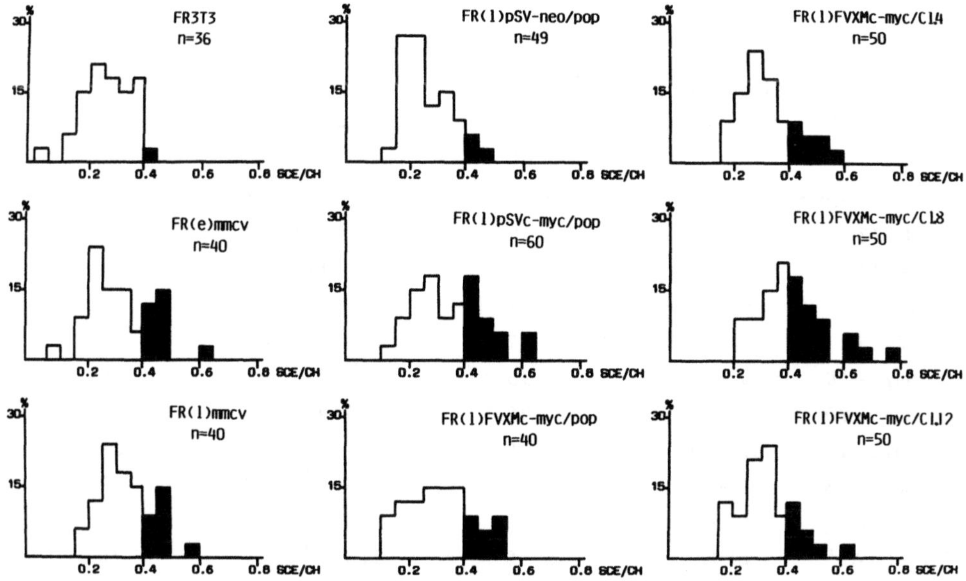

Fig. 2. SCE distribution pattern of FR3T3 derived lines expressing high levels of myc.
The high SCE fraction (percent of metaphases with more than 0.4 SCE per chromosome) correspond to the closed bars in each graph. The total number of metaphases studied (n) is indicated for each cell line. FR(e) and FR(l) indicate transfection of either early-passage or late-passage FR3T3. The frequencies of SCEs were determined in individual clones (Cl) and in populations (pop) consisting of about 200 clones.

Increase of SCE after transfer of "immortalising" oncogenes

We investigated whether the ability of the myc gene to increase SCE frequencies is restricted to this oncogene, or shared by functionally related genes. It was shown that a group of oncogenes including in addition to myc the polyoma virus plt (large T protein) and adenovirus E1A genes have a variety of properties in common (Rassoulzadegan et al. 1982, 1983; van den Elsen et al. 1982; Land et al. 1983; Ruley 1983; Mougneau et al. 1984): 1. they immortalize normal rodent cells in culture, 2. they reduce serum requirement in some rodent cells, and 3. they cooperate with other oncogenes (such as ras or polyoma pmt or adenovirus E1B) in the malignant transformation of normal rodent cells. Table 1 shows SCE frequencies of a series of early-passage FR3T3- and rat embryo fibroblast (REF) derived lines after transfer of different class I oncogenes. Clones were isolated by their ability to grow at low serum concentration (FR3T3-derived) or to have extended life span in culture (REF-derived). Details on these lines will be published elsewhere (Cerni et al. in preparation). All cell lines obtained by transfer of class I oncogenes had elevated SCEs with high SCE fractions amounting to as much as one third of the metaphases or more.

Cell line	Oncogene (plasmid)	Number of metaphases studied	SCE/Chrom. mean±SEM	High SCE fraction (%)
FR3T3	-	36	0.270±0.02	3
FR-LT1	pPYLT1	40	0.321±0.02	24
RAT-LT1	pPYLT1	54	0.431±0.02	47
RAT-LT2	pPYLT1	52	0.323±0.02	21
FR-cmyc-10	pSVc-myc-1	35	0.284±0.02	9
FR-cmyc-20	pSVc-myc-1	40	0.314±0.02	15
FR-vmyc-11	pSVv-myc	40	0.330±0.02	21
FR-vmyc-23	pSV-myc	50	0.341±0.02	32
RAT-vmyc3	pSV-myc	72	0.337±0.02	26
RAT-E1A3	pE1A	50	0.330±0.02	20

Table 1. SCE in rat cells after transfer of class I oncogenes. Individual immortalizing oncogenes were transfered either into FR3T3 (FR lines) or in REF (RAT lines).

SCE in rat cells after transfer of pmt or ras

FR3T3 cells were transfected with the pmt gene which codes for polyoma virus middle T antigen or with a mutated human ras gene (EJ6.6). SCE determination revealed that these genes, which convert FR3T3 into highly tumorigenic cells (1×10^6 cells injected into newborn syngeneic animals produce tumors detectable after 4 days, our unpublished observation), did not affect the SCE rates (Fig. 3).

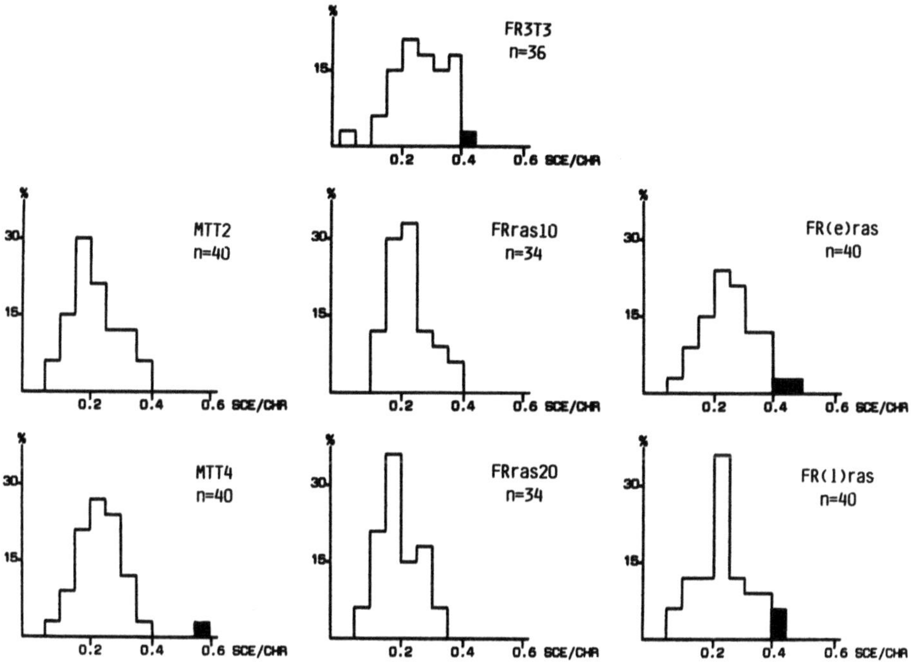

Fig. 3. SCE distribution patterns in cell lines expressing pmt or ras oncogenes. MTT4 and MTT2 express the pmt gene coding for polyoma middle T; FRras10 and 20 express a mutated human ras gene; FR(e)ras and FR(l)ras were derived from early and late passage FR3T3 cells by infection with a H-ras retrovirus vector (L.W. Stanton and K.B. Marcu, unpublished results).

SCE in cell lines carrying different oncogenes

We next investigated the SCE rates in cells transfected with both a class I oncogene and either pmt or ras.

MTT4-derived cell lines carrying either plt, myc or E1A were isolated by their ability to grow in low serum concentration, a property which is confered by these genes (Rassoulzadegan et al. 1982; Mougneau et al. 1984). As shown in Table 2, this "complementation" to a fully transformed phenotype hardly affects SCE compared to the parental MTT4 cells.

In another experiment, FR-LT1 and FR-vmyc-23 cells, both showing increased SCE rates, were transfected with the ras gene and clones were isolated on the basis of their focus forming ability. SCE determination in several clones revealed a reduction of SCE frequencies (Table 2).

Cell line	Complementing oncogene (plasmid)	Number of metaphases studied	SCE/Chrom. mean±SEM	High SCE fraction (%)
MTT4	-	40	0.216±0.02	0
MTT4-LT1	pPYLT1	50	0.251±0.02	6
MTT4-cmyc-1	pSVc-myc-1	40	0.247±0.02	3
MTT4-vmyc-6	pSVv-myc	40	0.233±0.02	8
MTT4-E1A7	pE1A	40	0.252±0.02	3
FR-LT1	-	40	0.321±0.02	24
FR-LT-ras1	pEJ6.6	50	0.255±0.01	2
FR-vmyc23	-	40	0.341±0.02	32
FR-vmyc-ras1	pEJ6.6	40	0.174±0.02	0
FR-vmyc-ras2	pEJ6.6	40	0.212±0.02	0
FR-vmyc-ras3	pEJ6.6	40	0.200±0.02	3

Table 2. SCE of MTT4 cells complemented with class I oncogenes and class I oncogene-transfected cells complemented with ras.

Abnormal karyotypes in the myc/plt group

The elevated SCEs in the myc/plt group indicated increased rearrangements. This observation was further substantiated by abnormal numbers of chromosomes invariably found in this group (Table 3). Only a few lines remained apparently diploid (2n=42), the others showed either slight (2n=40-44) or severe heteroploidy. This was never seen in the ras/pmt cells, which remained diploid in spite of profound morphological alterations and of a high degree of tumorigenicity.

	Number of cell lines studied	Karyotype 2n=42	2n=40-44	heteroploid
CLASS I ONCOGENES (*plt*, E1A, *myc*)	18	5	5	8
CLASS II ONCOGENES (*pmt*, *ras*)	7	7	-	-
CLASS II + I (MTT4 cells complemented by *plt*, E1A, *myc*)	9	7	2	-
CLASS I + II (FR-LT1 and FR-v-myc23 complemented by *ras*)	8	8	-	-

Table 3. Karyotypes in cell lines expressing individual oncogenes of class I and II or in combination.

CONCLUSION

Increased genomic instability mediated by legitimate or illegitimate recombination is generally considered an important aspect of oncogenic transformation (Cairns 1981). One of the few assays which is indicative for increased recombinational activities in eukaryotic cells on the chromosomal level, is determination of SCEs. Transfer into embryonic or established rat fibroblast cells of "immortalizing" oncogenes such as c-*myc*, v-*myc*, *plt* and E1A resulted in substantial increases of SCEs. This was not observed in cell lines which express one of the oncogenes responsible for the terminal stage of tumorigenic transformation (*pmt*, mutated *ras* genes), nor in cell lines carrying oncogenes of both types.

Data are provided which indicate that the first step in the tumorigenic transformation pathway, mediated by class I oncogenes, is associated with increased recombinational events. It is conceivable that the contribution of such genes to cellular transformation results at least partially from the induction of rearrangements. The conspicuous genomic destabilisation induced by these genes is further substantiated by the observation of abnormal karyotypes, exclusively found in the *myc*/*plt* group. This was never found in cell lines transformed with *ras* or *pmt*.

The significance of the low SCE values in the highly tumorigenic *pmt* or *ras* lines and the non-additivity of phenotypes corresponding to the expression of individual genes are less obvious. However, we observed on several occasions that tumor-derived re-established cell lines invariably have lower SCEs compared to the cells originally injected (Cerni, unpublished results). It could be that selective pressure for more efficiently growing cells, *in vivo* as well as *in vitro*, leads to progenies with new combinations of oncogenes where continuous increase in recombination frequencies and karyotypic abnormalities are no longer advantageous but rather deleterious. Experiments are in progress to investigate this possibility.

ACKNOWLEDGEMENTS

This work received support from "Medizinisch-Wissenschaftlicher Fonds des Bürgermeisters der Bundeshauptstadt Wien", awarded to CC, from "Association pour la Recherche sur le Cancer" (France), awarded to FC, and from the National Institutes of Health, awarded to KBM. KBM is a Research Carrier Development Awardee of the US National Institutes of Health.

REFERENCES

Adams, JM, Harris, AW, Pinkert, CA, Corcoran, LM, Alexander, WS, Cory, S, Palmiter, RD & Brinster, RL (1985) The c-*myc* oncogene driven by immunoglobuline enhancers induces lymphoid malignancy in transgenic mice. Nature 318: 533-538

Cairns, J (1981) The origin of human cancers. Nature 289: 353-357

Cerni, C & Mougneau, E (1984) Sister chromatid exchange (SCE) in FR3T3 rat fibroblasts transformed by simian virus 40. Exp Cell Res 154: 83-94

Cerni, C (1984) Effect of tissue culture variables on sister chromatid exchange in a nontransformed rat cell line. In Vitro 20: 305-313

Croce, CM, Thierfelder, W, Erikson, J, Nishikura, K, Finan, J, Lenoir, GM & Nowell, PC (1983) Transcriptional activation of an unrearranged and untranslocated c-*myc* oncogene by translocation of a C locus in Burkitt lymphoma cells. Proc Natl Acad Sci USA 80: 6922-6926

Dalla-Favera, R, Martinotti, S, Gallo, RC, Erikson, J & Croce, CM (1983) Translocation and rearrangements of the c-*myc* oncogene locus in human undifferentiated B-cell lymphomas. Science 219: 963-967

Klein, G & Klein, E (1985) Evolution of tumours and the impact of molecular oncology. Nature 315: 190-195

Land, H, Parada, LF & Weinberg, RA (1983) Tumorigenic conversion of primary embryo fibroblasts requires at least two cooperating oncogenes. Nature 304: 596-602

Mougneau, E, Lemieux, M, Rassoulzadegan, M & Cuzin, F (1984) Biological activities of the v-*myc* and of rearranged c-*myc* oncogenes in rat fibroblast cells in culture. Proc Natl Acad Sci USA 81: 5758-5762

Nau, MM, Brooks, BJ, Battey, J, Sausville, E, Gazdar, AF, Kirsch, IR, McBride, OW, Bertness, V, Hollis, GF & Minna, JD (1985) L-*myc*: a new *myc*-related gene amplified and expressed in human small cell lung cancer. Nature 318: 69-73

Rassoulzadegan, M, Cowie, A, Carr, A, Glaichenhaus, N, Kamen, R & Cuzin, F (1982) The roles of individual polyoma virus early proteins in oncogenic transformation. Nature 300: 713-718

Rassoulzadegan, M, Naghashfar, Z, Cowie, A, Carr, A, Grisoni, M, Kamen, R & Cuzin, F (1983) Expression of the large T protein of polyoma virus promotes the establishment in culture of "normal" rodent fibroblast cell lines. Proc Natl Acad Sci USA 80:4354-4358.

Ruley, HE (1983) Adenovirus early region 1A enables viral and cellular transforming genes to transform primary cells in culture. Nature 304: 602-606

Schwab, M (1985) Amplification of N-myc in human neuroblastomas. Trends Gen 1: 271-275

Seif, R & Cuzin, F (1977) Temperature-sensitive growth regulation in one type of transformed rat cells induced by the tsa mutant of polyoma virus. J Virol 24: 721-728

Stewart, TA, Pattengale, PK & Leder, P (1984) Spontaneous mammary adenocarcinomas in transgenic mice that carry and express MTV/myc fusion genes. Cell 38: 627-637

Van den Elsen, P, de Pater, S, Houweling, A, van de Veer & van der Eb, A (1982) The relationship between region Ela and Elb of human adenoviruses in cell transformation. Gene 18:175-185

Wagner, EF, Vanek, M & Vennström, B (1985) Transfer of genes into embryonal carcinoma cells by retrovirus infection: efficient expression from an internal promotor. The EMBO J. 4: 663-666

Wolff, S (1982) Sister chromatid exchange. Wiley & Sons, NY

Chromosomal Radiosensitivity During G_2 Phase and Susceptibility to Plasmacytoma Induction in Mice

K.K. Sanford, R. Parshad[1], M. Potter[2], G.M. Jones, R.P. Nordan[2], S.E. Brust[2], and F.M. Price

Laboratory of Cellular and Molecular Biology, National Cancer Institute, Bethesda, MD 20892

INTRODUCTION

Genetic differences in susceptibility to plasmacytoma induction among inbred strains of mice are well documented. Whether induced by i.p. implantation of plastic discs or injection of pristane, the BALB/c mouse, in contrast to most other commonly used inbred strains, is significantly more susceptible (Merwin and Redmon, 1963; Morse et al., 1980; Potter et al., 1984). The F_1 hybrid between BALB/c and a resistant strain such as DBA/2 is resistant. This and other findings on hybrid crosses suggest that specific genes for susceptibility and/or resistance determine tumor incidence (Potter et al., 1975; Potter and Wax, 1981). Studies are in progress to identify these genes through the development of congenic BALB/c sublines carrying genes from a resistant strain. Particularly useful in this endeavor is the BALB/cJ mouse, which was separated in 1937 from the BALB/cAn subline; although showing minimal genetic drift in most properties, the BALB/cJ mouse is resistant to plasmacytoma induction (Potter and Wax, 1981, 1985).

Mechanisms underlying genetic susceptibility to plasmacytomagenesis are largely unknown. However, our recent studies on human cells in culture in relation to cancer susceptibility have provided an approach for exploring this problem. Irradiation of human cells in culture during the G_2 period of the cell cycle with x-rays or fluorescent light (effective wavelength in the visible range, 405 nm) produces chromatid breaks and gaps seen in the first posttreatment metaphase. The metaphase chromosome consists of two chromatids joined at the centromere or spindle attachment site. Aberrations scored as breaks show chromatid discontinuity and misalignment with displacement of the broken segment to varying degrees. Since each chromatid is formed by coiling and folding of a fiber containing a single continuous DNA double strand associated with protein, a chromatid break represents an unrepaired DNA double strand break (Kihlman, 1971; Evans, 1977). Aberrations scored as chromatid gaps show an apparent discontinuity longer than the chromatid width with no misalignment or displacement of the segment distal to the lesion. Several lines of evidence indicate that radiation-induced chromatid gaps represent unrepaired DNA single-strand breaks (Bender et al., 1974; Natarajan et al., 1980; Parshad et al., 1985; Sanford et al., 1985).

In examining the influence of x-irradiation on cells in G_2 phase of the cell cycle, synchronization of cells is unnecessary since only metaphase cells are examined. In cultures x-irradiated, incubated for 0.5 h to allow mitotic cells to complete division, treated with Colcemid to accumulate cells in metaphase, and processed within

[1]Department of Pathology, Howard University College of Medicine, Washington, DC 20059
[2]Laboratory of Genetics, National Cancer Institute, Bethesda, MD 20892

Current Topics in Microbiology and Immunology, Vol. 132

1.5 h of irradiation, one can be assured that each metaphase cell examined was irradiated in late G_2 phase or within 1.5 h of metaphase. Under these conditions, we found that apparently normal skin fibroblasts from individuals with genetic disorders predisposing to a high risk of cancer, compared with skin fibroblasts from normal controls, showed a significantly higher incidence of chromatid aberrations (Parshad et al., 1983). Furthermore, apparently normal skin fibroblasts from individuals with diverse neoplasms and from families with a history of neoplastic disease showed a significantly higher incidence of chromatid breaks and gaps when irradiated during G_2 phase than cells from normal controls, 28 cell lines to date, derived from individuals ranging in age from 1 to 96 yrs (Parshad et al., 1985b and unpublished). Thus, enhanced G_2 chromatid radiosensitivity, resulting from deficient DNA repair during G_2 phase, is associated with genetic susceptibility to cancer.

Enhanced G_2 chromatid radiosensitivity also has a genetic basis. In human somatic cell hybrids between a tumor cell and a normal cell, the enhanced radiosensitivity, like tumorigenicity, is suppressed or complemented and segregates with the neoplastic phenotype in tumorigenic segregants (Sanford et al., 1986).

The DNA repair deficiency in cancer-prone individuals appears to be a prerequisite and driving force in carcinogenesis. DNA lesions induced in living cells by exogenous or endogenous insults, if unrepaired during G_2 phase, would accumulate with cell cycling and lead to the continuous emergence of new genetic variants. Certain of these variants with enhanced growth potential would be selected *in vivo* and are candidates for progression to a more autonomously proliferating cell type.

CHROMATID RADIOSENSITIVITY OF BALB/c AND DBA/2 MOUSE CELLS

These observations on chromatid radiosensitivity associated with deficient DNA repair in human cells suggested that a similar mechanism might account for the susceptibility of the BALB/c mouse to plasmacytomagenesis. Accordingly, we compared the G_2 chromatid radiosensitivity of BALB/c LPS-stimulated B-lymphocytes with those of a plasmacytoma-resistant DBA/2 mouse and the resistant F_1 hybrid, BALB/c x DBA/2 (CDF_1) (Fig. 1).

The frequencies of chromatid gaps and breaks induced by 100 R irradiation in cells from the two parental strains and their F_1 hybrid were initially similar when examined at 0.5 h post irradiation, an observation indicating no significant difference in susceptibility to irradiation-induced damage. Nor did they differ markedly in chromatid gap formation. A maximal response at 1.5 h post irradiation dropped to a plateau from 3 to 4.5 h. Frequencies of chromatid breaks for both plasmacytoma-resistant lines, DBA/2 and CDF_1, decreased at a similar rate with post-irradiation time. However, the response of BALB/c cells differed. Significantly more chromatid breaks remained in BALB/c cells at post-irradiation times of 2.5 h or more than in either of the resistant lines. Thus, the BALB/c cells appeared to repair the radiation-induced DNA double strand breaks more slowly than the plasmacytoma-resistant cells. Similar results were obtained following a 2 h exposure to fluorescent light (data not shown). Furthermore, as with human cells, the enhanced G_2 chromatid radiosensitivity of the BALB/c mouse appeared to behave as a recessive trait in the F_1 hybrid mouse.

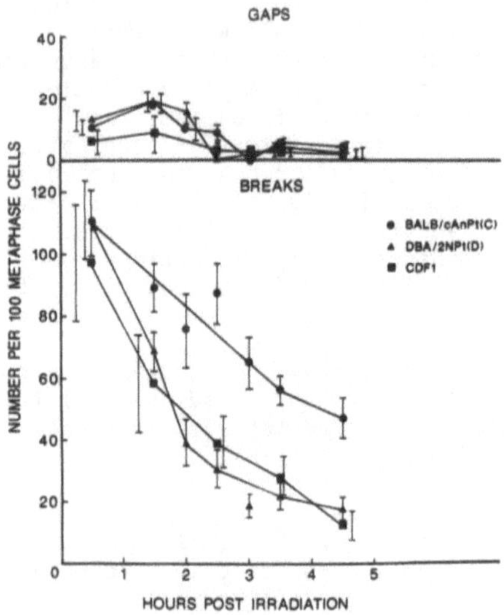

Fig. 1. Influence of time after x-irradiation (100R) on chromatid aberrations in B-lymphoblasts. Washed spleen cells, ~ 5 x 10^6, were inoculated into T-25 flasks in 5 ml DMEM with 10% fetal bovine serum, 5 x 10^{-5} M mercaptoethanol and 10 µg/ml lipopolysaccharide (LPS) to stimulate B-lymphocytes. After 48 to 96 h incubation at 37°C, cultures were x-irradiated. Those harvested at 0.5 h post irradiation received Colcemid (0.1 µg/ml) directly after irradiation. In all other cultures the irradiated medium was replaced directly after irradiation and Colcemid added 1 h before harvest. Cultures were incubated at 37°C until harvesting and processing for chromosome analysis. Data were pooled from several experiments following statistical evaluation. With few exceptions, each determination is based on more than 100 metaphase cells examined. Vertical bars represent standard errors of the mean.

To determine whether the enhanced radiosensitivity is a genetic trait affecting other tissues of the BALB/c mouse we examined the response of skin fibroblasts to x-irradiation during G_2 phase (Fig. 2). Cells from the BALB/c mouse again showed a significantly higher frequency of chromatid breaks than those from the DBA/2 mouse when examined 1.5 h after x-irradiation.

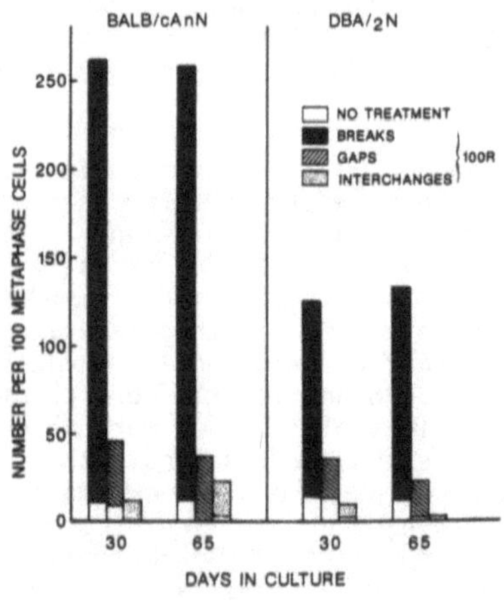

Fig. 2. Influence of x-irradiation (100R) during G_2 phase on chromatid damage in skin fibroblasts of 10-18 day-old mice. Skin freed of fur, minced, washed, digested with collagenase for 24 h was used to initiate cultures in T-25 flasks grown in DMEM with 10% fetal bovine serum and antibiotics. Cultures in the 6th and 10th passage were used for assay as described previously (Parshad et al., 1985b). Antibiotics were removed after the first 5 passages. Cells were fixed at 1.5 h after x-irradiation. Each determination is based on 31 to 100 metaphase cells examined.

As noted earlier, the BALB/cJ subline is relatively resistant to plasmacytoma induction but otherwise genetically very similar to the BALB/cAn subline. B-lymphoblasts from the BALB/cJ subline, like DBA/2 cells, showed a more rapid decrease in chromatid breaks with time after x-irradiation (100R), presumably from more efficient repair of radiation-induced DNA strand breaks, than B-lymphoblasts of BALB/cAnPt origin (Fig. 3). Spleen fibroblasts from these two sublines also reflected this difference in G_2 chromatid radiosensitivity when examined 1.5 h after x-irradiation (Fig. 4).

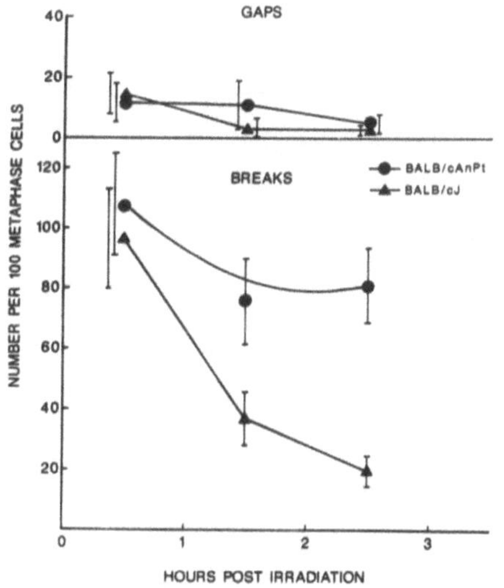

Fig. 3. Influence of time after x-irradiation (100R) on chromatid aberrations in B-lymphoblasts. For procedure, see legend Fig. 2. In this experiment, each determination is based on 26 to 76 metaphase cells examined.

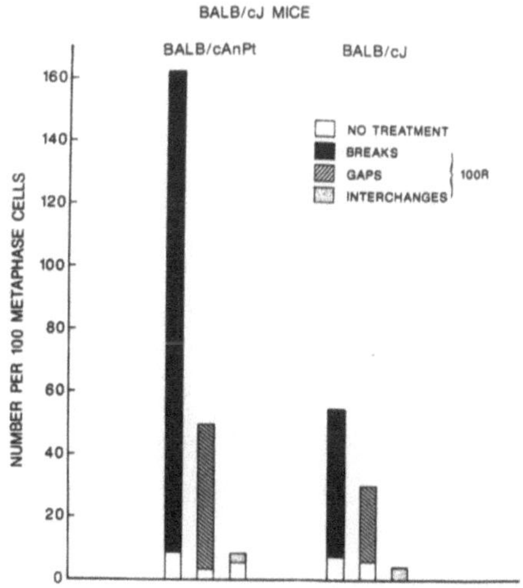

Fig. 4. Influence of x-irradiation (100R) during G_2 phase on chromatid damage in spleen fibroblasts of 1 to 2 mo-old mice. Cells were assayed after 2 to 4 passages, 19 to 47 days in culture. Cells grown in DMEM with 10% fetal bovine serum were fixed at 1.5 h after x-irradiation. Each determination is based on at least 50 metaphase cells examined.

These findings indicate an association between enhanced G_2 chromatid radiosensitivity, resulting from deficient DNA repair during G_2 phase, and susceptibility to plasmacytoma induction.

"SPONTANEOUS" CHROMOSOMAL TRANSLOCATIONS IN CULTURE

This deficiency in DNA repair may contribute to the formation of chromosomal translocations. As noted, DNA double strand breaks are repaired more slowly in the BALB/cAnPt mouse, leaving broken ends available for chromatid interchanges and subsequent chromosomal translocations. One type of translocation is metacentric chromosome formation. The mouse chromosome is normally acrocentric with the centromere near one end, whereas in the metacentric chromosome, the centromere is median. Metacentric chromosomes arise during G_1 phase by breaks in two chromosomes followed by an interchange or translocation between the broken segments (Parshad and Sanford, 1968). In populations of LPS-stimulated, nonirradiated B-lymphocytes examined at different intervals in culture, up to 96 h, increasing numbers of metacentric chromosomes appeared among BALB/cAnPt cells (Fig. 5). None were observed in DBA/2NPt and an intermediate number in the F_1 hybrid.

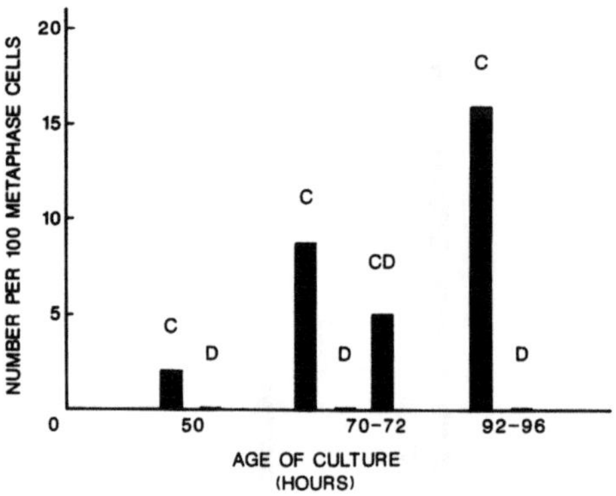

Fig. 5. "Spontaneous" incidence of metacentric chromosomes in B-lymphoblasts of BALB/cAnPt (C), DBA/2NPt (D) and (BALB/cAnPt x DBA/2NPt) F_1 (CD) mice.

Likewise, the deficiency in DNA repair in B-lymphocytes of the BALB/cAnPt mouse may contribute to the formation of the rcpt 12:15 and rcpt 6:15 chromosomal translocations that occur in over 98% of pristane-induced plasmacytomas (for review see Potter et al., 1984). These translocations deregulate or activate the c-myc oncogene, confer a strong proliferative stimulus and apparently play a critical role in plasmacytogenesis.

In the development of mineral oil or pristane-induced plasmacytomas, the foci of dividing plasma cells appear first in the inflammatory tissue or oil granuloma that forms in response to the oil (Potter et al., 1985). Phagocytes in inflammatory lesions enzymatically reduce oxygen to reactive metabolites including hydrogen peroxide, hydroxyl radicals and superoxide anions (Weitberg et al., 1983). These reactive species are known to damage DNA, causing chromatid breaks and chromosomal aberrations (Sanford et al., 1986; Jones et al., 1985). Active proliferation in the presence of this low to moderate DNA damage during the G_2 period of the cell cycle when the cells are deficient in DNA repair may so stress the cells capacity to maintain fidelity of DNA replication as to increase the probability of further mutations, genetic instability and cell heterogeneity. Thus the deficiency in G_2 DNA repair combined with activation of an oncogene stimulating proliferation or cell cycling may be the only critical ingredients required for progression to malignancy in plasmacytomagenesis.

SUMMARY AND CONCLUSIONS

1. We have presented evidence that susceptibility to plasmacytomagenesis in the BALB/cAnPt mouse is associated with enhanced chromatid radiosensitivity, resulting from deficient repair of DNA strand breaks during G_2 phase.

2. In the BALB/cAnPt mouse, DNA double strand breaks are repaired more slowly, leaving broken ends available for chromatid interchanges and subsequent chromosomal translocations; this deficiency in DNA repair thus provides a mechanism for the chromosomal translocations associated with plasmacytomas.

3. The deficiency in DNA repair during G_2 phase may be a prerequisite and driving force in plasmacytomagenesis, leading to the emergence of new genetic variants selected *in vivo* for their growth potential and autonomy.

4. From observations on the F_1 hybrid mice, both susceptibility to plasmacytomagenesis and enhanced G_2 chromatid radiosensitivity appear to behave as recessive traits.

ACKNOWLEDGEMENT

We are grateful to Dr. Robert E. Tarone, Biostatistics Branch, National Cancer Institute, for statistical analysis of data.

REFERENCES

Bender MA, Griggs HG, Bedford JS (1974) Mechanisms of chromosomal aberration production III. Chemicals and ionizing radiation. Mutat Res 23:197-212

Evans HJ (1977) Molecular mechanisms in the induction of chromosome aberrations. In: Scott D, Bridges BA, Sobels FH (eds) Progress in Genetic Toxicology. Elsevier/ North Holland Biomedical Press, Amsterdam pp 57-74

Kihlman BA (1971) Molecular mechanisms of chromosome breakage and rejoining. Adv Cell Mol Biol 1:59-107

Jones GM, Sanford KK, Parshad R, Gantt R, Price FM, Tarone RE (1985) Influence of added catalase on chromosome stability and neoplastic transformation of mouse cells in culture. Br J Cancer 52:583-590

Merwin RM, Redmon LW (1963) Induction of plasma cell tumors and sarcomas in mice by diffusion chambers placed in the peritoneal cavity. J Natl Cancer Inst 31:997-1017

Morse HC III, Hartley JW, Potter M (1980) Genetic considerations in plasmacytomas of BALB/c, NZB and (BALB/c x NZB) F_1 mice. In: Potter M (ed) Progress in Myeloma. Elsevier/North-Holland, Inc. pp 263-279

Natarajan AT, Obe G, van Zeeland AA, Palitti F, Meijers M, Verdegaal-Immerzeel EA (1980) Molecular mechanisms involved in the production of chromosomal aberrations. II. Utilization of neurospora endonuclease for the study of aberration production by x-rays in G_1 and G_2 studies of cell cycle. Mutat Res 69:293-305

Parshad R, Sanford KK (1968) Effect of horse serum, fetal calf serum, bovine serum and fetuin on neoplastic conversion and chromosomes of mouse embryo cells in vitro. J Natl Cancer Inst 41:767-779

Parshad R, Sanford KK, Jones GM (1983) Chromatid damage after G_2 phase x-irradiation of cells from cancer-prone individuals implicates deficiency in DNA repair. Proc Natl Acad Sci USA 80:5612-5616

Parshad R, Sanford KK, Jones GM (1985) Chromatid damage induced by fluorescent light during G_2 phase in normal and Gardner syndrome fibroblasts. Interpretation in terms of deficient DNA repair. Mutat Res 151:57-63

Parshad R, Sanford KK, Jones GM (1985b) Chromosomal radiosensitivity during the G_2 cell-cycle period of skin fibroblasts from individuals with familial cancer. Proc Natl Acad Sci USA 82:5400-5403

Potter M, Pumphrey JG, Bailey DW (1975) Genetics of susceptibility of plasmacytoma induction. I. BALB/cAnN (C), C57BL/6N (B6), C57BL/Ka (BK), and CXB6) F_1, (CXBK)F_1 and CXB recombinant inbred strains. J Natl Cancer Inst 54:1413-1417

Potter M, Wax JS (1981) Genetics of susceptibility to pristane-induced plasmacytomas in BALB/cAn: Reduced susceptibility in BALB/cJ with a brief description of pristane-induced arthritis. J Immunol 127:1591-1595

Potter M, Wax JS (1985) Role of genes in the susceptibility to plasmacytomas. In: Skamene E (ed) Progress in Leucocyte Biology: Genetic Control of Host Resistance to Infection and Malignancy. Alan R. Liss Inc., New York 3:793-804

Potter M, Wax JS, Anderson AO, Nordan RP (1985) Inhibition of plasmacytoma development in BALB/c mice by indomethacin. J Exp Med 161:996-1012

Potter M, Wiener F, Mushinski FJ (1984) Recent developments in plasmacytomagenesis in mice. In: Klein G (ed) Advances in Viral Oncology. Raven Press, New York 4: 139-162

Sanford KK, Parshad R, Gantt R (1985) Enhanced G_2 chromosomal radiosensitivity, susceptibility to cancer and neoplastic transformation. In: Skamene E (ed) Progress in Leucocyte Biology: Genetic Control of Host Resistance to Infection and Malignancy. Alan R Liss Inc., New York 3:811-820

Sanford KK, Parshad R, Gantt R (1986) Responses of human cells in culture to hydrogen peroxide and related free radicals generated by visible light: Relationship to cancer susceptibility. In: Johnson J (ed) Free Radicals, Aging and Degenerative Diseases. Alan R Liss Inc., New York, in press

Sanford KK, Parshad R, Stanbridge EJ, Frost JK, Jones GM, Wilkinson JE, Tarone RE (1986) Chromosomal radiosensitivity during the G_2 cell cycle period and cytopathology of human normal x tumor cell hybrids. Cancer Res 46:2045-2049

Weitberg AB, Weitzman SA, Destrempes M, Latt SA, Stossel TP (1983) Stimulated human phagocytes produce cytogenetic changes in cultured mammalian cells. New Engl J Med 308:26-30

Normal and Neoplastic B Cell Development in the Bursa of Fabricius

Craig B. Thompson*, Peter B. Challoner, and Paul E. Neiman

Fred Hutchinson Cancer Research Center, 1124 Columbia Street, Seattle, WA 98104

*Naval Medical Research Institute, Bethesda, MD 20814

INTRODUCTION

The bursa of Fabricius plays a central role in the development of B lymphocytes in avian species (Grossi 1976; Lydyard 1976; Ratcliffe 1985). The bursal anlage becomes populated with lymphoid stem cells between 8 to 14 days of embryogenesis. These cells begin to express histocompatibility class II antigens (Ia) from day 10 (Ewert 1984) and surface immunoglobulin (sIgM) from day 12 of embryonic life (Grossi 1976). By the time of hatching at day 21 of embryogenesis, nearly all (>95%) of bursal lymphocytes express the phenotype of a mature B cell (sIa^+, $sIgM^+$). After hatching, the bursa continues to increase in size as the number of cells in an individual follicle increases and B cells begin to seed to other organs. The bursa reaches its maximum size between 8 to 12 weeks of age and then begins to involute. By 6 months of age all that is left is a sclerotic remnant of the bursa. Several lines of evidence suggest that the bursa plays a central role in the development of B cells. Birds bursectomized at 17 days of embryogenesis fail to develop B cells and become completely agammaglobulinemic (Cooper 1969), suggesting that normally B cell differentiation occurs exclusively in the bursa. If, however, one ablates the bursal epithelium at 60 hours of incubation, the resulting chickens lack a bursa but do develop some circulating B cells and serum Ig (Jalkanen 1983). However, they remain unable to mount specific antibody response, are defective in their light chain diversity, and are markedly depleted of $sIgG^+$ cells (Jalkanen 1983, 1985). On the basis of these results, it appears that the bursal environment normally induces not only the differentiation of stem cells into B cells, but also the somatic diversification of the immune response, and the developmental switch of IgM to IgG and IgA producing cells.

In view of the central role the bursa plays in B-cell development, it is not surprising that the bursa is also a frequent site of neoplastic transformation of B cells. Among domestic chicken flocks, B-cell lymphomas arising within the bursa have presented a significant problem for animal husbandry. A viral etiology for this problem was suggested by the demonstration that, while typical bursal lymphomas can arise at low frequency in the absence of known exogenous viruses, bursal neoplasms arise at high frequency in chickens congenitally infected with avian leukosis viruses (ALV) (Crittenden 1979). The induction of bursal lymphomas by ALV has provided viral oncologists with a revealing experimental system with which to study the development of neoplasia. Infection of either embryonic chickens or chickens within 2 weeks of hatching with ALV results in the development of lymphomas in up to 50% of infected birds within 4-6 months (Baba and Humphries 1985). In contrast, infection after 2 weeks of age, rarely leads to the

Current Topics in Microbiology and Immunology, Vol. 132

development of lymphomas. The development of ALV-induced tumors also appears to follow an orderly progression which appears to require at least two independent transforming events (for review see Neiman 1980). Following infection of newly hatched chicks with ALV, a small percentage of bursal follicles take on an altered morphology with an increase in the number of cells within the follicle which have a lymphoblastic morphology. The early proliferative lesions, called transformed follicles, remain confined to the architecture of individual follicles, and appear to regress along with the normal bursal follicles during development. As such, they have been thought to represent a preneoplastic stage in tumor development. Tumor progression occurs when one (or rarely two) of these pre-neoplastic transformed follicles develops into an expanding nodule. These nodules are clonal growths as judged by ALV integration events and can appear as early as 10 weeks after infection. Within a number of weeks of their development, cells from the nodules begin to metastasize and lead to death of the chicken.

B Cell Developmental Stage Involved in ALV-Induced Bursal Lymphomas

The above data suggest that there may be a particular stage during B cell differentiation when B cells are susceptible to transformation and that several steps are required for complete neoplastic transformation. A candidate cell stage for the ALV-transforming event is the bursal stem cell. The bursal stem cell is a bursa-specific cell, present from day 12 of embryogenesis to 2 weeks post hatching, which expresses both sIg and sIa antigens (Ratcliffe 1985). These cells are transplantable and capable of reseeding the bursa and restoring antibody responses in birds whose bursas have been ablated with cyclophosphamide. The bursal stem cell may be analogous in development to the preprogenitor B cell that has been described in the mouse (Howard 1982). Consistent with these observations we have found that ALV-induced bursal lymphoma cells express both sIa and sIgM and lack expression of a common lymphoid antigen present on pre-bursal stem cells prior to their expression of surface Ig. The fact that ALV fails to induce lymphomas when birds are infected after the first two weeks post hatching suggests that post bursal B cells which contain a self renewing pool of sIgM+ cells which maintain the adult B cell repertoire are not involved in lymphomagenesis since they are maintained throughout a chicken's life. These cells which appear to be present in the bursa as well as elsewhere from just before birth until the bursa's involution at 6 months, appear to undergo selection and clonal expansion following activation by gut antigens encountered in the bursa.

Oncogenes Potentially Involved in the Development of Bursal Lymphomas

Avian leukosis viruses lack viral transforming genes and the mechanisms through which they initiated neoplastic transformation were unknown for many years. A major breakthrough came when Hayward et al. (1981) found that over 90% of ALV-induced metastatic bursal lymphomas contained ALV long terminal repeat (LTR) sequences integrated in close proximity to the c-*myc* gene. Subsequently it has been shown that these integrations act as either promoters and/or enhancers of c-*myc* transcription and lead to altered regulation and enhanced production of c-*myc* mRNA (Schubach and Groudine 1983). At the same time, Cooper and Neiman (1980) demonstrated that high molecular weight DNA from seven ALV-induced tumors efficiently transformed NIH/3T3 cells. They went on to demonstrate that these same tumors also contained LTR sequences integrated near c-myc, but that the NIH/3T3 transforming activity of DNA from these cells was not mediated by transfer of the altered c-myc genes (Cooper 1981). These observations lead to the hypothesis that at least two different cellular oncogenes with distinct oncogenic activity were activated by different mechanisms in ALV-induced bursal lymphomas. The concept that deregulation of at least 2 distinct oncogenes is generally required to induce neoplasia in normal cells has been supported by a number of subsequent studies (Land 1983). The involvement of two independent transforming events in the generation of bursal lymphomas is supported by studies concerning the kinetics of ALV-induced lymphomas, which demonstrate a log-log dependency with time (Neiman 1980).

The Effect of Unregulated myc Expression on Bursal Development

To dissect further the process of bursal lymphomagenesis, we have developed an *in vivo* assay to assess the effect of unregulated expression of the *myc* gene on bursal development (Neiman 1985). Chicken embryos are treated with cyclophosphamide on days 15,16, and 17 which causes ablation of the developing bursal lymphocytes. Bursal follicles can be reconstituted by infusion on day 18 with embryonic bursal cells containing bursal stem cells. Histologic examination of reconstituting bursal follicles showed that the first lymphocytes to appear are large pyrinophilic lymphoblasts which are in active proliferation and which appear to serve as progenitors of the bursal medullary lymphocytes. Normally, as bursal medullary cells increase in number many of them appear to develop into small resting lymphocytes. In the adult bursa only 20-30% of the cells in the bursa are in active proliferation at any one time. When the embryonic bursal cells used for transplantation are infected with a helper virus-dependent avian retrovirus, HB1, which expresses a high level of the v-myc oncogene (Enrietto 1983), the cells continue to home to the bursa. The initial layers of lymphoblasts appear to develop normally along the basement membrane. However, as the bursal medullary cells increase in number, normal differentiation processes that lead to the development of the small resting lymphocytes fail to occur. Instead, the individual follicles which develop from HB1-infected cells form preneoplastic transformed follicles indistinguishable from those which develop during the initial stages of bursal lymphomagenesis induced by ALV.

Careful cell cycle analysis of bursal cells from a 4 week old chick whose bursa was reconstituted with embryonic bursal cells of which only 5-10% were infected with HB1, has demonstrated that while resting bursal cells develop normally in follicles reconstituted with non-HB1-infected cells, the follicles which develop from HB1-infected cells are made up exclusively of cells in active proliferation. Based on these data, we conclude that the initial transforming event induced by ALV is deregulation of myc expression through adjacent integration. This event apparently fixes the bursal stem cell in a proliferative state and prevents the cell or its progeny from differentiating into a resting cell. This process is analogous to the block to mouse erythroleukemic cells (MEL) differentiation induced by high level c-myc expression when transcribed from the SV40 promoter (J. Coppola and M. Cole, personal communication). Under these conditions, MEL cells expressing a high level of exogenous c-*myc* maintain their proliferative capacity and fail to be induced to globin gene expression even under the normally potent differentiating influence of DMSO. Deregulation of *myc* gene expression, however, appears to be only the initial step to bursal lymphomagenesis. Recently, Baba and Humphries (1985) have shown that the development of transformed follicles is necessary but not sufficient to induce bursal lymphomas. Furthermore, unlike DNA from bursal lymphomas, DNA from bursas with greater than 90% HB1-transformed follicles fail to induce transformation of NIH/3T3 cells following transfection.

Potential Mechanisms for Activation of 2° Transforming Activity in Bursal Lymphomas

Based on the above data, one possible explanation of the ordered process of ALV-induced lymphomagenesis, would be to hypothesize that the immortalization of the bursal stem cell through deregulation of c-*myc* expression, fixes the cell in a state where it is at high risk for secondary genetic alteration. Two potential mechanisms for such alterations have been shown to exist in the bursal stem cells. Hope et al. (1986) have recently demonstrated that the embryonic bursa contains a high level of specific endonuclease required for immunoglobulin rearrangement. Whether this activity could also lead to rearrangement or translocation of other related sequences remains unknown. In addition, the chicken appears to generate all of its light chain diversity through somatic mutation of a single V region (Reynaud 1985). Normally, this high level of somatic mutation occurs between day 15 of embryogenesis and 2-4 weeks post hatching and apparently involves the cycling bursal stem cell. Again, this activity could lead to somatic mutations of other regions of DNA in addition to the variable region of the immunoglobulin gene. Whether either or both of these mechanisms of gene alteration contribute to the development of ALV-induced bursal lymphomas is unknown. To date, the genes involved in the NIH/3T3 transforming activity of bursal lymphomas have not been identified (Cooper 1986). Until these genes are cloned and sequenced, the mechanism of their activation, whether by rearrangement, mutation, or some other process, will remain open to speculation.

Conclusions

A great deal has been learned in recent years about the processes involved in ALV-induced bursal lymphomagenesis. ALV appears to induce a preneoplastic state in bursal stem cells by enhancing and deregulating c-*myc* gene expression through adjacent integration. This enhancement of c-*myc* expression apparently maintains the cells in a proliferative state and inhibits their differentiation to small resting lymphocytes (see Fig. 1).

The proliferating bursal stem cell has been demonstrated to have a high level of endonuclease activity apparently required for immunoglobulin gene rearrangement and undergoes a high rate of a somatic mutation of its expressed immunoglobulin gene. Both of these activities should they have effects on other sequences in the genome could lead to activation of other genes either through rearrangement or mutation. Should such events occur, they might lead to the generation of the NIH/3T3 transforming activity found in bursal lymphomas. Based on *in vitro* models of oncogenesis, the activation of an NIH/3T3 transforming gene in a cell already immortalized by ALV-induced c-myc deregulation would then lead to the cell's full neoplastic conversion. While by no means completely proven, these processes could entirely account for the generation of bursal lymphomas following embryonic or neonatal ALV infection.

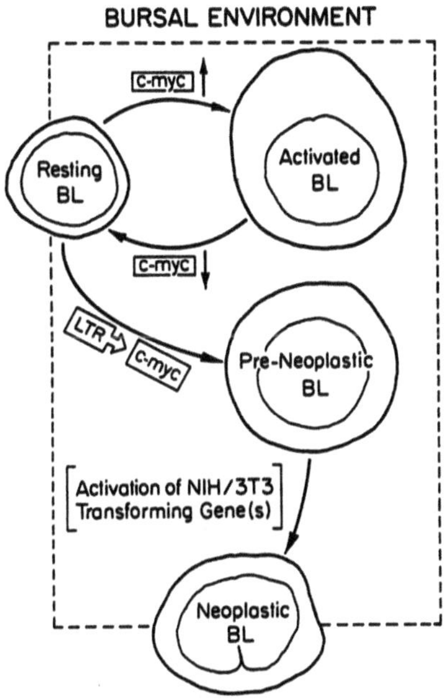

Figure 1. Schematic representation of the stages involved in ALV-induced bursal lymphomagenesis.

ACKNOWLEDGEMENTS

We thank our colleagues at the Fred Hutchinson Cancer Research Center for their thoughtful discussions, Louise Carlson and Angela Hein for their expert technical assistance, and Kay Shiozaki for her editorial assistance in preparing the manuscript. These investigations were supported by NCI grants CA20068 and CA 28151. P.C. is supported by NIH fellowship F32 HD06583. The opinions and assertions contained herein are those of the authors and are not to be construed as official or reflecting the views of the Navy Department of naval service at large.

REFERENCES

Baba TW, Humphries EH (1985) Formation of a transformed follicle is necessary but not sufficient for development of an avian leukosis virus-induced lymphomas. Proc Natl Acad Sci USA 82:213-216
Cooper GM, Neiman PE (1980) Transforming genes of neoplasms induced by avian lymphoid leukosis viruses. Nature 287:656-659

Cooper GM, Neiman PE (1981) Two distinct candidate transforming genes of lymphoid leukosis virus-induced neoplasms. Nature 292:857-858
Cooper CM, Goubin G, Diamond A, Neiman P (1986) Relationship of Blym oncogenes to repeated mouse sequences. Nature, in press
Cooper MD, Cain WA, VanAlten PJ, Good RA (1969) Development and function of the immunoglobulin producing system. I. Effect of bursectomy at different stages of development on germinal centers, plasma cells, immunoglobulins and antibody production. Int Arch Allergy Appl Immunol 35:242-252
Crittenden LB, Witter RL, Okazaki W, Neiman PE (1979) Lymphoid neoplasms in chicken flocks free of infection with exogenous avian tumor viruses. J Natl Cancer Inst 63:191-199
Enrietto PJ, Payne LN, Hayman MJ (1983) A recovered avian myelocytomatosis virus that induces lymphomas in chickens: pathogenic properties and their molecular basis. Cell 36:369-379
Ewert DL, Munchus MS, Chen CH, Cooper MD (1984) Analysis of structural properties and cellular distribution of avian Ia antigen by using monoclonal antibody to monomorphic determinants. J Immunol 132:2524-2530
Grossi CE, Lydyard PM, Cooper MD (1977) Ontogeny of B cells in the chicken. II. Changing patterns of cytoplasmic IgM expression and of modulation requirements for surface IgM by anti-μ antibodies. J Immunol 119:749-756
Grossi CE, Lydyard PM, Cooper MD (1976) B-cell ontogeny in the chicken. Ann Immunol (Inst Pasteur) 127:931-941
Hayward WS, Neel B, Astrin SM (1981) Activation of a cellular onc gene by promoter insertion in ALV-induced lymphoid leukosis. Nature 290:475-480
Hope TJ, Aguilera RJ, Minie ME, Sakano H (1986) Endonucleolytic activity that cleaves immunoglobulin recombination sequences. Science 231:1141-1145
Howard MC (1982) Antigen-induced B lymphocyte differentiation. In CRC critical reviews in immunology p 181-206
Jalkanen S, Granfors K, Jalkanen M, Toivanen P (1983) Immune capacity of the chicken bursectomized at 60 hr of incubation: surface immunoglobulin and B-L (Ia-like) antigen-bearing cells. J Immunol 130:2038-2041
Jalkanen S, Jalkanen M, Granfors K, Toivanen P (1984) Defect in the generation of light-chain diversity in bursectomized chickens. Nature 311:69-71
Land H, Parada LF, Weinberg RA (1983) Cellular oncogenes and multistep carcinogenesis. Science 222:771-778
Lydyard PM, Grossi CE, Cooper MD (1976) Ontogeny of B cells in the chicken. I. Sequential development of clonal diversity in the bursa. J Exp Med 144:79-97
Neiman PE, Jordan L, Weiss RA, Payne LN (1980) Malignant lymphoma of the bursa of Fabricius: Analysis of early transformation. In: Viruses in Naturally Occurring Cancers, Cold Spring Harbor Laboratory, Cold Spring Harbor, NY, p 519-527
Neiman, P, Wolf C, Enrietto PJ, Cooper GM (1985) A retroviral myc gene induces preneoplastic transformation of lymphocytes in a bursal transplantation assay. Proc Natl Acad Sci USA 82:222-226
Ratcliffe MJH (1985) The ontogeny and cloning of B cells in the bursa of Fabricius. Immu Today 6:224-227
Reynaud C-A, Anquez V, Dahan A, Weill J-C (1985) A single rearrangement event generates most of the chicken immunoglobulin light chain diversity. Cell 40:283-291
Schubach WS, Groudine M (1984) Alteration of c-myc chromatin structure by avian leukosis virus integration. Nature 307:702-708

Restrictions That Influence Avian Leukosis Virus-Induced Lymphoid Leukosis

Eric H. Humphries and Timothy W. Baba

Department of Microbiology, Southwestern Medical School, The University of Texas Health Science Center, 5323 Harry Hines Boulevard, Dallas, Texas 75235

INTRODUCTION

Infection of one day old White leghorn chicks with avian leukosis virus (ALV) usually results in the development of a bursal-dependent B-cell lymphoma (Purchase and Burmester, 1978). This tumor requires the bursal environment to develop and is characterized by the presence of cell surface immunoglobulin M (IgM) (Cooper et al., 1974). Integration of the ALV provirus within the normal c-myc locus of the target cell disrupts the expression of this locus and appears to be important in the development of the primary tumor (Hayward et al., 1981; Payne et al., 1982). However, alterations that influence the expression of the c-myc locus have been implicated in the development of a variety of lymphoid tumors in several species (Dalla-Favera et al., 1982; Shen-Ong et al., 1982; Corcoran et al., 1984; Levy et al., 1984). These lymphoid tumors exhibit considerable variation in their phenotype and include not only B-cell tumors that express IgM but also mature B-cell tumors that secrete IgG and T-cell tumors. It is not known why ALV infection produces such a restricted type of lymphoid tumor in the chicken. A variety of factors including (i) access of the virus to a particular type of target tissue, (ii) the abundance and proliferative capacity of different target cells at the time of virus replication and (iii) specific and non-specific host defense mechanisms could influence tumor development following ALV infection. Recent data from our laboratory indicate that such factors may indeed play a role in the tumor process. Results from studies of the SC White leghorn chicken indicate that there is very little persistent ALV integration in any lymphoid tissue except the bursal lymphocyte. Further, while integration within the bursal lymphocyte is associated with the development of transformed follicles, there appear to be situations in which progression of this preneoplastic lesion to the bursal lymphoma fails to occur. It seems likely, therefore, that as yet undefined genetic factors influence (i) the frequency of ALV integration in different lymphocytes and (ii) the progression of preneoplastic tissue in the bursa and so influence the development and specific character of ALV-induced neoplasia.

ALV INTEGRATION IS NOT OBSERVED IN ALL LYMPHOID TISSUES

One day old chicks were infected with RAV-1 and sacrificed at 1.5, 2.5, 5, and 9 weeks after infection. Following collection of sterile plasma samples, DNA was prepared from erythrocytes as well as bursal, splenic, thymic and peripheral blood lymphocytes.

Current Topics in Microbiology and Immunology, Vol. 132

Plasma samples were assayed for the presence of infectious virus and DNA samples were examined for the presence of integrated viral sequences. A standard Southern analysis was employed to detect a 2.1 kb DNA fragment specific for RAV-1 integration. The sensitivity in this assay is approximately 0.005 copies of RAV-1 per haploid genome or 1 infected cell in 100 uninfected cells.

In these and previous experiments (Baba and Humphries, 1984), injection of 1 day old SC chicks with 2×10^5 IU of RAV-1 produces viremia in greater than 95% of the birds. Nine weeks after infection, less than 10% of the birds were viremic. The data obtained from four separate experiments have been pooled and are presented in Table 1.

Table 1. Distribution of viral DNA sequences in lymphoid tissues from RAV-1-infected chickens

Weeks Post Infection	Copies of Integrated RAV-1 DNA Sequences/Haploid Genome[a] Erythrocytes	Bursa	Peripheral Blood	Spleen	Thymus
1.5	0.29 (5) ± 0.12	0.13 (5) ± 0.06	0.15 (4) ± 0.13	0.01 (5) ± 0.01	<0.005 (5) ----
2.5	0.42 (17) ± 0.25	0.09 (7) ± 0.11	0.05 (10) ± 0.04	<0.005 (9) ----	<0.005 (5) ----
5	0.09 (11) ± 0.05	0.06 (10) ± 0.08	<0.005 (6) ----	<0.005 (11) ----	<0.005 (5) ----
9	<0.005 (5) ----	0.04 (5) ± 0.05	ND[b]	<0.005 (5) ----	<0.005 (5) ----

[a]All values are calculated as arithmetic means ± standard deviation. The number of independent determinations is presented in parentheses.
[b]Not determined.

The data indicate that of the tissues examined, integrated viral sequences were most abundant in erythrocytes, with as many as 0.4 copies per haploid genome. Consistent with our earlier findings, no RAV-1 DNA was detected in erythrocytes 9 weeks after infection. Our results show further that integrated RAV-1 sequences were less abundant in bursal lymphocytes, 0.1 to 0.15 copies per haploid genome, suggesting that no more than 30% of this population were infected at any given time. The extent of integration detected in this experiment is 3 to 4-fold less than has been observed in bursal lymphocytes from line 7_1x$15I_5$ chickens infected with the same virus (Fung *et al.*, 1982) and may account for the lower incidence of tumors observed in the SC chicken (50% versus 100%). The data indicate that ALV integrated sequences persist in the bursal lymphocyte population so that the 2.1 kb fragment can still be detected 9 weeks after infection. In contrast, while integrated sequences are present at 0.15 copies per haploid genome in peripheral blood lymphocytes 1.5 weeks after infection, detectable sequences are absent 5 weeks after infection. The presence of viral sequences early after infection in these lymphocytes is consistent with the observation that infectious virus can be isolated from these cells (De Boer et al., 1981). Finally, with the exception of splenic lymphocytes examined 1.5 weeks after infection, sequences specific for integrated RAV-1 were not observed in cells prepared from either the spleen or the thymus, suggesting that less than 1 lymphocyte in 100 is infected in these tissues. The results from these experiments indicate that, even in chickens with high titers of circulating virus, among the lymphocytes examined in this study only the bursal population contained a detectable level of integrated viral sequences for an extended period of time.

THE TRANSFORMED FOLLICLE AND DEVELOPMENT OF THE BURSAL LYMPHOMA

Analysis of RAV-1-infected chickens has made it possible to follow three events important in the development of the bursal lymphoma. Figure 1 presents a summary of (i) the establishment of RAV-1 viremia, (ii) the appearance of integrated RAV-1 sequences, and (iii) the presence of the transformed follicle observed in the infected SC chicken.

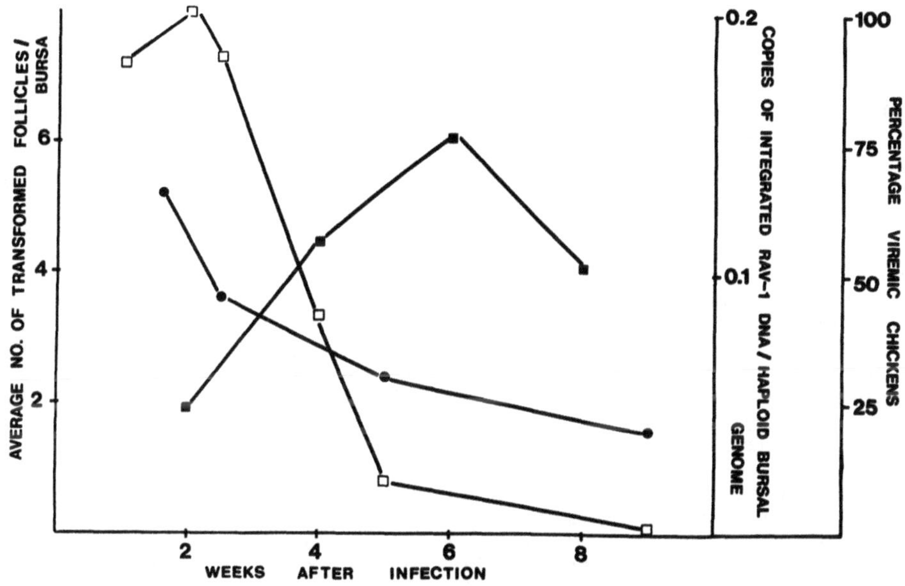

Fig. 1. One day old SC chicks were infected with RAV-1. At selected times after infection, chicks were sacrificed and assayed for circulating infectious virus (□), integrated viral DNA sequences present in bursal lymphocytes (●) and transformed follicles (■).

The picture that has emerged has established several observations. First, while all the chicks develop viremia, the virus seldom persists in the blood beyond 5 weeks post infection. Second, integrated viral sequences are detected in bursal lymphocytes early after infection. The number of viral copies per haploid genome does, however, decrease with time. Such sequences are generally not detectable in bursal lymphocytes 10 to 15 weeks after infection. Thirdly, the transformed follicle appears with the detection of integrated viral DNA. Unlike other markers of infection, there appears to be no decrease in the frequency of transformed follicles during the first 8 weeks of infection. The data presented in Fig. 1 are consistent with the hypothesis that viral integration next to c-myc is an early event in the development of the tumor and that such integration results in the development of the transformed follicle. With the gradual elimination of circulating infectious virus, new integration is prevented and the number of transformed follicles fails to increase with time.

We have argued elsewhere (Baba and Humphries, 1985), based upon an analysis of the development of the transformed follicle in two lines of chickens (one resistant to lymphoma development, the other sensitive), that the development of the transformed follicle is an event that is necessary but insufficient for the appearance of the bursal lymphoma. The suggestion is that the lesion persists until some additional event (or events) have occurred that alter the character of the lesion so that it becomes neoplastic. In the context of this hypothesis, several questions concerning the nature of the transformed follicle appear to be of particular relevance.

(1) Do transformed follicles persist (i) until they develop into tumors (or until the bursa undergoes physiological regression and atrophy) or (ii) can transformed follicles be eliminated by natural host defense mechanisms? Our study has revealed no decrease in the frequency of this lesion during the first 8 weeks of infection. It may be, however, that a more extensive study (analyzing more birds) or a more complete study (analyzing the first 15 weeks after infection) will reveal a gradual decrease in the incidence of this preneoplastic lesion with the passage of time. At present, however, it is clear that many more lesions develop than do tumors. Part of the explanation for the failure of a transformed follicle to become a tumor is certainly the result of the stochastic nature of tumor progression. However, the failure to observe lymphoma development in any Hyline FP chickens or in 50% of the Hyline SC chickens that possessed transformed follicles suggests that host genes may play a significant role in restricting the progression of the preneoplastic state.

(2) Are all transformed follicles genetically similar or do they represent different stages of tumor progression? In the absence of genetic markers, we do not know whether the transformed follicles present at 2 weeks after infection express the same genetic phenotype as the transformed follicles present 15 weeks after infection. While it seems certain that additional genetic alterations are required for emergence of the tumor, how many changes are required is unknown. The possibility exists, therefore, that, with the passage of time, genetic variation appears among the preneoplastic lesions and that this variation is accompanied by alterations in the phenotype of the cells within these follicles. The possibility that transformed follicles may be

eliminated by the host raises the issue of selection and continued progression of follicles resistant to host defenses. Such preneoplastic follicles would represent an altered stage of tumor development.

(3) What is the role of the bursal environment in the progression of the preneoplastic cell to a tumor cell? The staining properties of the transformed follicle suggests that the cells within these follicles are proliferating constitutively. As the average size of these preneoplastic lesions does not increase with time, these cells presumably leave the bursa or are eliminated. The role of the bursa in providing mature B-lymphocytes for the spleen suggests these cells may migrate from the bursal environment. Primary tumors, however, do not develop outside the bursa. It seems, therefore, that the bursa plays an essential role in tumor development in one or all of the following: (i) preventing elimination of preneoplastic cells by virtue of their presence in a privileged environment, (ii) supplying essential factor(s) for proliferation and survival of the preneoplastic B-cells and (iii) providing a special environment in which the acquisition of the additional genetic changes required for emergence of the lymphoma is favored.

SUMMARY

While elevated expression of the c-myc gene appears critical for the development of the ALV-induced lymphoma, additional genetic changes are required for the development of the malignant cell. We have provided evidence that genetic restrictions also play a role in tumor development. Specifically, viral integration in lymphoid tissue and progression of preneoplasia to neoplasia appear to be influenced by host cell factors.

ACKNOWLEDGMENTS

We thank Rae Allen for excellent technical assistance and Cindy Baselski for excellent secretarial assistance. The work was supported by Public Health Service grant CA32295 from the National Institutes of Health and grant I-962 from the Robert A. Welch Foundation.

REFERENCES

Baba TW, Humphries EH (1984) Avian leukosis virus infection: analysis of viremia and DNA integration in susceptible and resistant chicken lines. J Virol 51:123-130

Baba TW, Humphries EH (1985) Formation of a transformed follicle is necessary but not sufficient for development of an avian leukosis virus-induced lymphoma. Proc Natl Acad Sci USA 82:213-216

Cooper MD, Purchase HG, Bochman DE, Gathings WE (1974) Studies on the nature of the abnormality of B cell differentiation in avian lymphoid leukosis: Production of heterogeneous IgM by tumor cells. J Immunol 133:1210-1222

Corcoran LM, Adams JM, Dunn AR, Cory S (1984) Murine lymphomas in which the cellular myc oncogene has been activated by retroviral insertion. Cell 37:113-122

Dalla-Favera R, Bregni M, Erickson J, Patterson D, Gallo RC, Croce CM (1982) Human c-myc oncogene is located on the region of chromosome 8 that is translocated in Burkitt lymphoma cells. Proc Natl Acad Sci USA 79:7824-7828

De Boer GF, Maas HJL, Van Vloten J, Groenendal JE (1981) Horizontal transmission of lymphoid leukosis virus. Influence of age, maternal antibodies and degree of contact exposure. Avian Path 10:343-358

Fung Y-K, Fadley AM, Crittenden LB, Kung H-J (1982) Avian lymphoid leukosis virus infection and DNA integration in the preleukotic bursal tissues: a comparative study of susceptible and resistant lines. Virology 119:411-421

Hayward WS, Neel BG, Astrin SM (1981) Activation of a cellular onc gene by promoter insertion in ALV-induced lymphoid leukosis. Nature (London) 290:475-480

Levy LS, Gardner MB, Casey JW (1984) Isolation of a feline leukaemia provirus containing the oncogene myc from a feline lymphosarcoma. Nature (London) 308:853-856

Payne GS, Bishop JM, Varmus HE (1982) Multiple arrangements of viral DNA and an activated host oncogene in bursal lymphomas. Nature (London) 295:209-214

Purchase HG, Burmester BR (1978) Diseases of Poultry. Iowa State University Press, Iowa, p 418

Shen-Ong GCL, Keath EJ, Piccoli SP, Cole MD (1982) Novel myc oncogene RNA from abortive immunoglobulin-gene recombination in mouse plasmacytomas. Cell 31:443-452

Benign Monoclonal Gammapathy (BMG)

J. Radl

TNO Institute for Experimental Gerontology, Rijswijk, The Netherlands

HUMAN BMG

The term Idiopathic Paraproteinaemia or Benign Monoclonal Gammapathy (BMG) has been known to clinicians already for more than fourty years. It is used to denominate a condition characterized by the presence in serum of a homogeneous immunoglobulin (H-Ig) component persisting at a -more or less- constant concentration over many years, usually until the individual's death (for a review see Radl, 1982). The concentration of such a H-Ig component is usually less than 2 g/dl and the level of Ig classes and subclasses other than those of the H-Ig may be normal or decreased but never to such an extent as seen in multiple myeloma (MM) or Waldenström's macroglobulinaemia (WM). The class distribution of H-Ig is approximately 60%, 20% and 20% for IgG, IgA and IgM, respectively. Bence Jones proteinaemia and/or proteinuria, frequent in MM and WM, is very rare in BMG. When investigating the bone marrow cells, an increased monoclonal proliferation is found; however, these cells do not posses morphological abnormalities and they do not reach such a dominance as found in plasma cell malignancies. The benign character of this plasma cell proliferation is also reflected in the absence of bone destruction. The occurrence of BMG is clearly age-related: starting in the fourth decade, its frequency increases up to almost 20% in the tenth decade of life. The ratio of the incidence of malignant versus non-malignant monoclonal gammapathies (MG) can be estimated as about 1:200. Within the non-malignant MG, the BMG may represent about 50% of the cases. The other half represent MG of other categories, i.e., MG due to a T<B immunodeficiency and antigen driven MG (Radl, 1985). Suggestions that BMG may represent a pre-myeloma stage or an indolent MM are based on extremely rare observations of a terminal overt B-cell malignancy following a long-lasting stable MG of an unknown origin. In several long-lasting follow-up studies, however, BMG was shown to remain essentially benign in the vast majority of cases.

MOUSE MODEL OF BMG

In spite of the presence of a large body of clinical and laboratory data on several aspects of BMG, the etiology, pathogenesis and significance of this proliferative disorder have remained obscure. New clues for our understanding of BMG have recently been offered by results of experimental studies in an animal model. It has been shown that aging mice of the C57BL/KaLwRij strain develop MG in a high frequency. MG due to MM and WM-like lymphoma were found in about 0.5% of mice above two years of age. In about 10% of the cases the MG were transient. The majority of the remaining MG showed features very similar to those of human BMG (see review by Radl, 1981).
The results of subsequent studies revealed a number of new aspects of this mouse analogue (called idiopathic paraproteinaemia in the references) of the

human disorder:
1) Successful transplantation (Radl et al., 1979) of different individual BMG producing clones from old to young healthy mice of the same strain by bone marrow or spleen cell transfers (while maintaining their nonprogressive character) indicated that BMG represents an intrinsic B-cell abnormality with autonomous monoclonal proliferation. However, the further behaviour was different from that of MM or B-cell lymphoma. In following transplantations the "take" frequency of BMG in recipients gradually decreased and propagation of such a clone for more than three to four generations was not possible. In contrast, MM or B-cell lymphoma spontaneously appearing in the aging C57BL/KaLwRij mice (Radl et al., 1985) could be transplanted continuously, with a high "take" frequency, with progressive development of the MG and with shortened survival times of the recipient mice. This was the case also in a MM line which otherwise exhibited all features of a smoldering MM as observed and described in men (Kyle and Greipp, 1980). From this study it can be concluded that the mouse BMG is in its final stage an autonomous proliferative disorder, which, however, lacks the immortal and progressive components of the true B-cell malignancy.
2) Results from further studies on factors which may influence the development of BMG showed that a deficiency in the T immune system may play an important contributing role. Experiments in nude athymic mice (Radl et al., 1980a) and in adult- and/or neonatally thymectomized C57BL mice (Radl et al., 1980b) demonstrated a clear-cut correlation between the frequencies of age-related MG and the grade of the T immune system defect. Similar results were obtained in experiments with CBA mice with, however one exception: the numbers of MG which were transplantable were remarkably low. This indicates that genetic factors may be of basic importance in the pathogenesis of BMG.
3) The role of genetic factors in the development of BMG was indicated by:
  a) different frequencies and times of onset of MG in aging mice of different strains (Radl et al., 1978);
  b) the results of transplantation experiments in which B cells from a strain with a high BMG frequency led to the development of BMG in radiation chimeras of a strain with a low BMG frequency, but not vice versa (Radl et al., 1984);
  c) the high frequency of BMG of the IgG2a and IgD isotypes carrying the C57BL Ighb allotype in the F1 hybrid mice of the low CBA and high C57BL BMG frequency strains (Radl et al., 1985).

The last mentioned experiment indicated that genetic material associated with the Ig heavy chain locus can play a pathogenetic role in the development of BMG. In contrast, no association between the BMG frequencies and the H2 haplotypes was found in six congenic strains of C57BL and BALB origin (v.d. Akker et al., 1986).

THREE STAGE HYPOTHESIS

The results of studies performed in the C57BL mouse model support in principle the so called "three stage hypothesis" on the development of BMG (Radl., 1979). In this hypothesis, a gradual development of BMG -a benign B-cell neoplasia- in three stages has been postulated as a consequence of an age-related immunodeficiency. The first stage consists of an involution of the thymus, followed by a genetically determined selective decrease in certain T-cell subpopulations and an impairment especially of the regulatory T-cell function. The resulting imbalance in the T<B immune system network results in restriction of the heterogeneity of the antibody response and in excessive B cell clonal proliferations, i.e., MG of a transient nature (stage 2). These repeated mono- or oligoclonal expansions lead (on a susceptible genetic background) to a higher probability for a mutation; if it involves sequences which exert a negative

control on cell proliferation, the clone will continue to proliferate even after the original antigenic stimulation has disappeared (stage 3). The intrinsic defect in cell regulation in BMG is assumed to be different from that in B-cell malignancies.

BMG AND ONCOGENES

What can be the role of oncogenes in this disorder? It is tempting to speculate that a dysfunction of a given oncogene may lead to the development of BMG, while for the development of a malignancy two or probably more aberrant oncogene expressions will be necessary. The great difference in the incidence between these two proliferative disorders would indicate much more complex mechanisms in the case of the malignant as compared with the benign form. Another interesting question is whether the same oncogenes would be involved in the development of both neoplasias. Should this be the case, or should BMG be a pre-myeloma condition, MM would be expected to develop much more frequently from BMG than from normal clones. No evidence for this mechanism has been obtained so far either from investigations in men or from mouse studies. The implication is that either different oncogenes and their products are active in the benign and malignant neoplasias, or that the sequence of the activation of the oncogenes may be decisive for the form of the proliferative disorder which will develop.

REFERENCES

Kyle RA, Greipp PR (1980) Smoldering multiple myeloma. New Eng J Med 302: 1347-1349.

Radl J, Hollander CF, van den Berg P and de Glopper E (1978) Idiopathic paraproteinaemia I. Studies in an animal model - the ageing C57BL/KaLwRij mouse. Clin exp Immunol 33: 395-402.

Radl J, (1979) Idiopathic paraproteinemia - a consequence of an age-related deficiency in the T immune system. Three-stage development - a hypothesis. Clin Immunol Immunopathol 14: 251-255.

Radl J, de Glopper E, Schuit HRE, Zurcher C (1979) Idiopathic paraproteinemia II. Transplantation of the paraprotein producing clone from old to young C57BL/KaLwRij mice. J Immunol 122: 609-613.

Radl J, Mink, JG, van den Berg P, van Zwieten, MJ and Benner, R (1980a) Increased frequency of homogenous immunoglobulins in the sera of nude athymic mice with age. Clin Immunol Immunopathol 17: 469-476.

Radl J, de Glopper E, van den Berg P and van Zwieten M.J. (1980b) Idiopathic paraproteinemia. III. Increased frequency of paraproteinemia in thymectomized aging C57BL/KaLwRij and CBA/BrARij mice. J Immunol 125: 31-35.

Radl J (1981) Benign monoclonal gammopathy (Idiopathic paraproteinemia). Amer J Pathol 105: 91-93.

Radl J (1982) Effects of aging on immunoglobulins. In: Ritzman, SE, (ed) Pathology of immunoglobulins: Diagnostic and Clinical Aspects, Protein abnormalities, Vol. 2, , Alan R. Liss, Inc., New York, N.Y., p 55-69.

Radl J, Heidt PJ, Knaan-Shanzer S and van Zwieten MJ (1984) Idiopathic paraproteinaemia. IV. The role of genetic factors in the development of monoclonal B cell proliferative disorders - a study in the ageing C57BL/KaLwRij and CBA/BrARij mouse radiation chimeras. Clin exp Immunol 57: 213-216.

Radl J, van den Enden-Vieveen MHM, van de Akker TW, Benner R, Haaijman JJ and Zurcher C (1985) Idiopathic paraproteinaemia. V. Expression of Igh1 and Igh5 allotypes within the homogeneous immunoglobulins of ageing (C57BL/LiARij x CBA/BrARij)F1 mouse. Clin. Exp. Immunol. 62: 405-411

Radl, J (1985) Monoclonal Gammapathies - an attempt at a new classification. Neth J Med 28: 134-137.

Radl J, Croese JW, Zurcher C, Brondijk RJ and van den Enden-Vieveen MHM (1985) Spontaneous multiple myeloma with bone lesions in the aging C57BL/KaLwRij mouse as a natural model of human disease. In: Radl, J, Hijmans, W. and van Camp, B (eds) Monoclonal gammapathies, Clinical significance and basic mechanisms, EURAGE, Rijswijk, p. 191-194.

Van de Akker TW, Tio-Gillen AP, Benner R, Zurcher C, Radl J (1986) Idiopathic paraproteinaemia VI. The development of "Benign monoclonal gammapathy" in aging H2 congenic C57BL and BALB mice is independent on their H2 haptotype (in preparation).

DNA Rearrangement and Expression of the c-myc Gene in a Human Myeloma

G.F. Hollis, A.F. Gazdar, I.R. Kirsch

NCI-Navy Medical Oncology Branch, National Cancer Institute, National Institutes of Health, Bethesda, MD 20892

In both Burkitt's lymphomas and murine plasmacytomas there are specific disease-associated chromosomal translocations that bring into contiguity one of the immunoglobulin gene loci with the c-myc proto-oncogene (Klein 1983). These specific chromosomal translocations can occur 5' or 3' of the c-myc oncogene and are believed to cause deregulation of expression of c-myc. This is supported by the fact that in these tumors only the c-myc gene involved in the translocation is expressed (Taub 1984).

Because of the Burkitt's lymphoma and the murine plasmacytoma models, we were interested in determining whether the c-myc gene might also be activated by DNA rearrangement in a human myeloma. DNA and RNA were prepared from malignant plasma cells from an effusion occurring in a patient with IgAk myeloma and also from its corresponding cell line (NCI-H929). We examined the state of the c-myc proto-oncogene in this patient's tumor cells by Southern analysis and were able to demonstrate a DNA rearrangement close to or within c-myc (Gazdar 1986). Further analysis, based on Southern blotting and cloning experiments, indicates that the rearrangement has occurred on the 3' side of the c-myc gene as has been seen in the variant translocations of Burkitt's lymphoma. (Rearrangement 3' of c-myc has been established before in the variant translocations of Burkitt lymphoma (Hollis 1984, Denny 1985) and the DNA rearrangement appears to activate the expression of the c-myc gene.) We analyzed RNA from the tumor and cell line for c-myc transcripts and found that c-myc is more highly expressed in NCI-H929 than in a Burkitt's lymphoma. A detailed description of this work is being prepared for publication. The immunoglobulin and c-myc gene rearrangements, which are identical in the tumor and the cell line, form a molecular fingerprint of the NCI-H929 myeloma cell line (Gazdar 1986).

We analyzed DNA and RNA from bone marrow aspirates from 4 other patients with myeloma to determine whether DNA rearrangement and gene activation of the c-myc gene was common in human myeloma. We were unable to detect c-myc gene rearrangement or expression in these tissues.

Because we have been unable to demonstrate that c-myc gene alteration is a common feature of all human myelomas, it is important to consider what role it is playing in the NCI-H929 cell line and the original tumor cells. This patient was diagnosed as having myeloma, was treated with chemotherapy, and entered remission. After a few months the patient relapsed with an unusually aggressive tumor. It is possible that the c-myc gene rearrangement that has led to elevated levels of c-myc mRNA has caused this patient's tumor to progress to a more malignant state. This is consistent with our finding that in

Current Topics in Microbiology and Immunology, Vol. 132

the four "non-aggressive" myelomas we examined the c-myc gene was germline and unexpressed. Further studies of the c-myc gene and its expression will help to define its role in human myelomas.

REFERENCES

Denny CT, Hollis GF, Magrath IT, and Kirsch IR (1985) Burkitt lymphoma cell line carrying a variant translocation creates new DNA at the breakpoint and violates the hierarchy of immunoglobulin gene rearrangement. Molecular and Cellular Biology 5:3199-3207

Gazdar AF, Oie HK, Kirsch IR, and Hollis GF (1986) Establishment and characterization of a human plasma cell myeloma culture having rearranged cellular myc proto-oncogene. Blood (in press)

Hollis GF, Mitchell KF, Battey J, Potter H, Taub RA, Lenoir G, and Leder P (1984) A variant translocation places the lambda immunoglobulin genes 3' to the c-myc oncogene in Burkitt lymphoma. Nature 307:752-755

Klein G (1983) Specific chromosomal translocations and the genesis of B-cell derived tumors in mice and men. Cell 32:311-315

Taub R, Moulding C, Battey J, Murphy W, Vasicek T, Lenoir G, and Leder P (1984) Activation and somatic mutation of the translocated c-myc gene in Burkitt lymphoma cells. Cell 36:339-348

Inbred Strain Differences Influence the Focal Proliferation of Plasma Cells in Pristane Induced Oil Granuloma

M. Potter[1] and J.S. Wax[2]

[1]Laboratory of Genetics, National Cancer Institute, National Institutes of Health, Bethesda, MD, USA; [2]Hazleton Laboratories, Rockville, MD, USA

Plasmacytomas are inducible in a few genetically susceptible strains of mice (BALB/cAn, NZB) by the intraperitoneal injection of mineral oils (see Potter 1984 for refs). However, many other strains are resistant to plasma cell tumor formation (Potter et al. 1975, 1984; Potter and Wax 1981). Pristane (2,6,10,14 tetramethylpentadecane), a component of many mineral oils, also has a biogenic origin being produced by marine copepods from phytane. Pristane, like most of the components of mineral or paraffin oil, is not metabolized and its role as a plasmacytomagenic agent is not direct. When pristane and mineral oils are injected i.p., they induce the formation of a reactive tissue that forms on peritoneal surfaces, called oil granuloma (OG) (Potter and MacCardle 1964). The OG results from the phagocytosis of oil droplets by cells in the macrophage and myeloid series. A variety of configurations of oil droplets are seen in this tissue ranging from intracellular oil droplets to cystic structures onto which a variable number of macrophages and or neutrophils adhere. The oil laden phagocytes and the larger droplets surrounded by phagocytes adhere to mesothelial surfaces and become vascularized from underlying blood vessels and covered with mesothelium. The organized OG is invaded by other types of inflammatory cells and lymphocytes. Plasma cells can be found scattered throughout. OG formation begins very soon after the injection of pristane and is well developed by day 20.

The same process of peritoneal OG formation occurs in C57BL/6, DBA/2, BALB/cAn inbred and (BALB/c x DBA/2)F hybrid strains of mice that are resistant to plasmacytoma induction. In BALB/cAn mice some plasma cells begin proliferating in the OG tissue where they form various types of aggregations of plasma cells (Potter et al., 1985). These focal plasma cell proliferations, referred to here as foci (when they contained 50 or more cells in a 4 μ section) appear to be preneoplastic lesions in plasmacytoma formation. These are first seen as soon as 25 days after pristane infection. Foci increase in numbers of BALB/c mice during the latent period of plasmacytoma development (which is minimally 120 days, and on an average is 215 days). The number of foci (containing 50 or more) cells in individual mice also increases from day 50 onwards. In mice that have multiple foci, many of the foci appear to be derived from other foci. First, there are often multiple foci in a single sector of the mesenteric OG, suggesting that cells from one focus migrated into a new nearby region of the OG. Second, plasma cells from foci can probably spread across mesothelial linings to new sectors of the OG. Frequently two separate sectors of OG tissue that are neighbors contain foci near mesothelial surfaces suggesting the cells from one have

Current Topics in Microbiology and Immunology, Vol. 132

Table 1. Incidence of plasmacytomas (PCT) after three 0.5 ml injections of pristane

	no. PCT/total	Total PCT %		Reference
BALB/cAnPt	150/245	61.0%	1	Potter & Wax, 1983
BALB/cJax	33/358	9.2%	3	Potter & Wax, 1981
C576BL/6	3/47	6.4%	2	Potter *et al.*, 1975
C57BL/Ka	0/56	0%	2	Potter *et al.*, 1975
DBA/2	0/36	0%	1	Potter, 1984
(BALB/cAn x DBA/2)F_1	0/140	0%	1	Potter, 1984

invaded the other across the peritoneal space. Thus it is difficult to determine the number of clones of plasma cells that are present in a mouse with multiple foci. While some processes could be polyclonal, most of the multiple processes are probably monoclonal.

In the present study we have compared the development of foci in BALB/cAn and several strains of mice that are resistant to plasmacytoma development (PCT-R strains) (Table 1). All of the mice developed peritoneal OG tissue like BALB/cAn, but the OG tissues of the PCT-R strains contained many scattered plasma cells. There were two general differences that distinguished BALB/cAn from the PCT-R strains. First, the development of multiple foci was very low or absent in the PCT-R strains (Table 2). Second, while both BALB/c and PCT-R strains developed OG, i.e., a tissue containing oil droplets surrounded by or contained within macrophages and neutrophils, the degrees of infiltration of the OG with inflammatory cell types differed. In C57BL/6 and DBA/2, for example, the OG tissue contained many lymphoid aggregates and colonies of extramedullary myelopoiesis. The intercellular spaces were often crowded with a variety of cells of the myelomonocytic series. Also in C57BL/6 and DBA/2 the OG tissue after 150 days became necrotic and calcified. Similar processes could be seen in BALB/cAn but the effect was more striking in DBA/2 and C57BL/6. BALB/cAn and (BALB/CAn x DBA/2)F_1 mice developed intermediate types of OG tissue.

Plasma cells were found in abundance in DBA/2 and C57BL/6 mice and some of these infiltrates in C57BL/6 showed some tendencies towards clustering. This plasma cell infiltration was very striking around 150 days but diminished by 200 days. Typical plasmacytomas (overgrowth of the OG by plasma cells) were not found in DBA/2, C57BL/6 or CDF_1. One BALB/J mouse did have a plasmacytoma.

Table 2. Incidence of proliferative plasmacytic foci with 50 more cells in mice given 0.5 ml pristane on days 0, 60 and 120

Day	No. mice	% of mice with: 0 foci	1-4 foci	5-9 foci	10-19 foci	20+ foci	PCT cells in ascites
BALB/cAnPt							
146	25	20	28	12	12	28	12
150	25	32	40	4	8	16	16
156	20	0	25	20	35	20	10
162	25	10	44	12	12	16	28
BALB/cJ							
150	25	76	20	0	0	4	-
DBA/2							
150	25	84	16	0	0	0	-
156	22	77	22	0	0	0	-
226	25	96	4	0	0	0	-
(BALB/cAn x DBA/2)F1							
156	23	69	26	4	0	0	-
150	25	52	40	4	4	0	-
219	24	88	12	0	0	0	-
C57BL/6							
150	23	69	3	4	0	0	-
231	23	100	0	0	0	0	-

- = not done

In summary, the OG tissues of PCT-R strains contained plasma cells and occasionally infiltrates of plasma cells that were usually associated with the cellular inflammatory reaction. The PCT-R strains did not develop the progressive development of multiple foci nor plasmacytomas. In addition, the OG tissues of PCT-R strains appeared after 150 days to become necrotic and calcified, suggesting that the OG in these strains had in some way lost its inflammatory properties.

Susceptibility to plasmacytoma induction in mice is determined by specific genes that have not yet been identified. One clue about how susceptibility-resistance genes determine plasmacytoma development has come from experiments that have shown that chronic admin istration of the non-steroidal anti-inflammatory agent indomethacin strikingly inhibits plasmacytoma development but not OG formation (Potter et al. 1985). We have suggested that indomethacin may act by inhibiting the formation of radicals generated by the phagocytosis of pristane (Potter et al. 1985). The present study suggests that genetic differences that govern the nature of the response to pristane may be a factor in determining susceptibility or resistance. Sanford et al. (1986) have found that the B-lymphocytes (LPS blasts) of BALB/cAn mice are less efficient at repairing X-ray induced chromosome breakage that DBA/2, BALB/cJ and CDF_1. Since oxygen and lipid radicals can induce chromosome breakage (clastogenic effects) (Emerit and Cerutti 1982), it is possible that an inefficient repair process would increase mutations in plasma cells that permit progressive growth. This is a particularly attractive hypothesis since over 95% of BALB/cAn plasmacytomas have chromosomal translocations involving the c-*myc* locus in chr 15 (Ohno et al. 1979, 1984) with associated deregulations of c-*myc* transcription (Ohno et al. 1984).

REFERENCES

Emerit I, Cerutti PA (1982) Tumor promoter phorbol-12-myristate-13-acetate induces a clastogenic factor in human lymphocytes. Proc Natl Acad Sci USA 79:7509-7513

Ohno S, Babonits M, Wiener F, Spira J, Klein G, Potter M (1979) Non-random chromosome changes involving the Ig gene-carrying chromosomes 12 and 6 in pristane-induced mouse plasmacytomas. Cell 18:1001-1007

Ohno S, Migita S, Wiener F, Babonits M, Klein G, Mushinski JF, Potter M (1984) Chromosomal translocations activating *myc* sequences and transduction of v-*abl* are crtical events in the rapid induction of plasmacytomas by pristane and Abelson virus. J Exp Med 159:1762-1777

Potter M (1984) Genetics of susceptibility to plasmacytoma development in BALB/c mice. Cancer Surveys 3:247-264

Potter M, Hartley JW, Wax JS, Gallahan D (1984) Effect of MuLV-related genes on plasmacytomagenesis in BALB/c mice. J Exp Med 160:435-440

Potter M, MacCardle RC (1964) Histology of developing plasma cell neoplasia induced by mineral oil in BALB/c mice. J Natl Cancer Inst 33:497-515

Molecular Analysis of *myc* Gene Mutants

P. J. Enrietto

Department of Microbiology, State University of New York at Stony Brook, Stony Brook, New York 11794

INTRODUCTION

The myc gene was first identified as a specific cellular sequence in the avian acute leukemia virus MC29 (Mellon et al., 1978; Roussel et al., 1979). Analysis of this virus has led to an extensive characterization of this sequence, the cellular homologue from which it was derived, and the gene product encoded by the virus (Hayman, 1983). The myc gene as found in MC29 is closely related to the cellular sequence, c-myc (Watson et al., 1983). Only nine nucleotide changes are seen between MC29 v-myc and c-myc giving rise to seven amino acid changes. In addition v-myc contains ten base pairs of coding sequence at the 5' end not found in c-myc. The c-myc gene has three exons (two of which are coding exons) and two introns.

The protein products of the viral and cellular myc genes have been well characterized. In MC29 (Hayman, 1983) the protein is expressed as a fusion product between gag and myc sequences ($p110^{gag-myc}$). The products of c-myc in avian cells are 59,000 and 62,000 daltons (Hann et al., 1983). In each case the proteins are nuclear and highly phosphorylated (Abrams et al., 1982); they have long highly G-C rich stretches encoding prolines; and the amino acids at the carboxy terminus are very basic, a property reported to be required for nuclear transport (Kalderon et al., 1984).

The function of the myc gene is unknown although it has been implicated in several oncogenic processes in birds (for review, see Graf and Beug, 1978), mice and man (for review, see Robertson, 1983). One way to approach an understanding of the role of myc in the oncogenic process in the avian system is described in this paper. Mutants of MC29 in the myc gene and a variant of MC29 which exhibits altered target cell specificity have been characterized molecularly and pathologically to gain insight into the regions of the myc gene important in tumorigenesis.

RESULTS

Several years ago three mutants of MC29 (td10A, td10C, td10H) were isolated from a quail cell clone infected with wt MC29. While the mechanism by which the mutants were generated remains unclear, they proved to be very useful in analysis of the myc gene (Ramsay et al., 1980). One of the first parameters tested was the ability of the viruses to morphologically transform fibroblasts and to transform macrophages to increased growth in a bone marrow assay. As can be seen in Table 1, wildtype (wt) MC29 transforms both cell types while each of the mutants transforms fibroblasts but not macrophages. This result suggested that the mutation in the viruses rendered them transformation defective for macrophage transformation.

Table 1 Characterization of MC29 Deletion Mutants

Virus	Transformation Capacity: Macrophages	Transformation Capacity: Fibroblasts	Protein Product	Deletion size in Proviral DNA	Localization[a]	DNA binding[a]
td 10A	-	+	$p100^{gag\text{-}myc}$	200 bp	Nuclear	-
td 10C	-	+	$p95^{gag\text{-}myc}$	400 bp	Nuclear	-
td 10H	-	+	$p90^{gag\text{-}myc}$	600 bp	Nuclear	-
Wild type MC29	+	+	$p110^{gag\text{-}myc}$	-	Nuclear	+

Cumulative data

a) Taken from Abrams et al.(1982)and Donner et al. (1983)

Three approaches were taken to determine the nature of the mutation and characterize the viruses in more detail. In the first instance the proteins encoded by the mutants (Ramsay and Hayman, 1982) were analyzed and in each case found to be smaller than the wt protein $p110^{gag\text{-}myc}$. Table I lists the protein sizes. Oligonucleotide mapping of wt MC29 and mutant viral RNAs suggested that the mutant viral RNA was deleted, each lacking a specific set of myc oligonucleotides (Bister et al., 1982). Finally, the proviral DNA contained in fibroblasts transformed by the mutants was restriction mapped and compared to wt MC29 DNA (Enrietto et al., 1982). This analysis revealed that td10A had a deletion of 200 base pairs, ta10C a deletion of 400 base pairs and td10H a deletion of 600 base pairs. All of the deletions reside in the 3' half of the myc gene. However, all of the mutants retain the carboxy terminus of the protein since td10A, td10C, and td10H proteins can be immunoprecipitated by antiserum raised against the carboxy terminal portion of myc (Patchinsky et al., 1984). Table 1 summarizes the biochemical characterization of the deletion mutants including their localization and DNA binding ability and Fig. 1 is a schematic diagram of the restriction maps of each of the proviruses to demonstrate the position and extent of the deletions.

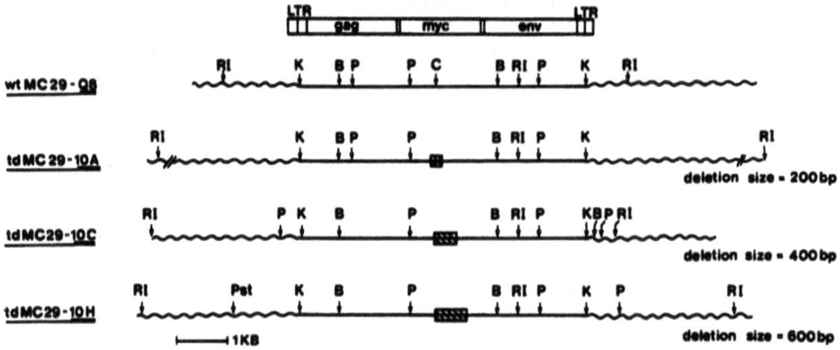

RESTRICTION ENZYME MAPPING OF MC29 MUTANTS

Fig 1

We were curious to know what effect these deletions had on the pathogenicity of MC29 (Enrietto et al., 1983). To examine this, one-day-old chickens were injected with wild type MC29, td10A, td10C and td10H. The results of these studies are shown in Table 2.

Table 2 **Pathogenicity of MC29 Deletion Mutants**

Virus	No. of Tumors	Type	Latency
Wild type MC29	9/9	Endotheliomas	66d
td 10A	2/10	Endothelioma & (a) Lymphoid leukosis	126d
td 10C	0/9		
td 10H	2/10	Lymphoid leukosis[a]	155d

a) Lymphoid leukosis were the result of helper virus integration near the c-*myc* locus.

As can be seen deletions in the 3' portion of *myc* effectively render the virus non-pathogenic. This study also revealed the relatively narrow pathogenic spectrum of the laboratory strain of MC29 now in use which only causes endotheliomas.

One of the interesting features of MC29 is the virus' ability to transform two cell types, macrophages and fibroblasts. The basis of this target cell specificity is unclear but we have attempted to approach this question by analyzing a variant of MC29 called HBI which has proven to have very interesting properties.

The procedure used to isolate this virus, its biological properties, structure and pathogenicity will now be described. One of the deletion mutants, td10H, proved to be unstable on passage in that proteins larger than the predicted $p90^{gag-myc}$ protein (see Table 1) could be detected. On the assumption that td10H was acquiring sequence during passage an attempt was made to select a virus which could transform macrophages from the td10H stock. To this end the td10H stock was used to infect chick bone marrow cells and three macrophage colonies resulted. From one of these colonies the HBI virus was rescued (Ramsay et al., 1982).

Because the HBI virus was isolated on the basis of its biological properties, it was of interest to examine its biochemical properties and determine if the ability to transform macrophages correlated with an acquisition or change in the structure of the provirus and its protein product. In the first instance, quail fibroblasts transformed by HBI were immunoprecipitated and a protein of 108,000 daltons was identified (in contrast to wt MC29 protein product of 110,000 daltons and the parental td10H protein product of 90,000 daltons). Obviously, this virus had acquired sequence which gave rise to an increased coding capacity. In order to identify the position of this sequence, restriction mapping of proviral DNA was carried out. Figure 2 shows the deduced restriction maps of wtMC29, td10H and HBI. As can be seen HBI seemed to have recovered *myc* sequence, presumably by recombination with c-*myc*. In addition, it had changes in *gag* (an additional PstI site) and the viral LTR (an EcoRI site instead of the KpN site found in wt MC29). These changes were thought to be the result of recombination with helper virus with which td10H was passaged (Ramsay et al., 1982).

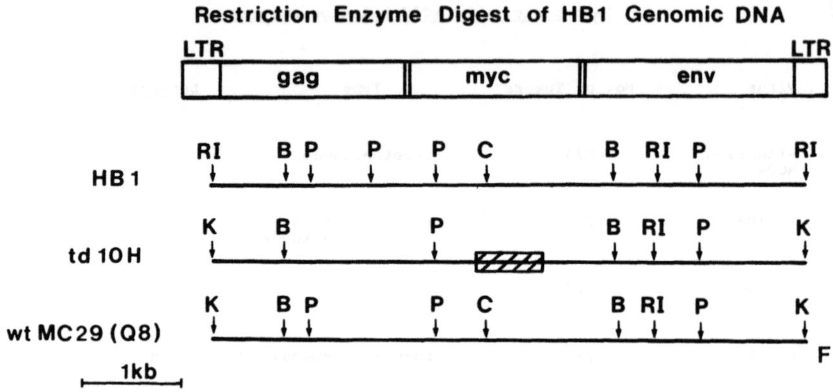

Fig2

Molecular cloning and sequencing of HBI has shown it to be a very unusual recombinant. Figure 3 is a schematic representation of the composition of HBI. As predicted the viral LTR and most of the <u>gag</u> gene appears to be derived from ring-neck pheasant virus, the helper with which td10H was passaged during the isolation of HBI. In addition HBI seems to be a "recovered" virus containing <u>c-myc</u>-specific nucleotides in the v-myc region, gained by recombination with the cellular locus (Smith et al., 1985).

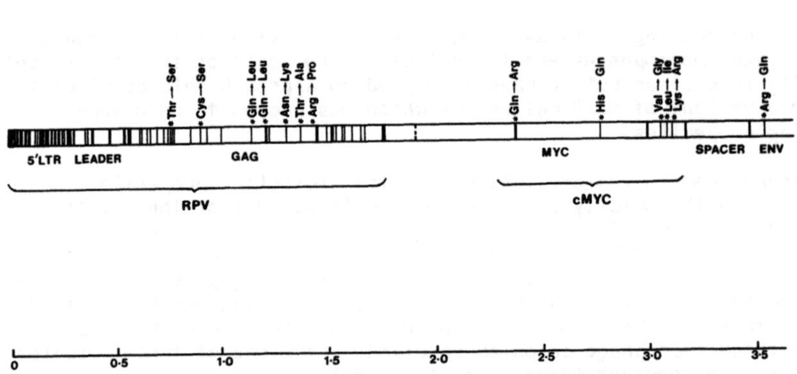

Fig3

It was clearly of interest to see what effect these changes had, if any, on the pathogenicity of HBI. One-day-old brown leghorn chickens were injected with HBI and examined for induction of tumors. A summary of our findings can be found in Table 3. As can be seen, the pathogenic spectrum of HBI is drastically altered: lymphomas were observed rather than endotheliomas (Enrietto et al., 1983). The lymphomas were of short latency (on average 101 days with some developing as early as 40 days post injection). The tumors were bursal-independent since bursectomized chicks developed lymphoid tumors at the same frequency as nonbursectomized chicks. The cell types involved were of both the T and B cell lineage as determined by staining tumors with antisera specific for B or T cells. In terms of the differentiation state tumors could be classed as lymphoblastoid, lymphocytic, and in some instances, plasmacytic. While lymphoid tumors were the predominant tumor type seen, as the virus dose was increased the spectrum of tumor types was broadened and occasionally a myelocytoma was found. This is the tumor type first attributed to infection by MC29 (for review, see Graf and Beug, 1978).

Table 3 Pathogenicity of HBI and wt MC29

Virus	No. of Tumors	Type	Latency	Bursal Dependence	Cell types involved
MC29	9/9	Endothelioma	66d	-	Histiocytes
HBI	8/12	Lymphoma	101d	-	T & B cells

To determine the mechanism by which these tumors arose, tumor tissue was analyzed by restriction enzyme digestion of high molecular weight DNA. In total 40 tumors were examined and in 39 of the 40 tumors, HBI proviral DNA could be identified without disruption of the *c-myc* locus. This result suggested that the presence of the HBI provirus was necessary for tumor maintenance. The provirus was expressed as well since tumor cells labeled with ^{35}S-methionine and immunoprecipitated were found to contain the HBI protein produced $p108^{gag-myc}$ (Enrietto et al., 1983).

In summary, the recombinant virus HBI is a novel MC29 virus in that it has regained *myc* sequences (from *c-myc*) lost by the parent td10H and has recombined with ring-neck pheasant virus resulting in the acquisition of a novel LTR and *gag* gene. These changes result in the generation of a different size protein product and a unique pathogenic spectrum.

DISCUSSION

The studies described in this paper suggest a system in which the oncogenic potential of *myc* can be dissected, altered, and related to changes in the viral genome and known *myc* functions. It has been possible to show that the avian *v-myc* gene has a relatively narrow pathogenic spectrum, inducing predominantly endotheliomas. When the 3' portion of the gene is deleted, no disease is induced in chickens. *In vitro* these defects manifest themselves as an inability to transform avian macrophages while retaining the ability to morphologically transform fibroblast. This data suggests that the *myc* protein has two functional domains: one responsible for macrophage transformation and one for fibroblast transformation.

The work with the recovered HBI virus suggests that recovery of 3' *myc* domain restores the ability of the virus to induce the proliferation of macrophages. *In vitro* this virus behaves in a manner very similar to wild type MC29. However, when examined *in vivo* the target cell specificity had altered significantly. We are now pursuing the sequence changes responsible for the altered target cell specificty by constructing chimeric viruses between wt MC29 and HBI.

In summary, this system allows us to approach two important questions: first, the function of the *myc* gene is a system where mutants are available to uncouple activities and characteristics of the gene: second, the ability of the virus to be targeted to a particular cell type and to transform that cell type in preference to others.

REFERENCES

Abram HD, Rohrschneider LR, Eisenman RN (1982) Nuclear location of the putative transforming protein of avian myelocytomatosis virus. Cell 29: 427-439

Bister K, Ramsay GM, Hayman MJ (1982) Deletion within the transformation-specific RNA sequences of acute leukemia virus MC29 give rise to partially transformation-defective mutants. J Virol 41: 754-766

Donner P, Bunte T, Greiser-Wilke I, Moelling K (1983) Decreased DNA binding ability of purified transformation-specific proteins from deletion mutants of the acute avian leukemia virus MC29. Proc Nat Acad Sci USA 80: 2861-2865

Enrietto PJ, Hayman MJ (1982) Restriction enzyme analysis of partially transformation defective mutants of acute leukemia virus MC29. J Virol 44: 711-715

Enrietto PJ, Hayman MJ, Ramsay GM, Wyke JA, Payne LN (1983) Altered pathogenicity of avian myelocytomatosis (MC29) viruses with mutations in the _v-myc_ gene. Virology 124: 164-172

Enrietto PJ, Payne LN, Hayman MJ (1983) A recovered avian myelocytomatosis virus which induces lymphomas in chickens: pathogenic properties and their molecular basis. Cell 35:369-379

Graf T and Beug H (1978) Avian leukemia viruses. Interaction with their target cells _in vivo_ and _in vitro_. Biochem Biophys Acta 516: 269-299

Hann SR, Abrams HD, Rohrschneider LR, Eisenman RN (1985) Proteins encoded by the _v-myc_ and _c-myc_ oncogenes: identification and location in acute leukemia virus transformants and bursal lymphoma lines. Cell 34: 789

Hayman MJ (1983) Avian acute leukemia viruses. Curr Top Microbiol Immunol 98: 109-116

Kalderon D, Richardson WD, Markham AF, Smith AE (1984) Sequence requirements for nuclear location of simian virus 40 large-T-antigen. Nature London 311: 33-38

Mellon P, Pawson A, Bister K, Martin GS, Duesberg PH (1978) Specific RNA sequences and gene products of MC29 avian acute leukemia virus. Proc Nat Acad Sci USA 75: 5874-5878

Patschinsky T, Watts G, Bister K (1984) Immunological analysis of _v-myc_ gene products using antibodies against _myc_ specific synthetic peptide. Virol 136: 348-385

Ramsay, GM, Hayman, MJ (1982) Isolation and biochemical characterization of partially transformation-defective mutants of avian myelocytomatosis virus strain MC29: localization of the mutation to the _myc_ domain of the 110,000 dalton gag-myc polypeptide. J Virol 41: 745-753

Ramsay, GM, Enrietto, PJ, Graf, T, Hayman, MJ (1982) Recovery of myc-specific sequences by a partially transformation defective mutant of avian myelocytomatosis virus, MC29, correlates with the restoration of transforming activity. Proc Nat Acad Sci USA 79: 6885-6889

Ramsay, GM, Graf, T, Hayman, MJ (1980) Mutants of avian myelocytomatosis virus MC29 with smaller gag gene related proteins have an altered transforming ability. Nature 288: 170-172

Robertson, M (1983) Paradox and paradigm: the message and meaning of myc. Nature 306: 733-736

Roussel, M, Saule, S, Lagrou, C, Rommens, C, Beug, N, Graf, T, Stehelin, D (1979) Three new types of viral oncogene of cellular origin specific for hematopoietic cell transformation. Nature 281: 452-455

Smith, DR, Vennstrom, B, Hayman, MJ, Enrietto, PJ (1985) Nucleotide sequence of HBI, a novel recombinant MC29 derivative with altered pathogenic properties. J Virol 56: 969-977

Watson, DK, Reddy, EP, Duesberg, PH, Papas, TS (1983) Nucleotide sequence analysis of the chicken c-myc locus reveals homologous and unique coding regions by comparison with the transforming gene of avian myelocytomatosis virus, MC 29. Proc Nat Acad Sci USA 80: 2146-2150

Induction of *fgr* Proto-oncogene mRNA in B Lymphocytes as a Consequence of Epstein-Barr Virus Infection

M.S.C. Cheah, T.J. Ley, S.R. Tronick, and K.C. Robbins

Laboratory of Cellular and Molecular Biology, National Cancer Institute and Clinical Hematology Branch, National Heart, Lung and Blood Institute Bethesda, MD 20205 USA

INTRODUCTION

The discovery that the v-sis oncogene was derived from a normal growth factor gene represented the first link between a transforming gene and a known cellular function. More recently, two additional retrovirus onc genes have been shown to be altered versions of normal cellular genes encoding cell surface receptors for other growth factors, namely epidermal growth factor (EGF) (Downward et al., 1984; Ullrich et al., 1984) and very likely colony stimulating factor-1 (CSF-1) (Sherr et al., 1985).

One of the first clues regarding onc gene function was provided by the observation that one onc gene, v-src, encoded a relatively rare enzymatic activity which catalyzed phosphorylation of tyrosine residues (Bishop, 1983). Moreover, receptors for normal growth factors such as EGF, insulin, and PDGF all respond to ligand binding by autophosphorylation of tyrosine residues present in their cytoplasmic domains. Thus, it is thought that tyrosine phosphorylation may be intimately associated with transmitting a proliferative signal to cells exposed to these growth factors. The fact that roughly half of the 20 or so oncogenes isolated to date encode tyrosine kinases suggests that additional links between oncogenes and growth factor receptors will be discovered. Taken together, these findings have strongly implicated the constitutive activation of growth factor-mediated stimulatory pathways in the malignant process.

The fgr Oncogene Encodes a Tyrosine Kinase

Gardner Rasheed feline sarcoma virus (GR-FeSV) is a sarcomagenic retrovirus initially isolated from a cat fibrosarcoma (Rasheed et al., 1982). The transforming protein of GR-FeSV is a 70,000 dalton molecule which possesses a kinase activity with specificity for tyrosine residues (Naharro et al., 1983). Nucleotide sequence analysis of GR-FeSV DNA has revealed that its transforming gene arose as a result of genetic recombination involving two distinct cellular genes, one encoding the cytoskeletal structural protein actin and the other a tyrosine-specific protein kinase. The molecular structure of this transforming gene, as well as the protein it specifies, are shown in Figure 1.

The presence of actin sequences near the amino terminal region of this transforming protein raises interesting questions. Actin is a highly conserved and abundant structural protein present in all eukaryotic cells. Six actin isoforms are known in vertebrates: four muscle types and two nonmuscle types. Each muscle-type actin is functionally involved in muscle contraction and is expressed only in particular muscle tissues. Conversely, cytoplasmic actins participate in a variety of functions, such as cell motility, mitosis, and maintenance of the cytoskeleton, and are expressed in all cell types. Stable alterations of cell shape and motility have been

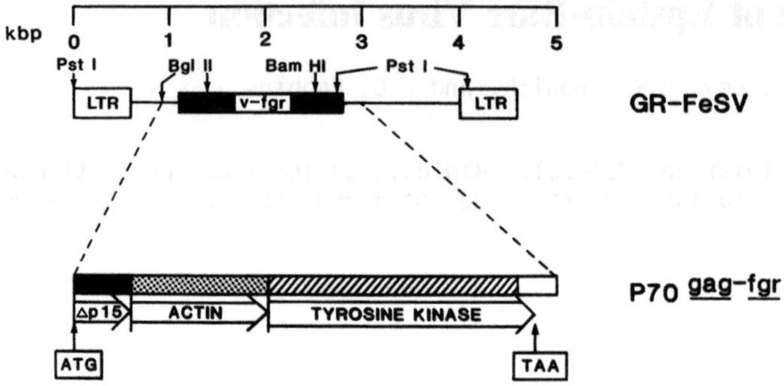

Fig. 1. Summary of the major structural features of the GR-FeSV genome. Important features of GR-FeSV genome including the open reading frame, important restriction enzyme cleavage sites, and the region of homology with FeLV p15, actin, and v-*yes* gene products are indicated. LTR, long terminal repeat; kbp, kilobase pairs.

considered as one of the phenotypic characteristics of transformed cells. There also appears to be some correlation between the presence of the variant actins and increased ability of these cells to produce tumors in nude mice. It is therefore possible that the GR-FeSV transforming protein P70$^{gag-fgr}$ which contains 134 out of actin's 375 amino acids represents an aberrant form of actin which interferes with the formation of proper cytoskeletal structure in cells transformed by GR-FeSV. Alternatively, the actin moiety of P70$^{gag-fgr}$ may serve to direct its tyrosine kinase to a limited set of cytoskeletal targets which would not normally be accessible for phosphorylation. Further investigation will be required to determine how the actin sequence relates to the oncogenic activity of this virus.

The other GR-FeSV cell-derived gene, designated v-*fgr*, was shown to specify a protein highly related to previously described *onc* gene-coded tyrosine kinases. By computer analysis, it was determined that the v-*fgr* gene product was 80% and 74% related in amino acid sequence to proteins specified by v-*yes* and v-*src* genes, respectively (Naharro *et al*., 1984). The highly conserved nature of the predicted products of feline-derived v-*fgr* and avian-derived v-*src* and v-*yes* raised the possibility that the *fgr* proto-oncogene was the cat homologue of either c-*src* or c-*yes* chicken proto-oncogenes. To address this question, human DNA was analyzed with v-*fgr*, v-*src* and v-*yes* probes. Although each probe detected related sequences in restriction enzyme treated DNA, none of the human DNA fragments hybridized by v-*src* or v-*yes* probes corresponded to those detected with *fgr* probes. Thus, the human genome must contain distinct proto-oncogenes related to each of these tyrosine kinase-encoding *onc* genes. These findings have implied a strong evolutionary pressure to conserve a similar structure and kinase function at three different human loci.

Detection of the *fgr* proto-oncogene in human DNA made it possible to isolate and characterize this sequence utilizing recombinant DNA techniques (Tronick *et al*., 1985). A small portion of the human *fgr* proto-oncogene sequence was then used to locate this gene within the human genome. The human *fgr* proto-oncogene was localized by in situ hybridization techniques to chromosome 1 at p36.1-36.2. Previous studies have shown that many forms of cancer, including solid and hematopoietic tumors (Gilbert et al., 1982), display alterations affecting chromosome 1 (Yunis, 1984). This chromosome is also known to contain a number of other genes that affect cell growth, including the oncogenes B-lym (p32) (Morton et al., 1985) and N-ras (p11-p13) (Rabin et al., 1984), as well as the gene encoding nerve growth factor (p21-p22) (Franke, 1983). Specific deletions involving 1p31-36 have been described in certain neuroblastomas and result in monosomies of the terminal region of 1p (Gilbert, 1983). Thus, it should now be possible to determine whether fgr proto-oncogene structure and/or expression is perturbed in human tumors possessing chromosome 1 alterations.

Expression of fgr Proto-oncogene mRNA in Normal and Malignant Cells

To investigate whether the fgr proto-oncogene was expressed in human tumor cells, RNAs were prepared from selected cell lines which represented a diverse spectrum of human cancers. After selection on oligo(dT) columns, poly(A)+ RNAs were examined for the presence of fgr proto-oncogene mRNA by Northern blotting. C-fgr transcripts were detected in 6 of 11 cell lines derived from myelo- or lymphoproliferative disorders but not in any of the 9 carcinoma or 6 sarcoma cell lines examined. In a representative experiment (Fig. 2) the fgr related mRNA detected was 3 kb long, which is in close agreement with the length of the transcript detected in normal human lung tissue (Tronick et al., 1985).

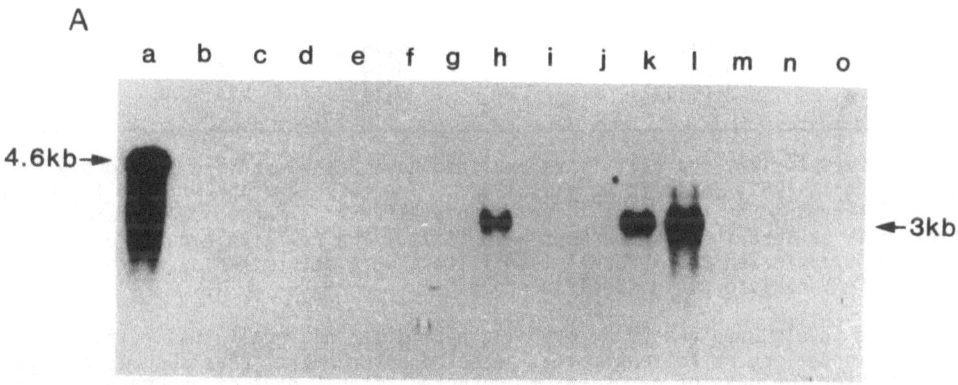

Fig 2. Survey of human tumor cell lines for expression of c-fgr-related RNA. Poly-(A)$^+$-containing RNA was prepared, as described (Adams et al., 1974), from human tumor cell lines and examined by the Northern technique using a v-fgr-specific DNA fragment as probe. Carcinoma derived cell lines, A2054, A549, A2182, A431, A1847, and A2199 (Giard et al., 1973; Aaronson and Ellmore, unpublished) (lanes b-g, respectively), lymphoma derived cell lines JI, MC116, JD38, RAJI and NAMALWA (lanes h-i, respectively), as well as sarcoma derived cell lines A375, A1632, and A2984 (lanes m-o, respectively), were examined. RNA from GR-FeSV-infected mink cells (lane a) was used as a control. The relative amounts of hybridizable RNA transferred to nitrocellulose filters were shown to be similar by rehybridization with a GR-FeSV-derived, actin-specific probe.

Detection of fgr Proto-oncogene mRNA in Burkitt's Lymphoma Cells Naturally Infected with EBV

Because our initial survey had indicated the presence of the c-*fgr* transcript in cell lines derived from lymphoproliferative disorders, our analysis was extended to include various B cell lines derived from African and American undifferentiated lymphomas of the Burkitt and non-Burkitt types. As summarized in Table 1, the c-*fgr* transcript was detected in approximately half of the lymphoma cell lines tested. All cell lines infected with EBV expressed detectable *fgr* mRNA. One non-Burkitt's lymphoma cell line that expressed detectable c-*fgr* mRNA was not nuclear antigen (EBNA) positive. These results revealed an association of *fgr* proto-oncogene mRNA with Burkitt's lymphoma cells which had been naturally infected with EBV.

Table 1. Detection of *fgr* proto-oncogene mRNA in cell lines derived from Burkitt's and non-Burkitt's undifferentiated lymphomas

Histopathology	Cell line	EBNA status	Chromosomal translocation	Geographical origin	Expression of v-*fgr** related transcript
Burkitt's lymphoma	Namalwa	+	8;14	Africa	+++
	Keeper	+	8;14	S. Africa	+++
	AG876	+	8;14	Africa	++
	JI	+	2;8	Europe	++
	Raji	+	8;14	Africa	++
	LY47	+	8;22	Africa	+
	BL2	-	8;22	Europe	-
	ST486	-	8;14	USA	-
	MC116	-	8;14	USA	-
	CA46	-	8;14	S. America	-
Non-Burkitt's lymphoma	EW36	-	8;14	USA	-
	DS179	-	8;14	USA	+
	JD38	-	8;14	USA	-
	JLPC119	-	8;14	USA	-

The characteristics of the cell lines examined have been described previously (Lenoir *et al.*, 1982; Benjamin *et al.*, 1982). The concentration of 3-kb *fgr*-related mRNA was determined by analyzing 10 μg of poly(A)$^+$ RNA in formamide-formaldehyde agarose gels as described (Lehrach *et al.*, 1977). The relative amounts of hybridizable RNA transferred to nitrocellulose filters were determined by rehybridization with a GR-FeSV-derived actin-specific probe.

*Detectable levels were graded by exposing hybridized nitrocellulose filters for varying time periods as follows: +++, detected after overnight exposure; ++, detected after two days of exposure; +, detected after 5 days of exposure; -, not detectable after 5 days of exposure.

EBV Infection of B Lymphocytes Results in Induction of fgr Proto-Oncogene mRNA

To further assess the association between expression of the fgr proto-oncogene and EBV infection, we examined RNAs prepared from normal umbilical cord or peripheral blood lymphocyte cell lines established as a result of EBV infection. Figure 3 shows that the fgr proto-oncogene transcript was expressed at detectable levels in each of these cell lines, providing further evidence that EBV infection was responsible for the increased concentration of fgr proto-oncogene transcripts detected in the lymphoid cells. Efforts to determine whether normal B lymphocytes express c-fgr mRNA have revealed that normal peripheral blood mononuclear cells contain this transcript. However recent experiments have revealed that c-fgr mRNA is not expressed in normal resting or mitogen activated B lymphocytes. In any case, the fact that normal lymphocytes become immortalized as stable cell lines in response to EBV infection but do not acquire fully neoplastic properties suggests that expression of c-fgr mRNA alone is not sufficient to induce the neoplastic state.

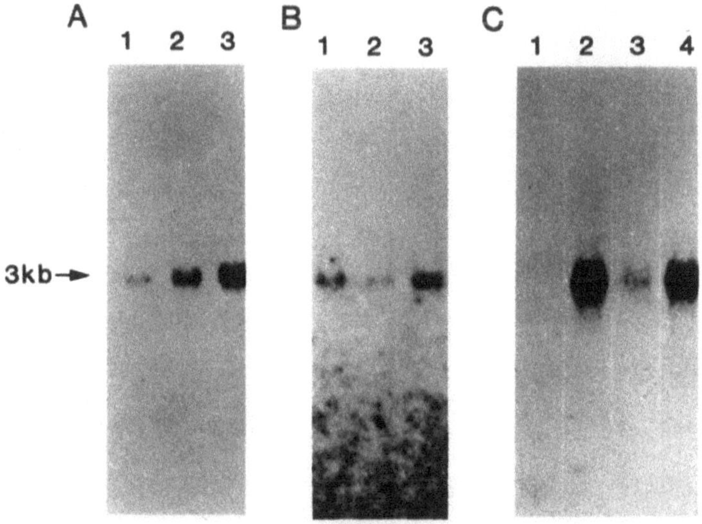

Fig 3. Expression of fgr-related mRNA in cells infected with EBV in vitro. Poly-$(A)^+$-containing RNAs prepared from EBV-infected normal peripheral (A) or umbilical cord (B) blood lymphocytes, as well as uninfected (C, lanes 1 and 3) or EBV-infected (C, lanes 2 and 4), BJAB (lanes 1 and 2) or RAMOS (lanes 3 and 4) Burkitt's lymphoma cell lines (Clements et al., 1975; Klein et al., 1975) was analyzed as described in Fig. 2 legend. Relative amounts of hybridizable RNA transferred to nitrocellulose filters were shown to be similar by rehybridization with a GR-FeSV-derived actin-specific probe.

We extended our analysis to EBV negative Burkitt's lymphoma cells which are susceptible to EBV infection. BJAB cells infected with a prototype EBV, B95-8 (Henle et al., 1967, Pope et al., 1968), which is capable of immortalizing normal B lymphocytes, or RAMOS cells infected with a non-transformimng derivative, P3HR1 (Miller et al., 1974), were examined for the presence of fgr transcripts. These converted cell lines are known to resemble their parental cell lines in morphology and with regard to karyotype and HLA and B antigen typing (Klein et al., 1976). As shown in Fig. 3, uninfected BJAB or RAMOS cell lines expressed little or no detectable c-fgr mRNA, whereas cells infected with either one of the two strains expressed the c-fgr transcript. We conclude from these results that the increase in c-fgr RNA concentration was a specific event associated with EBV infection. Moreover, as infection with either an immortalizing or a non-immortalizing EBV strain led to an increase in the steady state concentration of fgr mRNA, we suggest that altered c-fgr expression alone is insufficient for immortalization.

Steady-state fgr mRNA Concentration is Increased at Least 50 Fold in Response to EBV Infection

To assess the level of c-fgr transcript induction in response to EBV infection, DNA fragments containing a dihydrofolate reductase exon (dhfr) (Chen et al., 1984) or human c-fgr sequences (Tronick et al., 1985) were used as probes in quantitative S_1

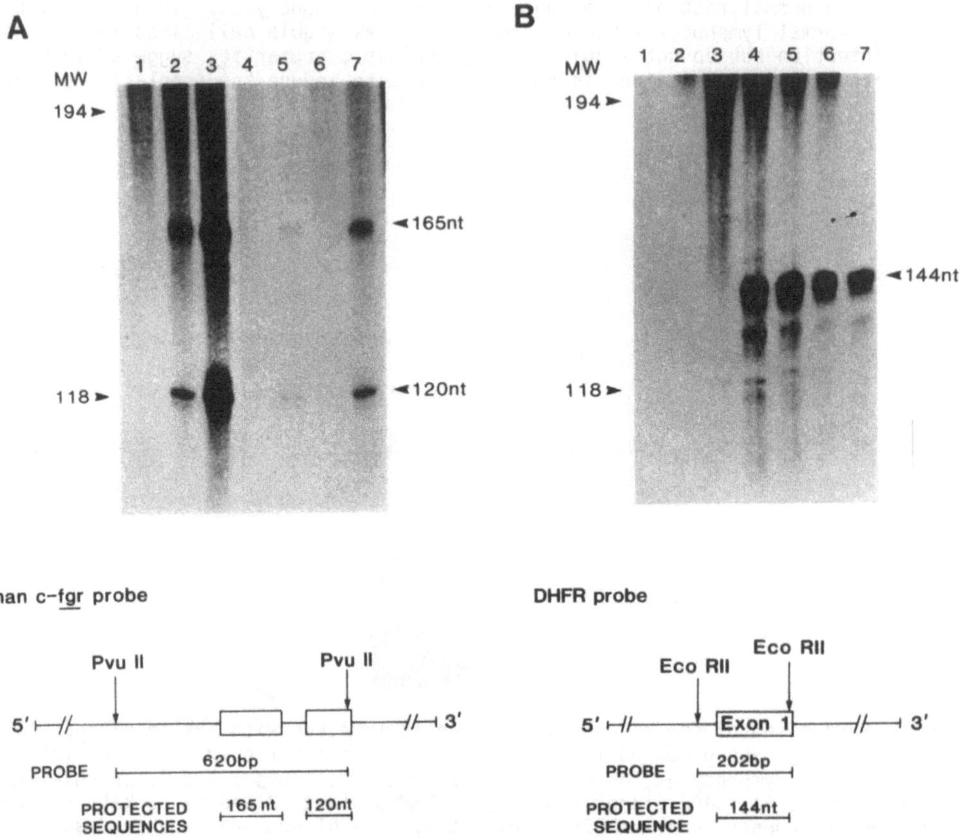

Fig. 4. Quantitation of fgr proto-oncogene mRNA induction in response to EBV infection. DNA fragments derived from the region of 6.0 to 6.62 kbp of the human fgr proto-oncogene (A) or the 5' end of the dihydrofolate reductase gene (B) were cloned into M13 phage vectors and used as templates for the synthesis of uniformly labeled anti-sense DNA. Conditions for hybridization of total cell RNA with the DNA probe, S1 nuclease digestion and polyacrylamide gel electrophoretic analysis of protected sequences were as described elsewhere (Berk and Sharp, 1977; Ley et al., 1982). Samples tested included 5 µg or 20 µg (lanes 3) total cellular RNA from normal human peripheral blood mononuclear cells, 20 µg from uninfected Ramos (lanes 4) or BJAB (lanes 6) as well as P3HR1-infected Ramos (lanes 5) or B95-8 infected BJAB (lanes 7) cell lines. Negative controls consisted of labelled probe hybridized in the absence of RNA and treated with S_1 nuclease (lanes 1). As expected, no dhfr mRNA was detected in peripheral blood mononuclear cells as these cells were not in cycle. The diagrams at the bottom of the figure show human c-fgr and dhfr exons and their protected sequences. The extent and locations of the human c-fgr exons shown were confirmed by nucleotide sequence analysis.

nuclease protection experiments. As a positive control for each probe, RNA prepared from normal human peripheral blood mononuclear cells was examined (Fig. 4). As expected, a major band of 144 nucleotides was protected with the dhfr probe in the cell lines that were in cell cycle. C-fgr DNA protected sequences of 165 and 120 nucleotides, sizes which were consistent with those of v-fgr related stretches present in the DNA fragment used as a probe (data not shown). The intensity of bands detected with each DNA probe increased as a function of RNA concentration, making it possible to quantitate the level of c-fgr mRNA induction. RNAs from uninfected or EBV infected cell lines contained silmilar amounts of dhfr mRNA as indicated by the intensity of the 144 nucleotide dhfr probe fragment (Fig. 4B). In contrast, c-fgr sequences of 165 and 120 nucleotides were protected by RNA from EBV infected but not uninfected BJAB or RAMOS cells. By varying the exposure times, we calculated that the steady state concentration of c-fgr mRNA increased by at least 50-fold in response to EBV infection. Based on other data obtained with probes of similar specific activity (Ley et al., 1984), we estimate that the EBV infected lines contain 20 copies of c-fgr mRNA per cell.

DISCUSSION

The correlation of increased fgr proto-oncogene expression with EBV infection of transformed lymphocytes was nearly absolute. Increased concentrations of c-fgr mRNA were detected in Burkitt's lymphoma cells whether infected naturally or deliberately in tissue culture. In addition, each of the umbilical cord or peripheral blood lymphocyte cell lines established by EBV infection expressed c-fgr mRNA. Increases in the levels of transcripts related to other mammalian tyrosine kinase-encoding onc genes (v-fms and v-fes) were also detected in some EBV infected Burkitt's lymphoma cell lines (data not shown), but these RNAs were not consistently detected in EBV infected cell lines and were in some cases detectable in uninfected cell lines. Taken together, these results establish a specific relationship between EBV infection and expression of the fgr proto-oncogene and suggest that EBV infection results in transcriptional activation of c-fgr. Further studies will be required to show whether increased transcriptional rates alone are responsible for the increase in steady-state concentration c-fgr mRNA.

Integration of EBV into host chromosomal DNA of Namalwa and IB4 cell lines has been described elsewhere (Henderson et al., 1983). In Namalwa cells the site of integration is close to the fgr proto-oncogene locus on chromosome 1 (Tronick et al., 1985; Henderson et al., 1983), whereas in IB4 cells the EBV genome integrates into chromosome 4. In the case of the Namalwa cell line, EBV may have a cis-acting effect on the expression of the fgr proto-oncogene. However, in most cases the influence of EBV on c-fgr is more likely to be trans, as the EBV genome typically exists in the host as an episome. Thus the isolation of EBV genes having specific functions may make it possible to identify the region of the EBV genome responsible for the increase in fgr proto-oncogene mRNA.

Several lines of evidence suggest that Burkitt's lymphoma results from a multi-step process involving the alteration of several genetic elements (Klein and Klein, 1985). Epidemiological data suggest that EBV has an important role in the etiology of African Burkitt's lymphoma (Gesner, 1982). Molecular studies have strongly implicated alterations of myc proto-oncogene expression in the process leading to American as well as African Burkitt's malignancies (Dalla-Favera, 1982; Taub, 1982). However there is no evidence to indicate that such genetic alterations are the only changes required to achieve lymphoid cell transformation. From the results of the present study we conclude that increased concentrations of c-fgr mRNA alone are not sufficient to induce malignant transformation of normal lymphocytes or even to immortalize them as continuous cell lines. Moreover, we have no direct evidence that

EBV induced immortalization involves c-fgr. Nevertheless, our results are consistent with the possibility that one step in EBV-induced B-cell immortalization involves transcriptional activation of the fgr proto-oncogene in response to an EBV encoded function.

ACKNOWLEDGEMENT

We thank N. Ellmore, L. Mickley, and C. Lengel for technical assistance; N. Raab-Traub, I.T. Magrath, and D. Ablashi for providing cell lines; T. Kawakami for making unpublished nucleotide sequence data available to us; T. Shimada and A. Nienhuis for the dhfr probe; and S. Aaronson for helpful discussions.

REFERENCES

Adams SL, Sobel ME, Howard BH, Olden K, Yamada KM, Crombrugghe BD, Pastan I (1977) Levels of translatable mRNAs for cell surface protein collagen precursors, and two membrane proteins are altered in Rous sarcoma virus-transformed chick embryo fibroblasts. Proc Natl Acad Sci USA 74:3399-3404

Benjamin D, Magrath IT, Maguire R, Janus C, Todd HD, Parsons RG (1982) Immunoglobulin secretion by cell lines derived from African and American undifferentiated lymphomas of Burkitt's and non-Burkitt's type. J Immun 129:1336-1342

Berk AJ, Sharp PA (1977) Sizing and mapping of early adenovirus mRNAs by gel electrophoresis of S_1 endonuclease-digested hybrids. Cell 12:721-732

Chen MJ, Shimada T, Moulton AD, Cline A, Humphries RK, Maizel J, Nienhuis AW (1984) The functional human dihydrofolate reductase gene. J Biol Chem 259:3933-3943

Clements GB, Klein G, Povey S (1975) Production by EBV infection of an EBNA positive subline from an EBNA-negative human lymphoma cell line without detectable EBV DNA. Int J Cancer 16:125-133

Dalla-Favera R, Bregni M, Erikson J, Patterson D, Gallo RC, Croce CM (1982) Human c-myc onc gene is located on the region of chromosome 8 that is translocated in Burkitt'slymphoma cells. Proc Natl Acad Sci USA 79:7824-7827

Downward J, Yarden Y, Mayes E, Scrace G, Totty N, Stockwell P, Ullrich A, Schlesinger J, Waterfield MD (1984) Close similarity of epidermal growth factor receptor and v-erbB oncogene protein sequences. Nature (London) 307:521-527

Geser A, deThe G, Lenoir G, Day NE, Williams EH (1982) Final case reporting from the Ugandan prospective study of the relationship between EBV and Burkitt's lymphoma. Int J Cancer 29:397-400

Giard DJ, Aaronson SA, Todaro GJ, Arnstein P, Kersey JH, Dosik H, Parks WP (1973) In vitro cultivation of human tumors: establishment of cell lines derived from a series of solid tumors. J Natl Cancer Inst 51:1417-1423

Henderson A, Ripley S, Heller M, Kieff E (1983) Human chromosome association of Epstein-Barr virus DNA in a Burkitt tumor cell line and in lymphocytes growth transformed in vitro. Proc Natl Acad Sci USA 80:1987-1991

Henle W, Diehl V, Kohn G, zur Hausen H, Henle G (1967) Herpes-type virus and chromosome marker in normal leukocytes after growth with irradiated Burkitt cells. Science 157:1064-1065

Klein G, Giovanella B, Westman A, Stehlin JS, Mumford D (1975) An EBV genome negative cell line established from an American Burkitt lymphoma, receptor characteristics, EBV infectibility and permanent conversion into EBV-positive sublines by in vitro infection. Intervirology 5:319-334

Klein G, Klein E (1985) Evolution of tumours and the impact of molecular oncology. Nature 315:190-195

Klein G, Zeuthen J, Terasaki P, Billing R, Honig R, Jonkal M, Westman A, Clements G (1976) Inducibility of the Epstein-Barr virus (EBV) cycle and surface marker properties of EBV-negative lymphoma lines and their in vitro EBV-converted sublines. Int J Cancer 18:639-652

Lehrach H, Diamond D, Wozney JM, Boedtker H (1977) RNA molecular weight determinations by gel electrophoresis under denaturing conditions, a critical reexamination. Biochemistry 16:4743-4751

Lenoir GM, Preud'Homme JL, Bernheim A, Berger R (1982) Correlation between immunoglobulin light chain expression and variant translocation in Burkitt's lymphoma. Nature 298:474-476

Ley TJ, Anagnou NP, Pepe G, Niehuis AW (1982) RNA processing errors in patients with B-thalassemia. Proc Natl Acad Sci USA 79:4775-4779

Ley T, Chiang YL, Haidario D, Anagnou NP, Wilson VL, Anderson WF (1984) DNA methylation and regulation of the human β-globin-like genes in mouse erythroleukemia cells containing human chromosome 11. Proc Natl Acad Sci USA 81:6618-6622

Miller G, Robinson J, Heston L, Lipman M (1974) Differences between laboratory strains of Epstein-Barr virus based on immortalization, abortive infection and interference. Proc Natl Acad Sci USA 71:4006-4010

Naharro G, Dunn CY, Robbins KC (1983) Analysis of the primary translational product and integrated DNA of a new feline sarcoma virus, GR-FeSV. Virology 125:502-507

Naharro G, Robbins KC, Reddy EP (1984) Gene product of v-<u>fgr</u> <u>onc</u>: hybrid protein containing a portion of actin and a tyrosne-specific <u>protein kinase</u>. Science 223: 63-66

Naharro G, Tronick SR, Rasheed S, Gardner MB, Aaronson SA, Robbins KC (1983) Molecular cloning of integrated Gardner-Rasheed feline sarcoma virus: Genetic structure of its cell-derived sequence differs from that of other tyrosine kinase coding <u>onc</u> genes. J Virol 47:611-619

Pope JH, Horne MK, Scott W (1968) Transformation of fetal human leukocytes <u>in vitro</u> by filtrates of a human leukemic cell line containing herpes-like virus. Int J Cancer 3:857-866

Rasheed S, Barbacid M, Aaronson SA, Gardner MB (1982) Origin and biological properties of a new feline sarcoma virus. Virology 117:238-244

Taub R, Kirsch I, Morton C, Lenoir G, Swan D, Tronick S, Aaronson SA, Leder P (1982) Translocation of the c-<u>myc</u> gene into the immunoglobulin heavy chain lcous in human Burkitt's lymphoma and murine plasmacytoma cells. Proc Natl Acad Sci USA 79:7837-7841

Tronick SR, Popescu NC, Cheah MSC, Swan DC, Amsbaugh SC, Lengel CR, DiPaolo JA, Robbins KC (1985) Isolation and chromosomal localization of the human <u>fgr</u> proto-oncogene, a distinct member of the tyrosine kinase gene family. Proc Natl Acad Sci USA 82:6595-6599

Ullrich A, Bell JR, Chen EY, Herrera R, Petruzzelli LM, Dull TJ, Gray A, Coussens L, Liao Y-C, Tsubokawa M, Mason A, Seeburg PH, Grunfeld C, Rosen OM, Ramachandran J (1985) Human insulin receptor and its relationship to the tyrosine kinase family of oncogenes. Nature 313:756-761

Epstein-Barr Virus Induced Differentiation of Early B-Lineage Cells

H. Kubagawa, P.D. Burrows, C.E. Grossi, and M.D. Cooper

Cellular Immunobiology Unit, Comprehensive Cancer Center, Depts. of Pathology, Microbiology and Pediatrics, University of Alabama at Birmingham, Birmingham, Alabama 35294.

INTRODUCTION

During their differentiation, members of a clone of B-lineage cells undergo a series of irreversible gene rearrangements involving the immunoglobulin (Ig) gene loci. The rearrangement process, though itself error-prone, proceeds in a programmed, normally well-regulated fashion (reviewed in Tonegawa 1983; Alt et al. 1984). It occurs first at the heavy chain locus, then at a light chain locus and, if successful, ultimately generates an antigen-specific IgM molecule. Subsequently some members of the clone can switch heavy chain isotypes, again by a process involving DNA deletion and Ig gene rearrangement (reviewed in Honjo 1983; Burrows and Cooper 1984). Much of the information concerning these events came initially from studies in the mouse of transformed cell lines thought to represent the various stages of differentiation along the B-lineage. We have been using Epstein-Barr virus (EBV) to examine the genetic events occurring in the early precursors of human B cells. This technique has allowed us to rescue cells with unusual Ig gene and Ig protein phenotypes, and has provided new data concerning the expression of J chain as a function of B cell maturation.

Rescue of early B-lineage cells with Epstein-Barr virus (EBV).

EBV is a lymphotropic herpes virus, capable of transforming human B cells *in vitro* into continuously proliferating lymphoblastoid cell lines (Henle et al. 1967). Although most B cells express receptors for EBV (see references in Fingeroth et al. 1984; Frade et al. 1985), it has been demonstrated that only certain subpopulations of B cells are successfully transformed and secrete Ig molecules after infection with EBV (see Tosato et al. 1985; Chan et al 1986). Transformation rates reported by several groups (Yarchoan et al. 1983; Martinez-Maza and Britton 1983; Chan et al. 1986) vary between 0.1 and ∿30% of the surface Ig-bearing (sIg^+) B cells. The nature of the target cells for EBV transformation is still poorly understood and is not solely associated with the amount of EBV/C3d receptors expressed. Marrow pre-B cells, which do not express sufficient EBV receptors to be detectable by immunofluorescence, have been successfully transformed after *in vitro* infection with EBV (Fu et al. 1980; Hansson et al. 1983; Katamine et al. 1984; Ernberg et al. 1986).

We have utilized EBV to transform bone marrow pre-B and B cells from normal fetuses and X-linked agammaglobulinemia (XLA) patients to explore early genetic events in B lineage differentiation. Since sIg^+ B cells are more easily transformed by infection with EBV than are their sIg^- precursors (our unpublished results), we performed EBV-transformation of the following cell populations: 1) normal fetal bone marrow mononuclear cells (MNC), from which surface IgM-bearing B cells had been depleted either by "panning" procedures or by fluorescence activated cell sorting, and 2) bone marrow MNC from XLA patients, whose marrow contained a normal number of pre-B cells but very few B cells (Pearl et al. 1978; Tedder et al. 1985).

Current Topics in Microbiology and Immunology, Vol. 132

The first notable observation was that all EBV-transformed cultures and subclones derived from samples enriched for bone marrow pre-B cells exhibited a spectrum of cell phenotypes ranging from lymphoblastoid to plasmacytoid cells. This suggested that EBV induced ongoing B-lineage differentiation. Immunofluorescence analysis of the transformed cell lines using a panel of mouse monoclonal antibodies to human Ig isotypic, V_H or J chain determinants revealed four major phenotypes in both normal and XLA samples: 1) lines containing mature cells which expressed J chains without Ig molecules (Ig^-J^+), 2) lines with mature cells which expressed J chains and μ heavy chains but no light chains ($\mu^+LC^-J^+$), 3) lines with cells expressing J chains and K light chains but no heavy chains ($K^+HC^-J^+$), and 4) lines with cells expressing J chains and both Ig heavy and light chains ($HC^+LC^+J^+$).

These phenotypic patterns of EBV-transformed cells would have been predicted with two notable exceptions. First, J chain expression occurred as a function of maturation of EBV-transformed cell lines, regardless of the states of Ig heavy chain or light chain expression. Second, the existence of K chain only cell lines would not have been predicted by current hypotheses.

Expression of J chains without Ig heavy and light chains.

J chain is a highly acid glycoprotein with molecular weight of 15,000 that is involved in the assembly of IgM and IgA polymers via disulfide bridges to the penultimate cysteine residues of μ and α chains (reviewed in Koshland 1974). The regulation of J chain expression during B cell development has been studied by several groups with conflicting results. In mice, J chains appear to be absent in pre-B cells and resting B cells but present in large amounts in mitogen-stimulated B cells and plasma cells, suggesting that J chain expression occurs at a late stage in the B cell differentiation pathway (Koshland 1983). In humans, J chain expression is also up-regulated as a function of plasma cell maturation (Mestecky et al. 1980). However, J chain expression may begin at an earlier stage of B cell differentiation, even before synthesis of Ig molecules (McCune et al. 1981; Hajdu et al. 1983; Max and Korsmeyer 1985). Our study of cell lines established by EBV transformation of early B lineage cells may provide new insight into this controversial issue.

Several cell lines obtained from bone marrow of both normal fetuses and XLA patients did not express Ig heavy or light chains that could be detected in the cytoplasm or on the cell surface by sensitive immunofluorescence and biosynthetic analyses. Both Ig heavy chain alleles in most of these Ig^- cell lines had undergone J_H rearrangements but the K light chain genes were found to be in germ line context. These cells may thus represent early members of the B cell lineage, having undergone DJ_H rearrangements on both alleles. Alternatively, they may be defective pre-B cells, rescued by EBV transformation, that have abortive V_HDJ_H rearrangements. In 1 of 6 Ig^- cell lines, analysis with both J_H and J_κ probes revealed that the majority of cells had both heavy and light chain genes in germ line configuration. All of these Ig^- cell lines were found to contain varying proportions of plasmacytoid cells which expressed J chains in their cytoplasm.

This suggests that J chain expression in human B lineage cells is not directly coupled to synthesis of Ig molecules, or even to rearrangements of Ig heavy chain genes. It is more likely that J chain expression is somehow linked with the stage of maturation achieved by the cells after EBV transformation. This idea is supported by the following findings. All EBV-transformed cell lines regardless of their Ig phenotypes displayed similar morphology with a spectrum of cell types from lymphoid to plasmacytoid within a clone. The proportion of J^+ cells among Ig^- and Ig^+ cell lines was correlated with that of cells having fully developed rough endoplasmic reticulum. No J chains could be detected in spontaneously transformed pre-B leukemia cell lines (PB-207 and PB-697) that were morphologically similar to normal pre-B cells and which did not contain well-developed rough endoplasmic reticulum. These findings suggest that EBV can rescue early B-lineage cells either before Ig gene rearrangement or after having undergone either DJ_H or abortive V_HDJ_H rearrangements, and can induce them to undergo sterile plasma cell differentiation accompanied solely by J chain expression. The mechanism for this could involve the synthesis of a transacting inducer capable of binding to the recently discovered conserved sequence in the promoter region 5' to the J chain gene. This sequence has remarkable homology to that of a conserved sequence detected in the promoter region of the K light chain gene (Matsuuchi et al 1986).

Ig gene rearrangement hierarchy, heavy chain before light chain.

In addition to the Ig^- cell lines, we have derived several EBV-transformed cell lines that express either μ chains without light chains (μ^+LC^-) or K light chains without heavy chains (K^+HC^-). The pre-B cell lines (μ^+LC^-) derived from both normal and XLA bone marrow samples were found to produce μ chains of normal size and glycosylation characteristics. Heavy chain gene rearrangements on both alleles were demonstrated in these pre-B cell lines except for one normal marrow-derived pre-B subclone which appeared to undergo a J_H rearrangement on only one allele. The pre-B cell lines from most XLA patients had their light chain genes in germ line context, as was also the case with the pre-B cell lines from normal fetuses. However, pre-B cell lines from one XLA patient consistently showed rearrangement of the K light chain locus in the absence of detectable K chain protein. These results are thus consistent with the hierarchy of Ig gene rearrangements, heavy chain before light chain, and implicate a defect in the process of light chain gene rearrangement in the pathogenesis of one form of XLA. Notably, J chains were expressed concommitantly with μ heavy chains in the cells that exhibited plasmacytoid morphology.

Expression of Kappa light chains without heavy chains.

Perhaps the most surprising phenotype of B-lineage cells rescued from bone marrow precursors by EBV transformation were the cells expressing K light chains only (K^+HC^-). These were found at a frequency of 0.5-20% in bulk cultures of EBV-transformed, B cell-depleted marrow, but were not observed in cultures of EBV-transformed normal blood cells, suggesting that this type of cell normally exists only in sites of B-cell generation.

In the one K^+HC^- cell line examined thus far for DNA rearrangements, the Ig heavy chain genes on the both alleles were rearranged as were the K light chain genes. Thus, the K only cell lines do not necessarily violate the hierarchy of Ig gene rearrangements, but suggest the possibility that K light chain gene rearrangement can occur in the absence of productive heavy chain gene rearrangements. J chains were expressed concommitantly with K light chains in these cell lines.

CONCLUSIONS

From our survey of EBV-transformed cells from bone marrow samples of both normal fetuses and XLA patients, we reached several conclusions. First, EBV can rescue early B-lineage cells even before the onset of Ig rearrangement and expression, and induce them to undergo "sterile" plasma cell differentiation accompanied solely by J chain expression. J chain expression does not appear to be directly coupled to Ig synthesis or even to Ig gene rearrangements. This is consistent with the notion that J chain is normally up-regulated as a function of plasma cell maturation. Secondly, most pre-B cell lines exhibit J_H gene rearrangements on both alleles but their light chain genes are germ line context. Thus, the EBV-cell lines maintain the hierarchy of Ig gene rearrangements, heavy chain before light chain. Unexpectedly, the pre-B cell lines derived from one particular XLA patient show abortive K chain gene rearrangements, implying a defect in the process of light chain gene rearrangement in the pathogenesis of this form of XLA. Thirdly, the most striking phenotype of early B-lineage cells rescued by EBV are the cells expressing K light chains without heavy chains. Ig gene analysis of one such cell line raises the possibility that K light chain gene rearrangement can occur in the absence of productive heavy chain gene rearrangements.

ACKNOWLEDGEMENTS

This work was supported by NIH grants CA 16673 and CA 13148. We thank Drs. J. Mestecky and G.L. Gartland for helpful suggestions, Nancy C. Martin and Virginia Hollinger for excellent technical assistance, and Ms. E. Ann Brookshire and Tami Rhinehart for preparing the manuscript.

REFERENCES

Alt FW, Yancopoulos GD, Blackwell TK, Wood C, Thomas E., Boss M., Coffman R., Rosenberg N., Tonegawa S., Baltimore D (1984) Ordered rearrangement of immunoglobulin heavy chain variable region segments. EMBO J 3:1209-1219

Burrows PD, Cooper MD (1984) The immunoglobulin heavy chain class switch. Mol Cell Biochem 63:97-111.

Chan MA, Stein LD, Dosh HM, Sigal NH (1986) Heterogeneity of EBV-transformable human B lymphocyte populations. J Immunol 136:106-112

Ernberg I, Falk K, Hansson M (1986) Progenitor and pre-B lymphocytes transformed by Epstein-Barr virus. Int J Cancer (in press)

Fingeroth JD, Weis JJ, Tedder TF, Strominger JL, Biro PA, Fearon DT (1984) Epstein Barr virus receptor of human B lymphocytes is the C3d receptor CR2. Proc Natl Acad Sci USA 81:4510-4514

Frade R, Barel M, Ehlin-Henriksson B, Klein G (1985) gp 140, the C3d receptor of human B lymphocytes, is also the Epstein-Barr virus receptor. Proc Natl Acad Sci USA 82:1490-1493

Fu SM, Hurley JN, McCune JM, Kunkel HG, Good RA (1980) Pre-B cells and other possible precursor lymphoid cell lines derived from patients with X-linked agammaglobulinemia. J Exp Med 152:1519-1526

Hajdu I, Moldoveanu Z, Cooper MD, Mestecky J (1983) Ultrastructural studies of human lymphoid cells: μ and J chain expression as a function of B cell differentiation. J Exp Med 158:1993-2006

Hansson M, Falk K, Ernberg I (1983) Epstein-Barr virus transformation of human pre-B cells. J Exp Med 158:616-622

Henle W, Diehl V, Kohn G, Hausen HZ, Henle G (1967) Herpes types virus and chromosome marker in normal leukocytes after growth with irradiated Burkitt's cells. Science 157:1064-1065
Honjo T (1983) Immunoglobulin genes. Ann Rev Immunol 1:499-528
Katamine S, Otsu M, Tada K, Tsuchiya S, Sato T, Ishida N, Honjo T, Ono Y (1984) Epstein-Barr virus transforms precursor B cells even before immunoglobulin gene rearrangements. Nature 309:369-372
Koshland ME (1974) Structure and function of the J chain. Adv Immunol 20:41-69
Koshland MD (1983) Presidential address: Molecular aspects of B cell differentiation. J Immunol 131:i-ix
Martinez-Maza O, Britton S (1983) Frequencies of the separate human B cell subsets activatable to Ig secretion by Epstein-Barr virus and pokeweed mitogen. J Exp Med 157:1808-1814
Matsuuchi L, Cann GM, Koshland ME (1986) Immunoglobulin J chain gene from the mouse. Proc Natl Acad Sci USA 83:456-460
Max E, Korsmeyer SJ (1985) Human J chain gene: Structure and expression in B lymphoid cells. J Exp Med 161:832-849
McCune JM, Fu SM, Kunkel HG (1981) J chain biosynthesis in pre-B cells and other possible precursor B cells. J Exp Med 154:138-145
Mestecky J, Preud'homme JL, Crago SS, Mihaesco E, Prchal JT, Okos AJ (1980) Presence of J chain in human lymphoid cells. Clin Exp Immunol 39:371-385
Pearl ER, Vogler LB, Okos AJ, Crist WM, Lawton AR, Cooper MD (1978) B lymphocyte precursors in human bone marrow: An analysis of normal individuals and patients with antibody-deficiency states. J Immunol 120:1169-1175
Tedder TF, Crain MJ, Kubagawa H, Clement LT, Cooper MD (1985) Evaluation of lymphocyte differentiation in primary and secondary immunodeficiency diseases. J Immunol 135:1786-1791
Tonegawa S (1983) Somatic generation of antibody diversity. Nature 302:575-581
Tosato G, Blaese RM, Yarchoan R (1985) Relationship between immunoglobulin production and immortalization by Epstein Barr virus. J Immunol 135:959-964
Yarchoan R, Tosato G, Blaese RM, Simon RM, Nelson DL (1983) Limiting dilution analysis of Epstein-Barr virus-induced immunoglobulin production by human B cells. J Exp Med 157:1-14

Epstein-Barr Virus Gene Expression During Primary B-Lymphocyte Infection, in Transformed and Burkitt Lymphoma-Derived Cell Lines

I. Ernberg, B. Kallin, J. Dillner

Department of Tumor Biology, Karolinska Institute, Box 60 400, 10401 Stockholm, Sweden

INTRODUCTION

Epstein-Barr virus (EBV) infection of resting human B-lymphocytes results in the establishment of transformed, continuously growing, virus genome carrying lymphoblastoid cell lines (LCL). This consequence of the virus infection is dependent on virus gene expression, as ultraviolet irradiation of EBV decreases the efficiency of transformation in a dose dependent manner. The early steps of the EBV infection shows many phenotypical parallels to B-lymphocyte activation obtained by mitogens and lymphokines in appropriate combinations. Thus EBV-induced B-lymphocyte activation defined as the first cell cycles after infection is one model from which conclusions can be made about signals involved in triggering of human B-lymphocytes. The expression and function of the virus coded proteins, which are present after EBV infection will be particularly usefool tools in providing knowledge about the significance of various steps in the B-lymphocyte activation. Some of these proteins may complement or replace cellular proteins that function in the physiologic, antigen induced lymphocyte activation. The cellular proteins cannot be identified so easily as those coded for by the virus, due to the availability of specific antibodies against the viral proteins.

Six virus coded proteins expressed in latently infected, transformed B-lymphocytes have been identified so far. Five of these are localized in the nucleus (Epstein-Barr virus nuclear antigens, EBNA 1-5;Reedman and Klein, 1973; Hennessy and Kieff, 1983; Hennessy and Kieff, 1984; Rymo and Klein, 1985; Hennessy et al, 1985; Kallin et al, 1986; Dillner et al, in press), and one has been found to be membrane associated (EBV latent membrane protein, LMP; Wang et al, 1985). The nuclear antigens appear within the first 24-48 hours after primary infection of the B-lymphocytes, that is during the first 48 hour long cell cycle. The time point for the appearence of the LMP has not been determined. To understand the role of these viral proteins in B-cell activation/ transformation we have studied their appearence during primary EBV-infection in relation to other events and their expression in latently infected, continuously growing cell lines of normal B-lymphocyte origin, LCL, and from virus carrying tumor derived cell lines, BL.

Current Topics in Microbiology and Immunology, Vol. 132

EBV-INFECTION OF HUMAN B-LYMPHOCYTES

Primary EBV-infection of human B-cells from blood results in induction of leukocyte migration inhibitory factor (LIF) (Masucci et al., submitted) and appearence of the BLAST-2 antigen (p45; Gordon et al., in press) within 6 hours. These two effects depend on the virus binding to its cell surface receptor (Complement receptor 2; CR 2) and do not require viral gene expression (Masucci et al., submitted). At the same time a small increase in RNA synthesis is seen, which is induced only by intact virus and presumably require virus gene expression. The first virus protein to be detected by immunofluorescence (IF) is EBNA 1, that appears between 5-10 hrs after infection (table 1). Human antiserum affinity purified with synthetic peptide 107, homologous to a part of this protein encoded by internal repeat 3 (IR 3) of the virus DNA, was used to detect the antigen. EBNA 2 appeared between 10 and 20 hrs after infection, as detected by IF with a human antiserum absorbed with EBNA 1+/EBNA 2- cells (Dillner et al.,1985). By immunoblotting EBNA 2 and trace amounts of EBNAs 1 and 3 were detected after 20 hrs (Kallin et al., in press). EBNA 4 could be detected after 48 hrs. After 72 hrs there was no relative change in the intensity of the blotting signals corresponding to the four antigens (Kallin et al., in press). EBNA 5 has just recently been detected as a 22-70 kD polyprotein, primarily identified by a rabbit antipeptide antiserum (Dillner et al., in press). It is encoded in part from the large internal repeats of the EBV genome (Bodescot et al.,1985). It was detected on day one after EBV-infection of tonsillar B-lymphocytes (Dillner et al., in press).

35 hours after infection there is a considerable increase in RNA synthesis of the B-lymphocytes and in parallel induction of immunoglobulin synthesis. The cells enter S phase 40 hrs after infection and the first mitoses can be seen 48 hrs after infection (Einhorn and Ernberg, 1978; Ernberg, 1979).

The known properties of the five nuclear antigens are summarized in table 2.

EXPRESSION OF EBNA 2 IN TRANSFORMED LCL AND BL-DERIVED CELL LINES

As mentioned above EBNA 2 is expressed 10-20 hours after virus infection. One EB virus variant, P3HR-I, has a deletion in the EBV genome area coding for EBNA 2, the Bam WYH region of EBV-DNA (Bornkamm et al, 1980). This virus strain cannot transform human B-lymphocytes. Because of this EBNA 2 has been suggested to play an important role in initiation of EBV induced transformation.

We collected 20 wild type isolates of EBV from patients with recent primary EBV infection and infectious mononucleosis (IM), either by collecting mouth washes or by establishing EBV-carrying LCLs from their blood. All these isolates induced EBNA 2. In contrast EBNA 2 was not detected in 60% of 27 BL-derived cell lines tested (table 3; Ernberg et al., subm for publication).

Those EBNA-2 negative cell lines were tested for the presence of the Bam WYH region coding for EBNA-2. In three of these lines a deletion was found, including the whole major open reading frame, like the one already described for P3HR-I, while in 9 of the lines the region was intact but with a variant sequence which resulted in a different restriction pattern. This variant sequence has been cloned from one of these cell lines, Jijoye, by Adldinger et al (1985). We obtained this cloned fragment from them and could show that all the cell lines with the variant sequence reacted with this probe. This variant sequence shows some 40% homology with the prototype EBNA-2 coding sequence , but does either not give rise to a protein, or more likely this protein is not recognized by any of our immunologic reagents, i.e. human sera from patients with virus strains with either prototype or variant sequence. Rowe et al (1985) have recently demonstrated a 70 kD protein in the Jijoye cell line that seems to be coded for by the variant open reading frame, by using carefully selected antisera from patients with chronic IM.

The recently detected EBNA 5 is only seen in lymphoblastoid cell lines, but not in tumor derived lines, which suggests a specific role in relation to the host cell differentiation stage (Dillner et al., in press).

DISCUSSION

Five nuclear , EB-virus encoded antigens, have been detected in EBV transformed cell lines. They all appear during the first cell cycle after primary virus infection of human B-lymphocytes from peripheral blood or tonsills. Their appearence does not seem to be coordinated. Thus EBNA 1 was the first protein that we could detect, closely followed in time by EBNA 2 and 3. The detection level of the EBNAs may vary with the different methods used, immunofluorescence and immunoblotting, and also due to differences in titers of the serologic reagents. The order of appearence was primarily determined by immunofluorescence, while in immunoblotting EBNA 2 gave a stronger signal than EBNA 1 when first analyzed 20 hrs after infection. The nuclear antigens appeared during the initial phase of this first cell cycle parallel to a small increase in cellular RNA synthesis and to an increase in cell size, during and after the shift from operationally defined G 0 to G 1 phase. One function has been implicated for EBNA 1, as it seems to interact with the only identified origin of virus DNA replication (oriP) and thus supports the maintenance of plasmid constructs carrying oriP in eukaryotic cells (Yates et al., 1984). Most likely it has a similar function in natural EBV-host cell interaction, maintaining the viral episomes in the transformed cells. This does not exclude other functions of this protein. EBNA 1 has a unique structure, as half of the protein is made up from glycine-alanine repeats, a polypeptide stretch that varies in length in different virus isolates (Hennessy and Kieff, 1983).

EBNA 2 also has a particular structure, being made up of 37 consecutive proline residues polyproline (Hennessy and Kieff, 1984). These structural pecularities may point to not yet identified specialized functions. There are strong reasons to believe that EBNA 2 is required for initiation of transformation, but not for maintenance, as the gene may be totally deleted in long term cultured tumor derived cell lines, but always is found intact in freshly transformed cell lines. Its function may be superfluous in the tumor cells due to secondary cellular genotypic changes, such as the translocation associated dysregulation of c-myc in these cell lines. One non-transforming virus strain has been shown to have the gene deleted. Another variation seen in this gene, is a variant sequence with only 40% homology to the prototype sequence.

Virus with the variant sequence is also transforming (Ragona et al., 1978;Hennessy and Kieff, 1984). The origin of the variant sequence virus types is not established. but it is most frequently seen in virus in cell lines from BL in the endemic African region.

EBNA 3, 4 and 5 were just recently described. Apart from EBNA 5 they have not been mapped to the viral genome. EBNA 3 and 4 are detected in all EBV carrying, transformed cell lines, while EBNA 5 was not detected in the tumor derived BL-lines, an observation which will focus the interest on this protein.

Although no human sera have been found reactive to the membrane protein, it has been detected by using immune rabbit serum to a fusion protein product between the hydrophilic part of the protein and beta-galactosidase of E.Coli (Wang et al,1985). It is associated with the inside of the cell membrane . Recently it was shown to have transforming potential in secondary rat embryo fibroblast cultures (Wang et al,1985). Its expression in tumor cells and LCLs has not yet been studied in great detail, and also it is not yet known when it appears during primary B-cell infection.

Functional and genetic studies of these six proteins encoded by the highly B-lymphocyte specialized EBV will provide important clues to molecular mechanisms involved in B-cell activation. It may also be important that two of them can be turned off in the tumor derived BL-lines (EBNA 2 and 5).

Table 1. Appearence of EBNA 1 and 2 after primary B-cell infection with EBV. Per cent positive cells in IF.

Antigen	Hrs p.i.: 5	10	14	17	21	26	32	40	48
EBNA 1[a]	20	-	16	28	27	22	32	46	76
EBNA 2[b]	0	0	0	17	16	25	30	20	56

a Detected by peptide affinity purified human serum in anti-complentary immunofluorescence(ACIF).
b Detected by human serum absorbed with EBNA 1+/EBNA 2- cells in ACIF.

Table 2. Properties of EBV encoded proteins in transformed cells.

Designation	Coding region	Expression	Apparent molecular weight(kD)	Function
EBNA 1	Bam K	LCL & BL	70-92	Episome maintenance
EBNA 2	Bam WYH	LCL,40% BL	80-85	Initiation of trsf.
EBNA 3	Bam CWLE?[a)]	LCL & BL	140-157	?
EBNA 4	?	LCL & BL	148-180	?
EBNA 5	Bam WYH	LCL	22-70	?
LMP	Bam N het	LCL & BL	58	Transformation

a)Bodescot et al., 1986

Table 3. Variation of EBNA 2.

Designation	Example	Frequency	Phenotype
Prototype (type A)	B 95-8	All LCL, 40 % BL	Transforming
Jijoye type (type B)	Jijoye M 13	40 % BL	Transforming
Deletion	P3HR-I	20 % BL	Non transforming

REFERENCES

Adldinger HK, Delius H, Freese U, Clark J, Bornkamm GW (1985) A putative transforming gene of Jijoye virus differs from that of Epstein-Barr virus prototypes. Virology 141: 221-234

Bodescot M, Chambraud B, Farrell P, Perricaudet M (1984) Spliced RNA from the IR1-U2 region of Epstein-Barr virus: presence of an open reading frame for a repetitive polepeptide. The EMBO J 3:1913-1917.

Bodescot M, Brinson O, Perricaudet M (1986) An Epstein-Barr virus transcription unit is at least 84 kB long. Nucl. Acids Res 14: 2611-2620.

Bornkamm GW, Delius H, Zimber U, Hudewentz J, Epstein MA (1980) Comparison of Epstein-Barr virus strains of different origin by analysis of the viral DNAs. J Virol 35: 603-618

Dillner J, Kallin B, Ehiln-Henriksson B, Timar L, Klein G (1985) Characterization of a second Epstein-Barr virus determined nuclear antigen associated with the Bam H I WYH region of EBV DNA. Int J Cancer 35: 359-366.

Dillner J, Sternås L, Kallin B, Alexander H, Ehlin-Henriksson B, Jörnvall H, Klein G, Lerner R (1984) Antibodies against a synthetic peptide identify the Epstein_abrr virus determined nuclear antigen. Proc Natl Acad Sci, USA 81: 4652-4656.

Dillner J, Kallin B, Alexander H, Ernberg I, Uno M, Ono Y, Klein G, Lerner R () A novel Epstein-Barr virus determined nuclear antigen (EBNA-5) partly encoded by the transformation-associated Bam WYH region of the EBV-DNA: differential expression in lymphoblastoid cell lines. Proc. Natl. Acad. Sci., in press.

Einhorn L, Ernberg I (1978) Induction of EBNA precedes the first cellular S phase after EBV infection of human lymphocytes. Int J Cancer 21: 157-160.

Ernberg I (1979) Epstein-Barr virus productive and non productive host cell interaction. Academic thesis, Karolinska Institutet, Stockholm.

Ernberg I, Kallin B, Dillner J, Falk K, Ehlin-Henriksson B, Hammarskjöld ML, Klein G ( ) Lymphoblastoid cell lines and Burkitt lymphoma derived cell lines differ in the expression of a second Epstein-Barr virus encodede nuclear antigen. Submiotted for publication.

Hennessy K, Kieff E (1983) One of two Epstein_abrr virus nuclear antigens contains a glycine-alanine copolymer domain. Proc Natl Acad Sci, USA 80: 5665-5669.

Hennessy K, Kieff E (1985) A second nuclear protein is encoded by Epstein-Barr virus in latent infection. Science 227: 1238-1240.

Hennessy K, Fennewald S, Kieff E (1985) A third viral nuclear protein in lymphoblasts immortalized by Epstein-Barr virus. Proc Natl Acad Sci 82: 5944-5948.

Kallin B, Dillner J, Ernberg I, Ehlin-Henriksson B, Rosen A, Henle W, Henle G, Klein G (1986) Four virally determined antigens are expressed in Epstein-Barr virus transformed cells. Proc Natl Acad Sci 86: in press.

Masucci M.G., Szigeti R., Ernberg,I., Hu C.-P., Torsteinsdottir S., Frade R., Klein E., Activation of B-lymphocytes by Epstein-Barr virus /CR 2 receptor interaction. Subm for publication.

Ragona G, Ernberg I, Klein G (1980) Induction and biological characterization of the Epstein-Barr virus (EBV) carried by the Jijoye lymphoma Virology 101, 553-557.

Reedman B, Klein G (1973) Cellular localization of an Epstein-Barr virus (EBV)-associated complement fixing antigen in producer and non-producer lymphoblastoid cell lines. Int J Cancer 11, 499-520.

Rowe D, Heston L, Hetlay J, Miller G (1985) Identification and expression of a nuclear antigen from the genomic region of the Jijoye strain of Epstein-Barr virus that is missing in its nonimmortalizing deletion mutant , P3HR-I. Proc Natl Acad Sci 82: 7429-7433.

Rymo L, Klein G, Ricksten A (1985) Expression of a second Epstein-Barr virus determined nuclear antigen in mouse cells after gene transfer with a cloned fragment of the viral genome. Proc Natl Acad Sci , USA 82: 3435-3439.

Wang D, Liebowitz D, Kieff E (1985) An EBV membrane protein expressed in immortalized lymphocytes transforms established rodent cells. Cell 43: 831-840.

Yates J, Warren N, Reisman D, Sugden B (1984) A cis-acting element from the Epstein-Barr viral genome that permits stable replication of recombinant plasmids in latently infected cells. Proc Natl Acad Sci, USA 81: 3806-3810.

Structure and Expression of Translocated c-myc Oncogenes: Specific Differences in Endemic, Sporadic and AIDS-Associated Forms of Burkitt Lymphomas

Luisa Lanfrancone, Pier-Giuseppe Pelicci and Riccardo Dalla-Favera

Dept. of Pathology and Kaplan Cancer Center, New York University School of Medicine, New York, NY 10016.

INTRODUCTION

Burkitt lymphomas (BL) are characterized by reciprocal chromosomal translocations which involve the c-myc oncogene locus on chromosome 8 and immunoglobulin (Ig) loci on either chromosome 2, 14 or 22 (Dalla-Favera et al. 1982, 1983; Taub et al. 1982; Leder et al. 1983; Croce et al. 1985). The consistent occurrence of these specific recombination events in BL and the presence of analogous recombinations involving c-myc in similar tumors in other species (Sheng-Ong 1982), suggests that the c-myc gene plays a role in the pathogenesis of BL. Despite their remarkable similarity at the cytogenetic level, these translocation events are extremely heterogeneous at the molecular level. In this study we report that chromosomal breakpoints and structural alterations of the c-myc locus differ in different subtypes of Burkitt lymphomas, namely endemic, sporadic BL and AIDS-associated undifferentiated B-cell lymphomas (AIDS-UBL). Chromosomal translocation is also associated with different levels of c-myc expression, and these levels directly correlate with the clonogenic and <u>in vivo</u> tumorigenic properties of BL cells.

RESULTS

<u>Structural Alterations of Translocated c-myc Genes.</u>

We have examined the position of the chromosomal breakpoints and the presence of other structural alterations relative to the c-myc locus in a large panel of fresh tumors and BL derived cell lines carrying the (8:14) chromosomal translocation. This panel is represented epidemiologically, phenotypically and pathogenetically distinct forms of BL, including: i) Endemic, African type BL (eBL) which are characterized by their restricted distribution in high incidence areas, namely Equatorial Africa and Papua New Guinea, and by its virtually complete association (96°/° of cases) with the Epstein-Barr virus (EVB); ii) Sporadic, American-type BL (sBL), which are characterized by a much lower incidence, their worldwide distribution, their different organ distribution and their only occasional association with EBV (Magrath 1985); iii) undifferentiated B-cell lymphomas associated with the acquired immunodeficiency syndrome (AIDS) (AIDS-UBL) (Ziegler et al. 1984).

Within these groups of BL cases, rearrangements or truncation of the c-myc locus can be readily detected by analysis of BL DNA with restriction enzymes, such as HindIII and EcoRI, which identify DNA regions containing the entire c-myc locus including the three

Current Topics in Microbiology and Immunology, Vol. 132

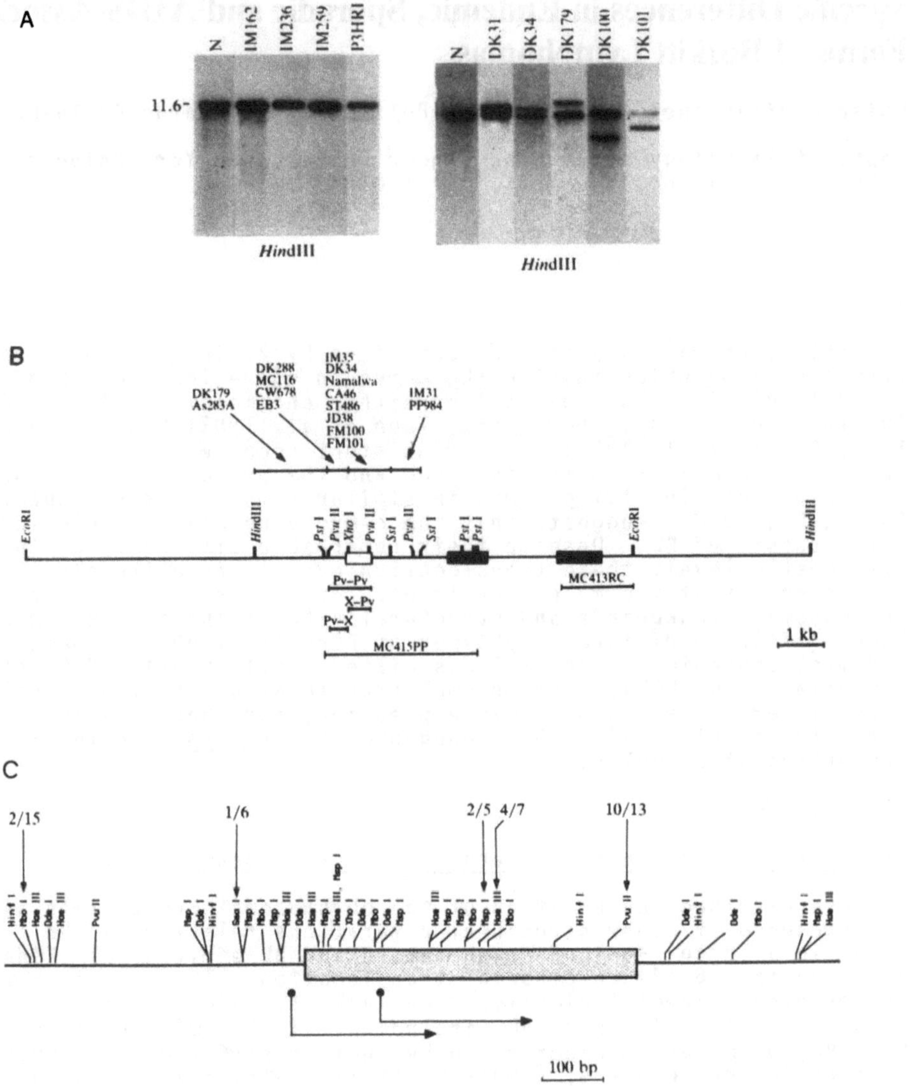

Fig. 1. Chromosomal breakpoints and structural alterations of the c-myc locus in eBL and sBL. Panel A = c-myc rearrangements in eBL and sBL. DNA samples from the indicated BL cases (left panel eBL, right panel, sBL and AIDS-UBL) and from normal human fibroblasts (lanes N) were digested with EcoRI or HindIII and hybridized with a PvPv-myc probe. Fragment sizes are given in kb. Panel B = Restriction enzyme map of the human c-myc locus: the non-coding exon is represented by an open box, and the coding exons by hatched boxes. Above the map, the approximate location of the breakpoints is indicated for each case. A schematic representation of the c-myc probes used is shown below the map. Panel C = Restriction enzyme map of the 5' flanking sequence, first exon (strippled box) and part of the first intron of c-myc. For polymorphic restriction enzyme sites, numbers indicate the frequency of polymorphism among the cases tested. The position of the two c-myc promoters and the direction of transcription (arrows) are indicated below the map.

Table 1: Frequency and type of structural alterations of the c-myc locus in eBL and sBL

	c-myc locus rearrangements[a]	5' restriction enzyme polymorphisms[b]
Endemic Cases		
Fresh samples	0/12	8/8
Cell lines	2/6	2/2
Sporadic Cases		
Fresh samples	7/7	0/3
Cell lines	7/7	1/7
AIDS UBL		
Fresh samples	8/10	NT

a Values express the relative frequency of rearrangements detectable by both EcoRI and Hind III restriction enzyme digestions.

b Values express the relative frequency of 5' restriction site polymorphisms detected by one or more of the following enzymes: Pvu II, Hae III, MboI, SmaI, MspI, DdeI, HinfI (see text and Fig. 1C for sites and relative frequencies for each enzyme).

c Not tested.

coding exons and evolutionarily conserved 5' and 3' flanking sequences of possible functional significance. Using this assay, all of the 12 freshly isolated eBL and 4 of 6 eBL cell lines displayed apparently unrearranged c-myc loci (see Fig. 1A for representative results and Table 1 for a summary of results in all the cases studied). By analogy, with previously reported studies, the chromosomal breakpoint in these 16 cases is assumed to be located at an undefined distance 5' to the c-myc gene in all cases carrying a t(8;14) translocation (Leder et al. 1983; Croce et al. 1985).

Conversely, in all 14 sBL fresh tumor samples and sBL cell lines, 8 out of 10 AIDS-UBL displayed rearrangements of one c-myc allele. The presence of rearranged alleles of different sizes indicate that in sBL the position of the breakpoint varies within the c-myc locus. We conclude that, while in most eBL the chromosomal breakpoint is located outside the c-myc locus, sBLs and AIDS-UBL are invariably characterized by rearrangements directly involving the c-myc gene or its immediately flanking sequences.

Mapping of Chromosomal Breakpoints in sBL and AIDS-UBL.

The c-myc rearrangements detectable in sBL can be further examined by Southern blot analysis using different restriction enzymes and probes enabling us to explore different segments of the c-myc locus. This approach allows an approximate mapping of the recombination sites corresponding to the breakpoints of a reciprocal chromosomal translocation. Using the combination of restriction enzymes and probes schematically illustrated in Fig. 1B, the approximate position of recombination sites was mapped in all sBL and AIDS-UBL cases. The results indicate that chromosomal breakpoints are clustered in a region of the c-myc locus spanning the first exon, first intron and 5' flanking sequences.

Table 2

CELL LINE	ORIGIN	EBV GENOME°	C-MYC mRNA LEVELS*	COLONY FORMATION IN AGAR^{x}	COLONY FORMATION IN AGAR AT 20%	10%	5% FCS Δ	TUMORIGENICITY IN NUDE MICE τ
Burkitt Lymphoma								
CW678	USA	-	3.9	+	NT	NT	NT	NT
RAMOS	USA	-	1.85	++	NT	NT	NT	+
MC116	North Am.	-	1.64	+++	+++	++	-	NT
PP984	USA	+	1.37	++	NT	NT	NT	NT
DAUDI	Africa	+	1.00	+++	+++	++	-	+
P3HR1	Africa	+	0.93	+++	+++	++	+	+
EW36	North Am.	-	0.86	+++	NT	NT	NT	NT
AG876	Africa	+	0.70	++	NT	NT	NT	NT
JD38	North Am.	-	0.59	+	+	-	-	+
CA46	South Am.	-	0.53	+	+	-	-	+
ST486	North Am.	-	0.15	-	-	-	-	-
PA682	Europe	+	0.13	+	+	-	-	-
Lymphoblastoid								
EBV1	-	+	0.20	-	-	-	-	NT
EBV2	-	+	0.43	-	-	-	-	NT
EBV3	-	+	0.70	-	-	-	-	NT
EBV4	-	+	0.35	-	-	-	-	NT
EBV5	-	+	0.18	-	-	-	-	NT

° Presence of Epstein-Barr virus genome

* Relative amounts of c-myc mRNA were measured by densitometric scanning of x-ray films and relative values are expressed assuming a value of 1 for the Daudi cell line and normalized against β-tubulin and β2-microglobulin (not shown) hybridization bands used as internal controls.

x (-) = No colony formation at 10^2, $5x10^2$ and 10^3 cells/plate; colony formation is expressed as (+) = 1-5%; (++) = 5-15%; (+++) => 15%

τ - = no tumor growth within 14 weeks of observation
+ =100% tumor growth in 1-3 weeks from the injection

Δ Colony formation has been observed in the presence of 20%, 10% and 5% fetal calf serum (FCS) in the semisolid medium.

The 5' Region of Unrearranged c-myc Loci Contains Mutations in eBL.

Several reports have demonstrated the occurrence of point mutations or other small internal rearrangements in the c-myc locus (Rabbits et al. 1984; Wiman et al. 1984; Taub et al. 1984). We sought to analyze the frequency and the approximate position of these structural alterations in our collection of eBL, particularly in those displaying c-myc loci which appeared intact by EcoRI and HindIII restriction analysis. As an alternative to determining the entire nucleotide sequences of the c-myc loci, an impractical approach for the analysis of so many cases, we analyzed parts of the c-myc locus by Southern blot hybridization, using a combination of restriction enzymes cutting within these genomic areas and thereby allowing an overall, albeit approximate, estimation of the frequency and position of mutations. No deviation from the normal pattern was observed using PvuII, HaeIII, MboI, MspI, DdeI, SmaI, HindIII restriction endonucleases in combination with a third exon probe (MC413RC) (data not shown). However, several alterations were detectable with several of the restriction enzymes using probes specific for the 5' region of the gene. The restriction sites involved and the relative frequency of involvement are schematically illustrated in Fig. 1C. A summary of the data for all the BL cases tested are reported in Table 1.

These alterations: i) have not been detected in a survey of sixty DNA samples from either normal individuals (peripheral blood lymphocytes, 15 cases tested) or from tumors other than B-cell neoplasias (45 cases tested); ii) vary from case to case, involving the loss of a site and the generation of a new one, and appear to be invariably monoallelic, since no homozygosity for an altered PvuII fragment has been detected; iii) are not detected in DNA from BL in which the chromosomal translocation truncates the c-myc locus leaving the first exon on chromosome 8. We therefore conclude that mutations and/or small internal rearrangements represent a specific and frequent feature of translocated c-myc alleles in eBL.

Effects of Translocation on c-myc Gene Expression: Correlations with Growth Characteristic of BL Cells.

Next the effects of the described structural alterations on c-myc gene expression were tested by comparing myc mRNA levels in our panel of BL cell lines. From several previous studies it is known that, in BL carrying a t(8:14) chromosomal translocation, RNA transcribed from the translocated c-myc allele, whereas the allele studied is almost invariable silent. We then studied myc mRNA levels in BL cells, using probes which would detect transcripts containing the coding portions of the translocated, rearranged or normal alleles. Representative results are shown in Fig. 2 and a summary is reported in Table 2.

No clear correlation was found between the degree of BL, i.e. eBL, sBL, or AIDS UBL, the type of structural alteration affecting the c-myc locus, i.e. translocation vs. mutation, or the presence of the Epstein Barr virus genome. A significant correlation was instead found between levels of myc RNA and several growth parameters including doubling time (not shown), clonogenic ability in semisolid media, serum dependency and in vivo tumorigenicity (data are summarized in Table 2). These data suggest that the c-myc gene is involved in the control of proliferation of BL cells. More recently, this notion has been directly tested by gene transfer experiments involving the introduction into BL cells, namely BL cells expressing low levels of c-myc mRNA, of plasmid vectors containing c-myc gene under the control of promoter elements strongly active in B-cells. In preliminary experiments the high constitutive expression of c-myc gene driven by the SV40 promoter-enhancer element leads to a significant increase of the clonogenic properties of BL cell lines which were originally expressing low levels of myc mRNA. Further experiments involving other cell lines and studies on the in vivo tumorigenicity of myc-transfected lines are currently in progress.

DISCUSSION

The first notion emerging from our survey of a large panel of BL is that in all BL cases structural alterations can be detected within a region spanning the first exon, first intron and 5' flanking sequences of the translocated c-myc locus. A regulatory role for this region has been repeatedly suggested (Siebenlist et al. 1984) and a negatively regulatory element has been preliminary identified 5' to the first c-myc exon both in mouse and man (Lanfrancone et al. unpublished work; K. Marcu, personal communication). While further studies are needed to define the functional role of these sequences, their consistent involvement in structural alterations following chromosomal translocation suggest that the disruption of the 5' regulatory elements of the c-myc gene is a necessary, if not sufficient event in the mechanism of c-myc activation in BL.

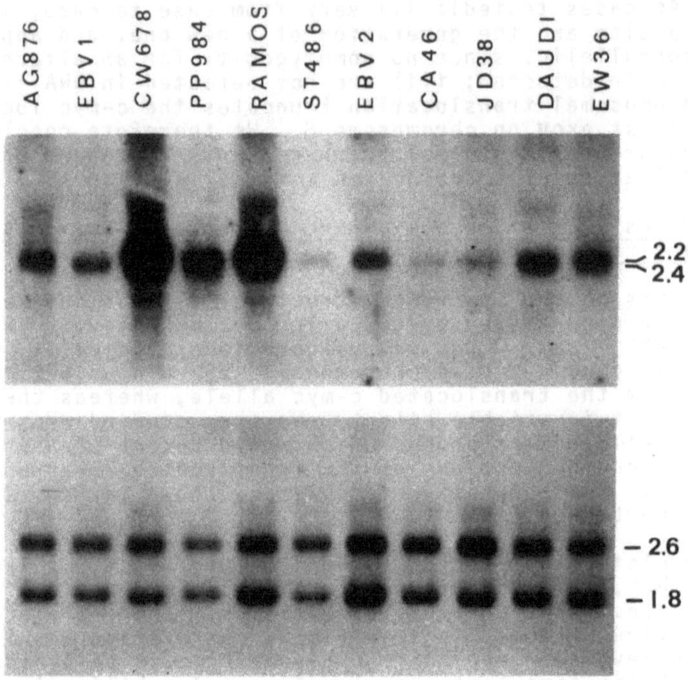

Fig. 2 Northern blot analysis of steady-state levels of c-myc mRNA in BLs. 15 μg of total RNA have been hybridized to c-myc exon III probe (upper panel). β-tubulin probe, used as an internal control for the amount of RNA loaded on the gel, has been hybridized to the same filter (bottom panel). BL cell lines are representative of eBL and sBL cases (see Table 1). EBV1 and EBV2 are EBV-infected-lymphoblastoid cell lines. Molecular weights are expressed in kb.

A strict correlation has also emerged between the different sites of chromosomal breakpoint and the different pathogenetic forms of BL. 16 out of 18 eBL displayed an unrearranged myc gene indicating that the chromosomal breakpoint lies outside the myc locus, while in 14 out of 14 sBL and 8 out of 10 AIDS-UBL the chromosomal breakpoint is variably located in the 5' portion of the gene or in its immediately flanking sequences. In this context it is important to consider several studies suggesting that eBL and sBL may derive from lymphocytes precursors at different stages along the B-cell differentiation pathway (Benjamin et al. 1982; Favrot et al. 1984). Most notably, most eBL, but not sBL, express Fc, C_3 and EBV receptors and sBL are characterized by significant amount of IgM secretion which is virtually undetectable in eBL (Benjamin et al. 1982). In our panel of cases no IgM secretion was detectable in eBL, with the exception of the two cases, (cell lines, Namalwa and EB3), which displayed the truncated version of the c-myc gene typical of sBL.

Conversely, significant amounts of secreted IgM were detectable in all sBL. These obervations suggest that a correlation may exist between the site of the chromosmal breakpoint and the stage of B-cell differentiation; and that in this respect, Ig secreting sBL, and AIDS-UBL carrying truncated c-myc loci, may represent more mature cells. Consistent with this notion mouse plasmacytomas, which represent relatively more mature, Ig-secreting cells, most often carry truncated c-myc genes (Harris et al. 1982). It is possible that translocations may be mediated by mistakes in Ig V-D-J joining or later occurring heavy-chain "switch" mechanisms in eBL and sBL, respectively. Preliminary data from Ig gene analysis of several BL appear to confirm this model.

In addition to the well-known association of c-myc translocations with eBL and sBL, our studies point-toward a remarkable association between the same translocations and AIDS-UBL. It is important to note that, despite their clinical and histopathologic heterogeneity, including both Burkitt and non-Burkitt types, these tumors appear unusually homogeneous with respect to oncogene activation. This observation suggests that the biological alterations present in AIDS may favor the development of lymphomas carrying activated c-myc oncogenes. The conditions of chronic EBV infection and immunosuppression present in AIDS are reminiscent of analogous conditions (EBV infection and immunosuppression related to malaria) present in eBL suggesting that eBL and AIDS-UBL may share common pathogenetic aspects. However, AIDS-UBL resemble more sBL in their pattern of c-myc gene rearrangements secretion IgM, suggesting that a more mature, B-cell is selected in AIDS-UBL than in eBL.

An additional element of heterogeneity in BL is provided by the significantly different levels of myc mRNA. The lack of an immediatley apparent correlation between the type and/or site of structural alterations and the levels of expression is likely to reflect the combined effects of multiple regulatory regions within the c-myc locus and the contribution of Ig regulatory elements which are either distant or variably juxtaposed to the c-myc gene in different BL cases (Leder et al. 1983; Croce et al. 1985). It is, however, clear that at least in BL cell lines the steady-state levels of myc mRNA expression, and presumably of the myc protein product, are involved in the control of cell proliferation. The correlation between myc gene expression and a more aggressive growth pattern in BL cell lines is reminiscent of changes in growth pattern observed in small cell lung carcinoma cell lines where levels of c-myc expression are increased due to gene amplification (Little et al. 1983). Preliminary experiments suggest that the induction of high levels of c-myc expression in c-myc transfected BL cells lead to changes in the growth phenotype suggesting that these cells may be used for the identification of genes directly or indirectly regulated by c-myc. Finally, the different biological behavior of BL cell lines _in vitro_ suggest that different levels of c-myc expresion may correlate with the different aggressivity of different BL cases _in vivo_.

ACKNOWLEDGEMENTS

We acknowledge the contributions of Drs. Ian Magrath and Daniel Knowles who provided all the clinical samples and cell lines used in these studies. We are grateful to Dianne Nazario and Linda Skillen for the careful editing of the manuscript. This work is supported by NIH grants CA37165 and CA37295. RDF is a recipient of a Senior AIDS Fellowship from the Kaplan Cancer Center and is a Scholar of the Leukemia Society of America.

REFERENCES

Benjamin, D., Magrath, I., Magure, R., Janus, C., Todd, H.D. a Parsons, R.G. (1982) Immunoglobulin secretion by cell lines derived from African and American undifferentiated lymphomas of Burkitt's and non Burkitt's type. J Immunol 129:1336-1342

Croce, C.M. a Nowell, P.C. (1985) Molecular basis of human B cell neoplasia. Blood 65:1-7

Dalla-Favera, R., Bregni, M., Erikson, J., Patterson, D., Gallo, R.C. a Croce, C.M. (1982) Human c-myc onc gene is located on the region of chromosome 8 that is translocated in Burkitt lymphoma cells. Proc Natl Acad Sci USA 79:7824-7827

Dalla-Favera, R., Martinotti, S., Gallo, R.C., Erikson, J. a Croce, C.M. (1983) Translocation and rearrangement of the c-myc oncogene locus in human undifferentiated B-cell lymphomas. Science 219:963-967

Favrot, M.C., Philip, I., Phillip, T., Dore, J.F. a Lenoir, G.M. (1984) Possible duality in Burkitt lymphoma origin. Lancet i:745-746

Harris, L.J., Lang, R.B. a Marcu, K.B. (1982) Non-immunoglobulin-associated DNA rearrangements in mouse plasmacytomas. Proc Natl Acad Sci USA 79:4175-4179

Lanfrancone, L., Pelicci, P.G., Cesarman, E. a Dalla-Favera, R. (1984) Mechanisms of oncogene activation in human hemotopoietic tumors. In New Trends in Experimental Hematology, eds. Peschle, C. a Rizzoli, C. (Serono Symposia, Rome), pp. 196-203

Leder, P., Battey, J., Lenoir, G., Moulding, C., Murphy, W., Potter, H., Steward, T. a Taub, R. (1983) Translocations among antibody genes in human cancer. Science 222:765-771

Little, C.D., Nau, M.N., Carney, D.N., Gazdar, A.F. a Minna, J.D. (1983) Amplification and expression of the c-myc oncogene in human lung cancer cell lines. Nature (London) 306:194-196

Rabbits, T.H., Forster, A., Hamlyn, P. a Baer, R. (1984) Effect of somatic mutations within translocated c-myc genes in Burkitt's lymphomas. Nature (London) 309:592-597

Siebenlist, U., Hennighausen, L., Battey, J. a Leder, P. (1984) Chromatin structure and protein binding in the putative regulatory region of the c-myc gene in Burkitt lymphoma. Cell 37:380-390

Sheng-Ong, G.L.C., Keath, E.J., Piccoli, S.P. a Cole, N.D. (1982) Novel myc oncogene RNA from abortive immunoglobulin-gene recombination. Cell 31:443-452

Taub, R., Kirsch, I., Morton, C., Lenoir, G., Swan, D., Tronick, S., Aaronson, S. a Leder, P. (1982) Translocation of the c-myc gene into the immunoglobulin heavy chain locus in human Burkitt's lymphoma and murine plasmacytomas cells. Proc Natl Acad Sci USA 79:7837-7841

Taub, R., Kelly, K., Battey, J., Latt, S., Lenoir, G.M., Tantravaki, V., Tu, Z. a Leder, P. (1984) A novel alteration in the structure of an activated c-myc gene in a variant t(2;8) Burkitt lymphoma. Cell 37:511-520

Wiman, K.G., Clarkson, B., Hayday, A.C. Saito, M., Tonegawa, S. a Hayward, W.S. (1984) Activation of a translocated c-myc gene: role of structural alteration in the upstream region. Proc Natl Acad Sci USA 81:6798-6802

Ziegler, J.L., et. al. (1984) Non-Hodgkin's lymphoma in 90 homosexual men: relation to generalized lymphadenopathy and the acquired immunodeficiency syndrome. N Eng J Med 311:565-570

EBV-Activation of Human B-Lymphocytes

P. Åman, N. Lewin, M. Nordström, G. Klein.

Dep. of Tumor Biology Karolinska Institute
10401 Stockholm Sweden

The Epstein-Barr virus (EBV) is a human herpes virus originally discovered in Burkitt lymphoma cell lines. The virus was found to specifically infect a subpopulation of B-lymphocytes. In vitro infected B-cells are transformed into immortalized but non-tumorigenic lymphoblastoid cell lines (LCL). The cell lines maintain the genome in a latent form with only limited parts of the genome expressed and none or very little virus is produced (Menezes 1976). Some of the latently transcribed EBV genes code for different components of the EBV nuclear antigens (EBNA) expressed in the cell nucleus of all EBV-carrying cells (Reedman 1973).

Characterization of Target Cells

A prerequisite for investigation of the cellular responses in primary infected B-lymphocytes was to characterize the EBV-target cells. In our first approach we used density gradient fractionation to purify B-cells of different sizes and activation stages. Using both blood and tonsil derived B-cell preparations, we found that only high to intermediate density B-cells produced EBV viral antigens after infection (Åman 1984 a). (TABLE 1). Although low density, large, activated B-cells bound and were penetrated by the virus, no EBNA-production was detected. These results suggest that EBV-infection and immortalization of B-lymphocytes are dependent both on the presence of a virus receptor and on intracellular complex interactions between cellular and viral functions.

TABLE 1

VIRUSBINDING, UPTAKE AND EBNA-PRODUCTION IN DENSITY FRACTIONATED B-CELL POPULATIONS.

DONOR	BINDING (CPM)	UPTAKE (%)	PER CENT EBNA POSITIVE CELLS
1			
HIGH DENSITY	5337	90	36
INTERMEDIATE	7098	68	3
LOW DENSITY	9622	62	0
2			
HIGH DENSITY	4899	83	23
INTERMEDIATE	5232	81	0
LOW DENSITY	5107	78	0
CONTROLS			
Raji	9842	37	
P3HR-1	889	63	

Density-fractionated B-cell-populations were incubated with H-thymidine labeled virus or nonlabeled virus for 1 hour at 37 C and then washed in medium. The samples were split in two and one part was trypsinized and washed to remove external virus particles. The cell-pellet associated radioactivity was counted. Uptake is presented as per cent of bound radioactivity present after trypsin-treatment. Per cent EBNA-positive cells were determined by an anti-complement immuno-fluorescens method.

In our density studies of normal B-lymphocytes we found that a large proportion (60-80%) of the high density cells spontanously shifted to lower density during the first 12 hours after explantation. To investigate the relationship between the spontaneous density shift and EBV-susceptibility, we

Current Topics in Microbiology and Immunology, Vol. 132

infected purified high density B-cells, cultured them for 9 hours, separated them again into density shifted and non-shifted populations and investigated the EBNA-expression after another 36 hours of incubation (FIGURE 1). EBNA-producing cells were only seen in the subpopulation that had shifted to lower density during the first 9 hours of incubation. The number of density shifting cells during the first 9 hours was, however, identical in the infected and noninfected cultures excluding EBV induced influence at this point. It is possible that cellular mechanisms associated with the spontaneous density shift may be essential for the virus.

1. HIGH DENSITY B-CELLS ------------- INCUBATE 9 HOURS

DENSITY FRACTIONATION

HIGH DENSITY FRACTION LOW DENSITY FRACTION

INCUBATE ANOTHER 36 HOURS
EBNA STAINING
EBNA NEGATIVE EBNA POSITIVE

The reason for the spontaneous density shift is not known. It is not a simple osmotic phenomenon and it is independent of serum source or presence of serum. The spontaneous density shift may be inhibited by coculturing with autologous T-cells, or, less efficiently by low density B-cells. Therefore the spontanous density shift in purified high density B-cells may reflect an activation like response after release from suppressing factors or cells present among T-cells and low density B-cells. T-cell mediated inhibition of EBV-infection (Tosato 1982) may be associated with inhibition of the spontaneous density shift.

TABLE 2
MEMBRANE MARKERS ON EBV-SUSCEPTIBLE HIGH DENSITY B-CELLS

	POPULATION	EBV-susceptiblility
	IgM+	Yes
	IgM-	Yes
	IgD+	Yes
mIg	IgD-	Yes
	IgG+	No
	IgG-	Yes
	B2+	Yes
	B2-	No
	BB1+	Yes
	BB1-	Yes
Activation markers.	BB2+	No
	BB2-	Yes
	38-13+	Yes
	38-13-	Yes

Purified high density B-cells were fluorescence labelled with different antibodies specific for the indicated markers. Positive and negative populations were FACS sorted and EBV-infected. EBV-susceptibility was studied by EBNA-expression 60 hours after infection and by outgrowth in long term cultures.

In our second approach to characterize EBV-target cells we utilized the fluorescence activated cell sorter (FACS) to sort out subpopulations of B-cells with different marker phenotypes and test them for EBV susceptibility. High density B-cells were labelled with different conventional or monoclonal fluorescent antibodies and sorted into strongly negative and positive populations. Intermediate staining cells were excluded. The sorted populations were infected with EBV and investigated for EBNA-production and outgrowth (TABLE 2).
We found that both IgM and IgD positive and negative cells were transformed by EBV, whereas only IgG-negative cells but not IgG-positives were EBV-susceptible.

Cells that were labelled with the activation marker detecting monoclonal antibodies BB1 and BB2 (Yokoshi 1982, Murray,1984), were respectively partly and totally resistant to EBV. The BB2 marker was present only on germinal center cells in vivo. Another germinal center marker was detected by the 38-13 monoclonal (Murray 1985) present on most Burkitt lymphomas. Both 38-13 positive and negative cells were susceptible to EBV-infection.

EBV-Induced B-cell Activation
EBV-infection of B-lymphocytes was reported to be followed by EBNA-production, cellular DNA-synthesis and proliferation, and Ig-secretion in this order (Menezes 1976, Bird 1979). We were particularly interested in the first events of EBV-induced activation and distinct marker changes compared to B-cells activated by other mitogens.

The first difference between EBV-infected and control cultured B-cells was a strong aggregation of the infected cells already 10 to 15 minutes after exposure to the virus. The aggregation was not affected by low temperature or UV-inactivation of the virus. Therefore it was probably mediated directly by the virions or fast membrane changes elicited by the virus-receptor interaction. If B-cells were infected in very diluted cultures to prevent cell to cell contact, the EBV induced EBNA-production and immortalization were inhibited (TABLE 3).

TABLE 3
EBNA-PRODUCTION AND OUTGROWTH IN B-CELL POPULATIONS EBV-INFECTED AT DIFFERENT CELL DENSITY

CELL DENSITY (MILLIONS/ml)	PER CENT EBNA POSITIVE CELLS	OUTGROWTH
1	18	+++
0.1	2	-
1	24	+++
0.1	<1	-
1	8	+++
0.1	2	+

High density tonsil B-cells were infected with purified virus preparations and incubated at different cell density for 60 hours at 37C. After this incubation, the cells were tested for EBNA-production and resuspended at a density of 0.3 millins/ml. Outgrowth was studied during three weeks. Results from thre experiments are shown.

These findings are interesting since EBV immortalized normal B-cells normally grow in large aggregates. Recently, it was reported that the proliferation is dependent on cell to cell contact (Gordon et al in press). These observations suggest that cell to cell contact is essential both for the primary activation and long term growth of EBV-infected B-lymphocytes.
It is interesting to notice that tonsil derived B-cells aggregated within minutes after EBV-exposure, while blood B-cells usually aggregated several hours after infection. This difference suggests that the aggregation is not mediated by the virus-particle itself, but by virus induced membrane changes.

Decreased IgD-expression is well known as an early activation response in mitogen stimulated B-cells. The expression of IgD decreased within 5 hours after EBV-infection (TABLE 4). This response was also seen with UV-inactivated virus indicating that it was independent of virus coded protein synthesis. Receptor mediated triggering or factors carried in the virions are possible explanations for this phenomenon.

TABLE 4
mIgD AND EBNA EXPRESSION FROM 0 TO 12 HOURS FOLLOWING INFECTION WITH ACTIVE OR UV-INACTIVATED EBV.

EXPERIMENT		PER CENT m-IgD POSITIVE CELLS		
		HOURS OF INCUBATION		
	0	5	8	12
1				
+EBV	52	28	23	28
+IRRADIATED EBV		22	22	20
CONTROL		45	48	45
		PER CENT EBNA POSITIVE CELLS.		
+EBV	0	0	0	6
2		PER CENT mIgD POSITIVE CELLS		
		HOURS AFTER INFECTION		
	0	5	8	12
+EBV	39	22	22	24
+IRRADIATED EBV		18	24	24
CONTROL		34	35	32
		PER CENT EBNA POSITIVE CELLS		
+EBV		ND	ND	4
+IRRADIATED EBV		ND	ND	0

Samples were stained for IgD and EBNA at indicated incubation times after infection and investigated on a immunofluorescence microscope.

The CR2-binding C3d fragment was recently reported to be a growth factor for B-cells (Melchers 1985). It is possible that EBV has evolved to utilize this receptor and induce a first activation signal as the virions bind to and penetrate into the cell. Evidence for an important function of the virion-cell interaction during primary infection have recently been reported by Volsky et al (Volsky 1984). They found that EBV-DNA microinjected into normal B-cells was activated to EBNA production only if the cells were stimulated by irradiated virions. We were interested in marker changes appearing after the first EBNA production that could be associated with the immortalization. We have compared the marker changes in EBV-infected B-cells and B-cells stimulated by the phorbol ester TPA. Both these agents induce DNA-synthesis and Ig-secretion in tonsilar B-cells.

Both TPA and EBV induced an increased expression of the monoclonal antibody detected activation markers BB1, BB2, and, (Åman 1984b,Åman in press) from 36 hours after stimulation. The expression of these markers was stable during long term culture of EBV-immortalized cells.

The B2 monoclonal antibody reacts with an epitope on the CR2-EBV-receptor complex in human B-lymphocytes. We detected a transiently increased expression of B2 in TPA activated cells and a return to control levels after 60 hours. Similar results have been reported when B-cells have been stimulated by other mitogens.

TABLE 5

B2 AND mIgD-EXPRESSION IN EBV-INFECTED AND TPA STIMULATED B-LYMPHOCYTES

HOURS OF INCUBATION	PER CENT FLUORESCENT CELLS					
	CONTROL		EBV		TPA	
	IgD	B2	IgD	B2	IgD	B2
DONOR 1						
0	52	72				
36	32	34	30	37	2	73
60	23	18	33	53	1	13
120	ND	ND	34	73	0	8
DONOR 2						
0	46	69				
36	40	47	33	45	0	89
60	18	11	35	45	0	22
120	ND	ND	31	67	ND	ND

Cells were stained with the B2 and IgD antibodies at indicated incubation times and investigated on a fluorescence microscope.

The EBV-infected cells showed a distinct pattern with no initial changes in B2 expression but a strong increase 60 hours after infection (TABLE 5).

Both TPA and EBV induced a rapid decrease in IgD-expression. The TPA-stimulated cells remained IgD-negative, whereas the EBV-infected cells re-expressed this marker from 60 hours after infection. The IgD-expression was stable for several weeks. The stable B2 and IgD-expression in EBV-immortalized B-cells suggests that the cells initially are trapped in a stage of maturation or activation that are characterized by these markers.

SUMMARY. In purified B-cell populations with no feeder cells, only small resting B-cells were susceptible to EBV-immortalization. The membrane marker profile of the target cells were IgM+or-, IgD+or-, IgG-, B2+, BB1-or+ with a strong preference for BB1-, BB2-, 38-13+or-.

EBV-infected B-cells were aggregated after infection and the cell to cell contact was important for the activation and EBNA-production. A rapid decrease in IgD-expression was elicited by UV-irradiated or viable EBV-particles. The rapid response in absence of virus coded protein production suggests that it was elicited through a receptor signal.

Like other mitogens, EBV induced a strong expression of the activation markers BB1, BB2, and LB1.

Elevated B2-expression and re-expression of IgD was detected from 60 hours after infection. These marker changes were distinct from the pattern in mitogen-stimulated B-cells and probably reflect the maturation and activation arrest associated with the immortalization.

REFERENCES

Åman, P., Ehlin-Henriksson, B. and Klein, G. (1984). Epstein-Barr-virus susceptibility of Human B-lymphocyte populations. J.Exp.Med, 159: 208-220

Åman, P., Gordon, J. and Klein, G. (1984). TPA-activation of human B-lymphocytes. Immunology, 51: 27-34

Bird, G. and Britton, S. (1979). A new approach to study human B-lymphocyte function using an indirect plaque assay. Immunol., 45: 41-52

Melchers, F., Erdei, A., Schulz, T. and Dierich, M.P. (1985). Growth control of activated murine B-cells by the C3d-fragment of human complement. Nature, 317: 264-265

Menezes, J., Jondal, M., Leibold, W. and Dorval, G. (1976). Epstein-Barr virus interaction with human lymphocyte populations. Infection and Immunology, 13: 303.

Murray, L.J., Swerdlow, S.H. and Habeshaw, J.A. (1984). Distribution of B-lymphocyte subsets in normal tissue. Clin.Exp.Immunol, 56: 399-412

Murray, L.J., Habeshaw, J.A., Wiels, J. and Greaves, M.F. (1985). Expression of Burkitt lymphoma associated antigen on both normal and malignant germinal centers. Int.J.Cancer, 36: 561-570

Reedman, B. and Klein, G. (1973). Cellular localization of an EBV-associated complement fixing antigen in producer and nonproducer lymphoblastoid lines. Int.J.Cancer, 11: 499-507

Tosato, G., Magrath, I. and Blease, M. (1982). T-cell mediated regulation of EBV-induced B-cell activation. J.Immunol., 128: 575-584

Volsky, D., Bartzatt, J.R., Kuszynski, C., Sinangil, F. and Gross, T. (1984). Transformation of human cord blood lymphocytes by coinfection with UV-inactivated Epstein-Barr virus and purified EBV-DNA. Book: Herpesvirus Allan R. Liss Inc. 497.

Yokoshi, T., Holly, R.D. and Clark, E.A. (1982). B-lymphoblast antigen BB1 expressed on EBV-associated B-cell blasts,B-lymphoblastoid cell lines and Burkitt lymphomas. J.Immunol., 128: 823-830

Myc Expression *in vivo* During Human Embryogenesis

Rolf I. Ohlsson and Susan Pfeifer-Ohlsson
Department of Oncology, University of Umea, S-901 87 Umea Sweden

INTRODUCTION

The postulated involvement of the myc oncogene in human neoplasia (Klein 1983, Adams 1985, Little 1984) lends considerable support from work on the retroviral myc oncogene. Thus, the v-myc oncogene promotes, directly or indirectly, immortalization of target cells, evasion from normal regulatory growth controls in addition to tumorigenic behaviour of transformed cells injected into syngeneic animals (Rapp 1985, Blasi 1985, Pfeifer-Ohlsson 1983).

The transiently expressed 'pseudomalignant' phenotype of early human placenta may therefore result from regulated expression of the corresponding proto-oncogene. Thus, following the first few weeks postimplantation, the trophoblastic components of early human placenta display rapid cell proliferation kinetics as well as controlled invasiveness into maternal uterine lining (Hamilton 1977). This behaviour is eventually terminated during the latter part of the first trimester, probably due to massive differentiation by fusion of proliferative mononuclear cytotrophoblasts into non-proliferative multinuclear syncytiotrophoblasts (Hamilton 1977).

We have investigated the pattern of c-myc gene expression during these early phases of placental development. Since we deal with active in vivo expression of the c-myc gene in homeostatic balance with its microenvironment, the initial finding of close association between active c-myc gene expression and cell proliferation (Pfeifer-Ohlsson 1984) has developed our objectives into defining the cell cycle kinetics and growth factor-promoted regulatory pathways associated with the c-myc specific function (Kelly 1983, Campisi 1984, Goustin 1985, Smeland 1985).

EXPRESSION OF THE C-MYC GENE IN EARLY HUMAN PLACENTA

Steady-State Levels of C-myc Products are Temporally and Spatially Controlled.

Total cellular RNA was extracted from legally aborted placentae at Umea county hospital. In Figure 1 is shown the pattern of c-myc gene expression as analyzed by Northern blots. In contrast to the constant steady-state levels of cognate HSP 70 mRNA, the c-myc transcripts are most abundant in the early placentas. The down-regulation of cytoplasmic myc mRNA at the end of first trimester associates closely with loss of the proliferative phenotype of the developing placenta. The spatial distribution of c-myc transcripts in the early placenta was examined further by employing in situ hybridization techniques. 125I-labeled c-myc probes were thus hybridized to thin sections of formalin-fixed

Current Topics in Microbiology and Immunology, Vol. 132

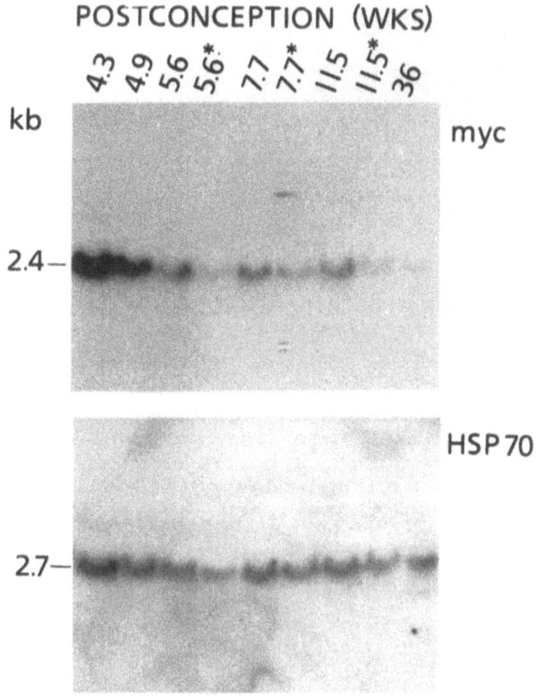

Figure 1. Northern blot analysis of the developmental profile of c-myc gene expression in human placenta. Twenty ug of total cellular RNA, extracted from placentae with known conception, was applied in each lane. The blot was probed with radioactively labeled c-myc (pMC 41 3RC) and HSP 70 plasmids, respectively.

placental tissue (Pfeifer-Ohlsson 1984). In Figure 2 is shown that c-myc expression at the transcriptional level occurs primarily in the proliferative cytotrophoblasts. At later stages of placental development the frequency of myc-positive cells significantly decreases, thus parallelling the pattern of c-myc gene expression as shown in Fig. 1 (Pfeifer-Ohlsson 1984).

In a collaborative effort with Dr R. Watt, we have confirmed this result at the protein level. Immunohistochemical staining of formalin-fixed placental sections, using a monospecific polyclonal antiserum against a recombinant myc protein (Watt 1985), show that the pattern of c-myc protein expression closely parallells the distribution of the myc transcript (Figure 2).

We therefore propose that the c-myc gene is involved in cytotrophoblast proliferation and that the downregulation of c-myc expression prior to differentiation of cytotrophoblasts into syncytiotrophoblasts reflects a developmental aspect of the placental ontogeny.

GROWTH FACTOR-CONTROLLED TROPHOBLAST PROLIFERATION

Platelet-Derived Growth Factor (PDGF) as a Major Embryonic Growth Factor

A central issue in comparing the growth of early placenta to that of a rapidly growing tumour relates to growth factor availabi-

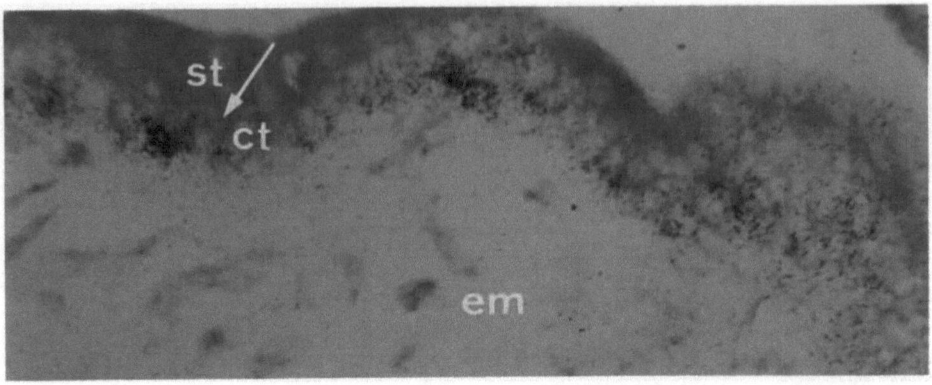

Figure 2. Spatial distribution of c-myc RNA in human placenta. *In situ* hybridization was applied to formalin-fixed thin sections of a 21 days old placenta (Pfeifer-Ohlsson 1984). A borderline between proliferative cytotrophoblasts (ct) and non-proliferative syncytiotrophoblasts (st) is demarcated with an arrow.

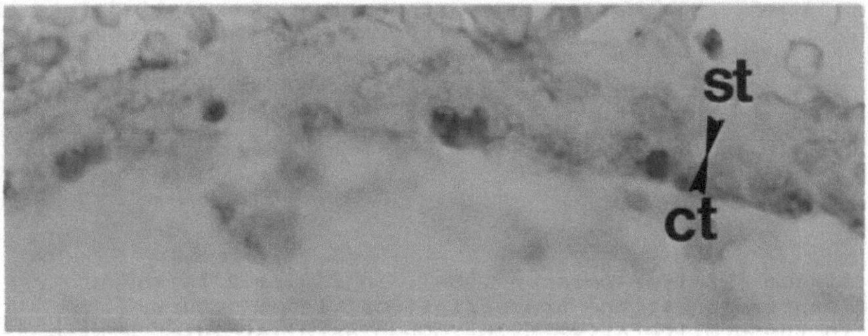

Figure 3. Immunohistochemical analysis of myc protein expression in early human placenta. Thin sections of a 26 days old human placenta were probed with a polyclonal myc antiserum (Watt 1985). The borderline between cytotrophoblasts (ct) and syncytiotrophoblasts (st) is demarcated with arrows.

lity. An autocrine mode of cellular growth has been associated with development of malignant phenotypes and acquisition of autonomy (Sporn 1981). We have, in collaboration with Dr B. Westermark and colleagues, earlier provided evidence that PDGF may function as a major embryonic growth factor (Goustin 1985). Coexpression of the c-sis (coding for PDGF B chain) (Doolittle 1983) and c-myc genes suggests that the proliferative phenotype of cytotrophoblasts during during early phases of human embryogenesis may be explained by an autocrine mechanism involving PDGF (Goustin 1985). Since these cells are most probably exposed to submitogenic levels of PDGF and related growth factors, a relevant question, regarding the 'pseudomalignant' phenotype of the early placenta, remains; are cytotrophoblasts continuously cycling or frequently entering in vivo resting state prior to each new round of cell cycle progression?

TGFβ as a Modulator of PDGF

TGFβ has by others been shown to inhibit PDGF-mediated cell proliferation of embryonic rat cells (Anzano 1986). In a collaborative effort with Drs R. Derynck and H. Moses we are assessing the role of TGFβ in placental development. A preliminary account of this study can be seen in Figure 4, which shows that PDGF is able to induce TGFβ expression in cultured trophoblasts. This result, taken together with preliminary accounts of in situ hybridization of TGFβ expression, suggests that PDGF-mediated placental growth is controlled by an autocrine antagonist of continuous proliferation.

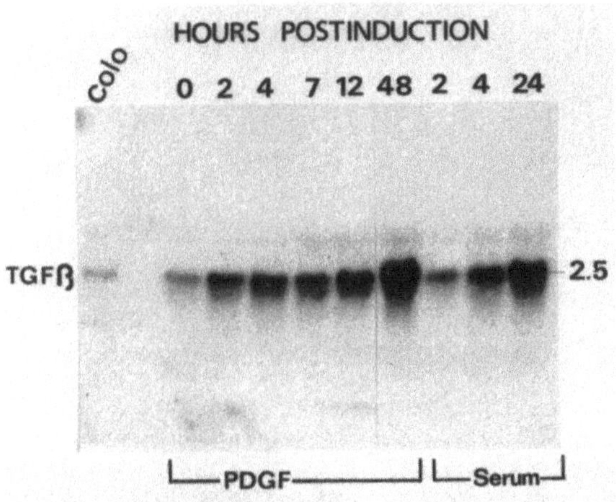

Figure 4. Northern blot analysis of PDGF-induction of TGFβ expression in cultured tropho blast cell line CF 1212. Ten μg of total cellular RNA was applied to each lane.

Cell Cycle-Specific in Vivo Expression of the c-myc Gene in First Trimester Placentas.

In vitro cell cultures, maintained in 10 % fetal calf serum, are continuously exposed to an excess of a variety of growth-promoting activities. C-myc expression has, under such circumstances, been found invariant throughout the cell cycle. Conversely, cells entering the cell cycle in vivo, conceivably respond to accumulated signals of growth factor threshold levels. To assess possible in vivo functions of the c-myc gene it is essential to describe its expression pattern in situ. In collaboration with Dr R. Watt, we have addressed this question by incubating explants, of late first trimester pregnancies, in medium RPMI 1640, supplemented with 10 % fetal calf sera and 50 μCI/ml (methyl-3H)-thymidine, for 6 hours. Since the G1 phase of proliferating cytotrophoblasts is 7-8 hours (Gerbie 1968), cells which have entered S phase, as monitored by autoradiography, must have entered the cell cycle in vivo. Thus, by analyzing the cellular distribution of the myc protein by immunohistochemistry and subsequent autoradiography of formalin-fixed tissue sections, a visual overview will demonstrate whether the c-myc protein is expressed in the S-phase in situ. In Figure 5 is shown a selection of motifs where myc-positive cells and S phase cells coappear. In only a few cases could we monitor S phase cytotrophoblast expressing the myc protein. In contrast, the vast majority of myc-positive cells did not display any evidence of the S phase parameter. Since the numbers of myc-positive cells amounted to only 5-10 % in comparison with S phase cells, we conclude that the myc protein is only transiently expressed in moderatly proliferative tissue (late first trimester placenta).

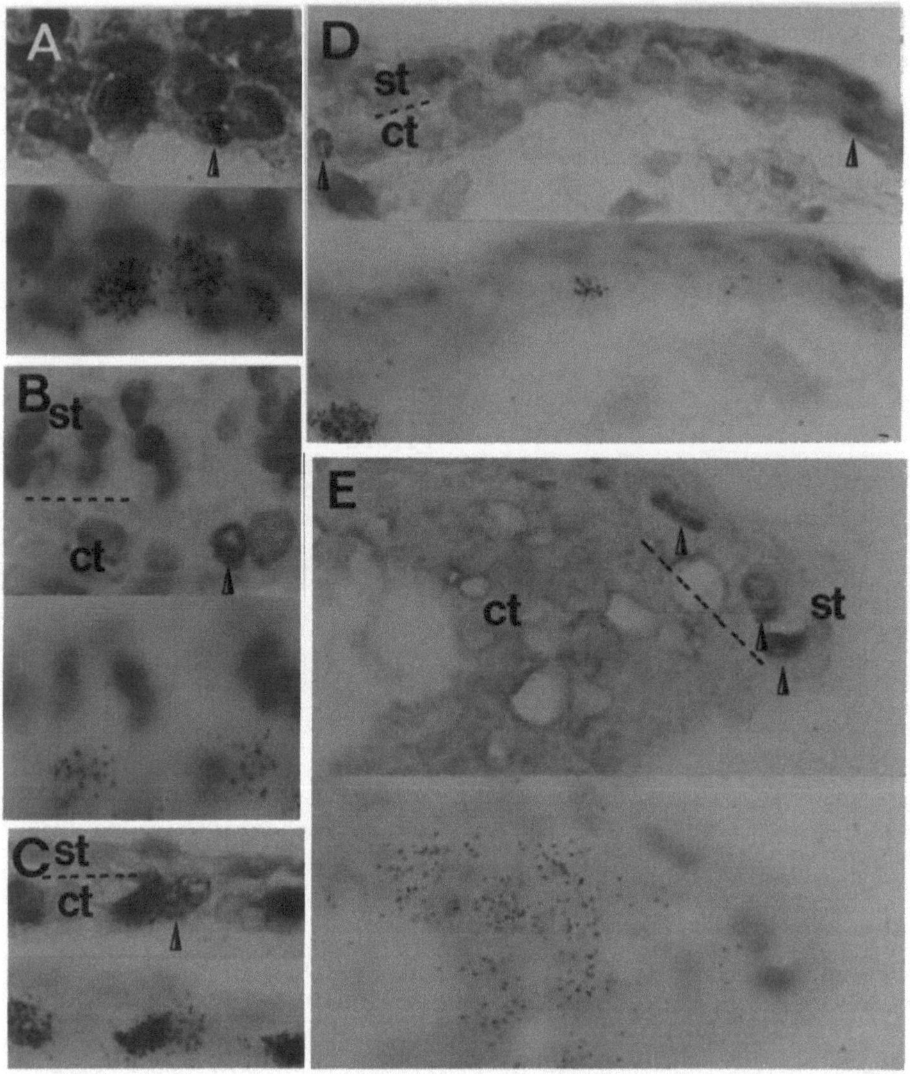

Figure 5. Cell cycle-specific c-myc expression in placental explants in situ. The photographs are displayed in two different focal planes to facilitate interpretation. Arrows denote myc-positive cells. Silver grains depict cells which, during the incubation period of 6 hours, progress through the S phase. In panels A, B, and D, are shown that the c-myc protein is not expressed in the S-phase, in contrast to the sole exception (out of 64 scored myc positive cells) represented in panel C, in placental explants incubated for 6 hours. In longer incubations (24 hours), the syncytiotrophoblast c-myc gene can be activated, apperently not leading to S phase entry (panel E).

CONCLUDING REMARKS

Myc Expression in Vivo and in Vitro

A deregulation of c-*myc* gene expression has been considered to be important in some tumorigenic processes and could result from either genetic lesions and/or autocrine production of growth factors. The maintenance of *in vitro* cell cultures in rich medium, usually containing high levels of exogenous growth factors, may, however, also promote unscheduled expression of the c-*myc* gene. Therefore, the differences between normal and neoplastic phenotypes with regard to cell cycle kinetics may in such culture conditions be superficially be distorted. An example of unscheduled c-*myc* expression, induced by external aministration of culture medium rich in growth-stimulating activities, is provided by placental syncytiotrophoblasts, which do not express the c-*myc* gene in vivo. Exposure of placental explants to a medium, containing RPMI 1640 and 10 % fetal calf serum, for 24 hours induce expression of the syncytiotrophoblast *c-myc* gene but without any concomitant entry into S phase (not shown). It therefore appears that the *in vivo* expression of the c-*myc* protein is transient in its nature, due to tightly controlled expression of growth factors and/or growth factor receptors.

Relevance to B Cell Neoplasia

Our result bears on B cell neoplasia in primarily one aspect. Thus, in analogy to placenta, B cell proliferation in lymph nodes may use the *myc* function only transiently and in a restricted part of the cycle. Therefore, other pleiotropic agonistic or antagonistic events, associated with the c-*myc* function should be assessed in relation to the architecture of the tissue for additional knowledge of the mechanisms involved in the development of B cell neoplasia.

The last point concerns the existence of several c-*myc* related genes. Notably, we have earlier presented data that the c-*myc* gene is cell type-specifically expressed (Pfeifer-Ohlsson 1985). Recently, Zimmerman (1986) have shown that the L-*myc*, N-*myc* and c-*myc* genes are expressed differentially during mouse embryogenesis and thus probably regulated through different mechanisms. The close homology between these genes of the *myc* family suggest related functions (Nau 1985, Stanton 1986, Schwab 1985). Since the c-*myc* expression appears to be transient, possibly related to cell cycle transitions, why should, in certain instances, a deregulation of c-*myc* gene expression so profoundly influence the phenotype? We propose that a deregulated expression of the c-*myc* could overlap with the functions of other *myc* related protein products, under the control of other promoters and therefore interfere with feed-back controls associated with regulated cell proliferation.

REFERENCES

Anzano MA, Roberts AB, Sporn M (1986) Anchorage-independent growth of primary rat embryo cells is induced by platelet-derived growth factor and inhibited by type-beta transforming growth factor J Cell Phys 126:312-318

Adams JM, Harris AW, Pinkert CA, Corcoran LM, Alexander WS, Cory S, Palmiter RD, Brinster RL (1985) The c-myc oncogene driven by immunoglobulin enhancers induces lymphoid malignancy in transgenic mice Nature 318:533-538

Blasi E, Mathieson BJ, Varesio L, Cleveland JL, Borchert PA, Rapp UR (1985) Selective immortalization of murine macrophages from fresh bone marrow by a raf/myc recombinant murine retro virus Nature 318:667-670

Campisi J, Gray HE, Pardee AB, Dean M, Sonenshein G (1984) Cell-cycle control of c-myc but not c-ras expression is lost following chemical transformation Cell 36:241-247

Doolittle RF, Hunkapiller MW, Hood LE, Devare SG, Robbins KL, Aaronson SA, Antoniades HN (1983) Simian sarcoma virus onc gene, v-sis, is derived from the gene (or genes) encoding the platelet-derived growth factor Science 221:275-277

Gerbie AB, Hathway HH, Brewer JI (1968) Autoradiographic analysis of normal trophoblast proliferation Am J Obst Gyn 100:640-650

Goustin AS, Betsholtz C, Pfeifer-Ohlsson SB, Persson H, Rydnert J, Bywater M, Holmgren G, Heldin C-H, Westermark B, Ohlsson R (1985) Coexpression of the sis and myc proto-oncogenes in developing human placenta suggests autocrine control of trophoblast growth Cell 41:301-312

Hamilton WJ, Hamilton DV (1977) Development of the human placenta, Scientific foundations of obstretics and gynecology. Heinemann, London

Hann SR, Thompson CB, Eisenman RN (1985) C-myc oncogene protein synthesis is independent of the cell cycle in human and avian cells Nature 314:366-369

Kelly K, Cochran BH, Stiles CD, Leder P (1983) Cell-specific regulation of the c-myc gene by lymphocyte mitogens and platelet-derived growth factor Cell 35:603-610

Klein G (1983) Specific chromosomal variations and the genesis of B cell-derived tumours in mice and men Cell 32:771-778

Stanton, L, Schwab, M, Bishop, JM (1986) Nucleotide sequence of the human N-myc gene Proc Nat Acad Sci USA 83, 1772-1776

Little CD, Nau MN, Carney DN, Gazdar AF, Minna JD (1983) Amplification and expression of the c-myc oncogene in human lung cancer cell lines Nature 306:194-197

Nau MN, Brooks BJ, Battey J, Sausville E, Gazdar AF, Kirsch IR, McBride OW, Bertness V, Hollis GF, Minna JD (1985) L-myc, a new myc-related gene amplified and expressed in human small cell lung cancer Nature 318:69-73

Pfeifer-Ohlsson (1984) OK10-transformed cell lines: viral component generation and tumorigenecity Intervir. 21:121-133

Pfeifer-Ohlsson SB, Goustin AS, Rydnert J, Wahlstrom T, Bjersing L, Stehelin D, Ohlsson R (1984) Spatial and temporal pattern of cellular myc oncogene in developing human placenta: implica tions for embryonic proliferation Cell 38:585-596

Pfeifer-Ohlsson SB, Rydnert J, Goustin AS, Larsson E, Betsholtz C, Ohlsson R. Cell-type-specific pattern of myc protooncogene expression in developing human embryos Proc Nat Acad Sci USA 82:5050-5054

Rapp UR, Cleveland JL, Brightman K, Scott A, Ihle JN (1985) Abrogration of IL-3 and IL-2 dependence by recombinant retroviruses expressing v-myc oncogenes Nature 317, 434-437

Smeland E, Godal T, Ruud E, Beiske K, Funderud S, Clark E, Pfeifer-Ohlsson S, Ohlsson R (1985) The specific induction of myc protooncogene expression in human B cells is not a sufficient event for acquisition of competence to proliferate Proc Nat Acad Sci USA 82:6255-6259

Sporn M, Todaro G (1980) Autocrine secretion and malignant transformation of cells N Engl J Med 303:878-880

Thompson CB, Challoner PB, Neiman PE, Groudine M (1985) Levels of c-myc oncogene mRNA are invariant throughout the cell cycle Nature 314:363-366

Watt RA, Shatzman AR, Rosenberg M (1985) Mol Cell Biol 5:448-456

Schwab, M, Varmus, HE, and Bishop, JM (1985) Nature 316, 160-162

Zimmerman KA, Yancopolous GD, Collum RG, Smith RK, Kohl NE, Denis KA, Nau MM, Witte ON, Toran-Allerand D, Gee CE, Minna JD, Alt F (1986) Differential expression of myc family genes during murine development Nature 319:780-783

Expression of c-*myc* and c-*fos* During Phorbol Ester Induced Differentiation of B-type Chronic Lymphocytic Leukemia Cells

K. Nilsson, L.-G. Larsson, M. Carlsson, A. Danersund, K. Forsbeck, L. Hellman, T. Tötterman, and U. Pettersson

Department of Pathology and Department of Medical Genetics, University of Uppsala, Uppsala, Sweden

INTRODUCTION

The development of the various functionally specialized cell types within the hematopoietic system involves not only stepwise, cell lineage specific phenotypic alterations towards the fully mature end cells, but also proliferation to allow for the necessary expansion of the stem cell progeny (Mak and McCulloch 1982). The two processes appear to be regulated by two independent but coupled genetic programs. In malignant hematopoietic cell clones, in contrast, cells often are arrested at a particular stage of differentiation (Greaves 1979). This arrest was until recently assumed to be irreversible. However, it is now clear from many studies in vitro of mouse and human leukemia/lymphoma cells that further, and in the case of some myelo-monocytic human tumor cell lines, even terminal differentiation may be induced by several inducers including phorbol esters (i.e. TPA), dimethylsulphoxide (DMSO), vitamin D3 and retinoic acid (Sachs 1980, Huberman and Callaham 1979, Nilsson et al. 1980).

The nature of the apparent deregulation of the gene programs for growth and differentiation in malignant hematopoietic cells is virtually unknown. However, in the case of Burkitt lymphoma (BL) the finding of the regular translocation of c-myc to either of the loci for immunoglobulin (Ig) heavy- or light chains suggests an important role of this oncogene in the transformation of the BL progenitor B-lymphocyte (Klein and Klein 1985).

That activated oncogenes may be involved in the pathogenesis of tumors of the hematopoietic system is also suggested by the findings that several proto-oncogenes appear to be involved in the control of normal growth and differentiation - the two processes assumed to be deranged in leukemia/lymphoma cells (Bishop 1985). Most of the information on hematopoietic cells in this regard concerns the c-myc proto-oncogene expression during a proliferative response. Thus, for normal B- and T-cells a transient increase in c-myc mRNA was found after mitogen stimulation (Kelly et al. 1983) and recently, Smeland et al. (1985) reported a similar finding in B-cells activated by anti-μ-chain. In none of these studies markers to indicate induced differentiation was examined. The reaction of c-myc expression to the differentiation process has therefore not been documented in normal hematopoietic cells. However, from studies on established hematopoietic cell lines capable of undergoing terminal differentiation when induced by DMSO or TPA (e.g. HL-60 and U-937) further information is available about the differentiation associated c-myc and c-fos proto-oncogene expres-

Current Topics in Microbiology and Immunology, Vol. 132

sion. A decrease in the c-myc mRNA has been reported to preceed or parallel the decrease in proliferation as the mature phenotype gradually develops during the differentiation process (reviewed by Nilsson et al. 1985). The view has therefore been put forward that the c-myc expression has to be downregulated to allow the genetic program for differentiation to be executed. However, contrasting to these findings is the result of Benjamin et al. (1984) in their study of a B-lymphoma cell line which suggests that further differentiation may be induced without the downregulation of c-myc expression. c-fos expression in human differentiating hematopoietic cell systems has been subject to but a few studies so far. The results have been intepreted to suggest that continued expression of this gene is necessary for monocyte-macrophage differentiation to occur.

In this paper we summarize our studies of the relationship of the proto-oncogenes c-myc and c-fos to the differentiation process in a selected case of human chronic lymphocytic leukemia of B-cell type (B-CLL), designated I-73 (Larsson et al. 1986). The differentiation induced by TPA in I-73 cells proceeds without concomitant proliferation. As a basis for the studies of the expression of these oncogenes we have also determined the cell-cycle position of the fresh, resting I-73 cells. We followed their cell-cycle transition after TPA treatment using flow cytometry to quantitate RNA, DNA, cell volume and immunofluorescence to determine the expression of selected cell-cycle associated B-cell surface antigens (Carlsson et al. 1986). The results suggest 1. that the I-73 B-CLL clone represent a homogeneous cell clone resting in the G0 phase of the cell cycle, which upon TPA exposure becomes activated and traverse synchronously to the G1A phase of the cell cycle, 2. that c-myc mRNA expression and translation increase during the G0 to G1 transition and thus do not prevent the differentiation process as was suggested from the studies of the HL-60 and U-937 systems and 3. that c-fos is expressed in uninduced cells and transiently increases its expression after TPA exposure.

CLL AS A DIFFERENTIATING TUMOR CELL SYSTEM

B-CLL is a heterogeneous disease, reflected not only by the variability in clinical behaviour but also by the variability in cellular phenotype. However, in the majority of the cases the cellular characteristics correspond roughly to those of slightly immature, resting blood B-cells. In recent years it has been demonstrated that the leukemic cells from the majority of the cases can be induced to differentiate by TPA and to a less regular degree also by T- and B-cell mitogens (for a review see Nilsson 1985 b). TPA has been found to be by far the most effective inducer of differentiation. The induced phenotypic changes of the cells include a) morphological changes of 80-90 % of the cells which transform into lymphoblasts and plasmablasts, b) increase in cytoplasmic β-glucuronidase, c) altered (increased or decreased) expression of several B-cell differentiation associated surface antigens, d) decreased expression of surface IgD and IgM and mouse erythrocyte- and Fcγ-receptors and e) the aquisition of capacity for secretion of pentameric IgM. Taken together the findings suggest that TPA inducible B-CLL populations undergo changes similar to those observed in normal B-cells when activated to maturation into Ig secretory cells.

More detailed studies of the most important functional hallmark of B-cell differentiation - Ig production - also agree that B-CLL cells probably follow the same differentiation pathway as normal B-cells. Thus, a recent study on the biosynthesis of cytoplasmic and surface μ-chains and the corresponding mRNA levels demonstrated that the B-cell differentiation process proceeds in several steps similar to what has been described for mouse cells (Forsbeck et al. 1986). Non-induced B-CLL cells expressed about equal amounts of mRNA for membrane associated (μm mRNA) and secretory μ-chains (μs mRNA). The μm RNA was translated, and the protein was expressed at the cell surface. However, although the μs mRNA message was translated to cytoplasmic μ-chains no pentameric, secretory IgM was assembled and exported. When induced to differentiate by TPA the total level of μ-chain mRNA was not increased but the ratio μs/μm RNA increased around 4 times. This contrasts to the marked downregulation of surface IgM and the development of a high capacity for Ig secretion. The findings thus suggest that aquisition of capacity for Ig secretion to the most part was the result of an increase in translation and probably post-translational modification of the Ig molecules.

The maturation of CLL cells usually proceeds with but minimal proliferation in most of the cases. In these cases the proliferating cells are T-cells contaminating the B-CLL population by 5-10 %. In rare cases, however, proliferation has been demonstrated to occur concomitant with the differentiation process in the B-CLL cells. In the non-proliferative type of B-CLL we have shown that the mechanism of action of TPA is both direct, by activating protein kinase C (Nilsson et al. 1985 b), and indirect by inducing the T-cells to proliferation and production of B-cell differentiation-inducing lymphokines (Danersund et al. 1985). Also with respect to responsiveness to physiological differentiation factors B-CLL cells thus appear to be similar to normal B-cells.

ACTIVATION AND CELL CYCLE TRANSITION (G0 TO G1) OF I-73 B-CLL CELLS DURING TPA INDUCED DIFFERENTIATION

As depicted in Fig. 1 non-induced I-73 cells (Fig. 1 A) have RNA and DNA values similar to normal resting peripheral blood lymphocytes (PBL:s Fig. 1 C), when analyzed by flow cytometry using the method of Darzynkiewicz et al. (1979), and should accordingly be regarded as G0 cells. Upon TPA treatment the cell population homogenously increased the amount of RNA but not DNA within 24 hours (Fig. 1 B). This contrasts to the behavior of the control PBL:s in which the RNA content continued to increase even further with time. A sizeable fraction of these cells also had increased DNA values at 72 hours post induction (Fig. 1 D). With the behavior of normal PBL:s as a reference the data thus demonstrate that most I-73 cells traverse to the G1A phase of the cell cycle, according to the terminology of Darzynkiewicz et al. (1979).

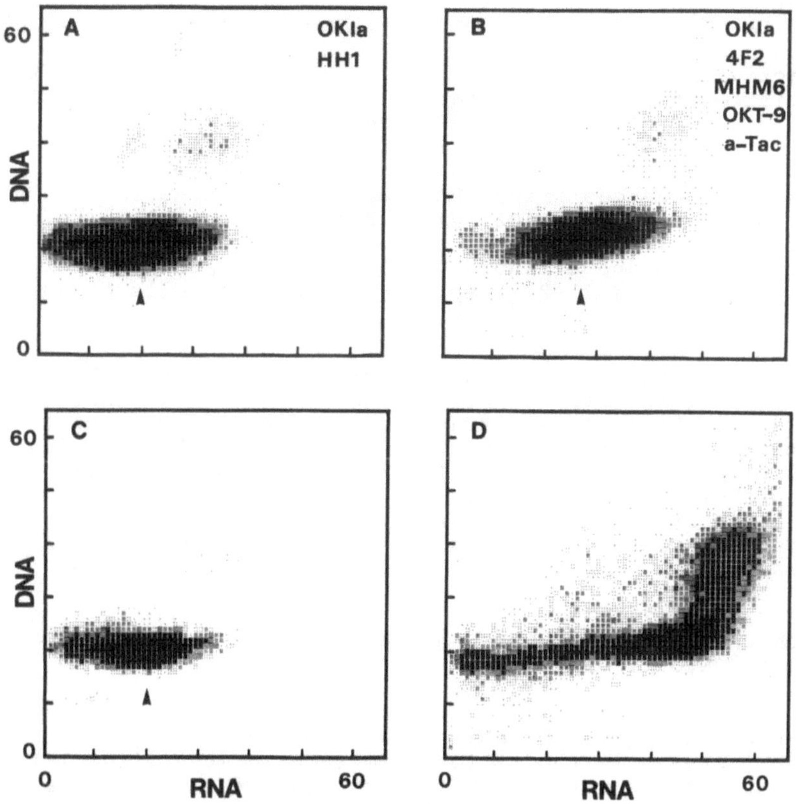

<u>Fig. 1.</u> A density plot presentation of acridine orange stained B-CLL cells and normal peripheral blood lymphocytes measured in 64-channels as a green fluorescence for DNA (F530nm) and as red fluorescence for RNA (F 600 nm, logaritmically amplified).
A: uninduced I-73 cells; B: I-73 cells induced with TPA for 72 hours. No spontaneous transition was observed when the cells were cultivated in absence of TPA. The arrows indicate the approximate position of the peak values. As control uninduced and 72 hours PHA-induced peripheral blood lymphocytes are shown in Fig C and D, respectively.

To increase the resolution of the analysis of possible induction of DNA synthesis in the I-73 cells after TPA exposure experiments were performed with cells labelled in vitro by 3H-thymidine (3H-TdR) after 72 hours TPA treatment. Cells expressing a late G1 marker, the transferrin receptor were sorted out, characterized for T-cell marker and analyzed by autoradiography for 3H-TdR uptake. The proliferating cells, representing around 2 % of the total I-73 cell population, were almost exclusively T-cells.

To further analyze the G0 to G1 transition several monoclonal antibodies (OKIa, HH1, 4F2, MHM6, OKT-9, a-Tac, Ki-67; for references see Carlsson et al. 1986) were employed to determine a) early lymphocyte activation antigen (4F2), b) early (HH1) and late (MHM6) differentiation antigens, c) late G1 antigens (OKT-9; transferrin receptor) and a-Tac antigen (Il-2 receptor), and d) an antigen expressed throughout the cell cycle in T-cells (Ki-67) (except during G0 to early G1 activation). The findings demonstrate (Fig. 1A, 1B) drastic changes after TPA exposure in expression of HH1, which disappeared, and in 4F2, which became detectable within 12 hours. Around 50 % of the cells became positive for the lymphoblast antigen MHM6 and a minority (10-25 %) aquired transferrin receptors (OKT-9) and Il-2 receptors (a-Tac). No cells became Ki-67 positive.

Taken together, the antigen studies agree with the RNA/DNA data that the I-73 represents G0 cells which during the TPA induced differentiation homogenously traverse into the G1 phase of the cell cycle. They also add to this picture that, while the majority of the cells become arrested in early G1, 10-15 % of the cells will proceed further to late G1. Later in the differential process (24-48 hours), the absence of Ki-67 reactivity also agrees that the differentiation process is not associated with proliferation.

EXPRESSION OF SECRETED/MEMBRANE μ-CHAIN mRNA DURING TPA INDUCED DIFFERENTIATION OF I-73 CELLS

Northern blot analysis of μ-chain mRNA expression (Fig. 2) demonstrated an increase in the ratio μs/μm μ-chain mRNA (from 1:1 to 4:1). This shift was very rapid and preceeded the earliest antigenic changes and the increase in RNA content, as described above, and the uridine synthesis (Larsson et al. 1986). During the first 4 hours a transient decrease in μ-chain mRNA expression was noted. Similar results have been published by Cossman et al. (1984) studying TPA induced differentiation of a B-CLL population. That the switch in μm to μs mRNA occurred earlier than the increase in RNA synthesis (Larsson et al. 1986) and in actin gene expression (Fig. 2) suggests that the μ-chain gene is rapidly regulated with a relative selectivity during the early activation/differentiation process.

EXPRESSION OF c-*myc* AND c-*fos* PROTO-ONCOGENES DURING TPA INDUCED DIFFERENTIATION OF I-73 B-CLL CELLS

The expression of c-myc

Fig. 3 shows that, as determined by northern blot analysis, the levels of c-*myc* mRNA was drastically increased simultaneously with the μs/μm mRNA shift but prior to the increase in RNA, protein synthesis and Ig secretion. The level started to increase 2 hours post TPA induction and peaked at 4 hours. At later time points (12-72 hours) the c-*myc* mRNA expression remained constant.

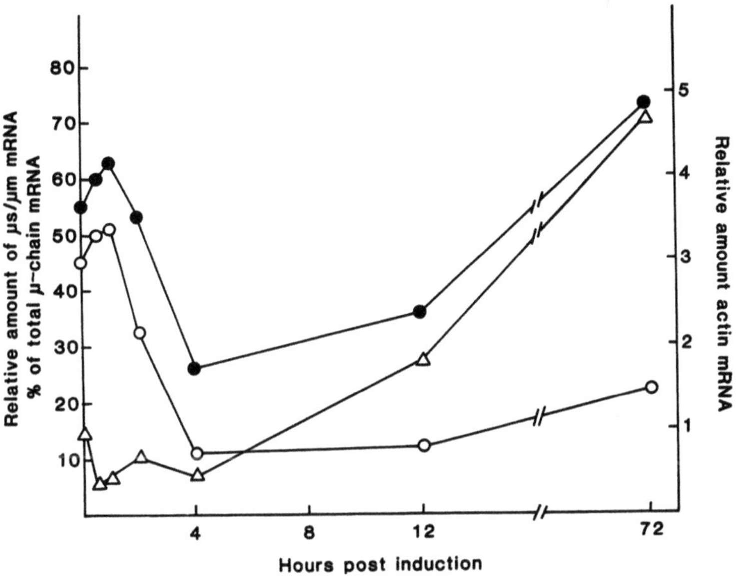

Fig. 2. Northern blot analysis of µ-chain mRNA and actin mRNA expression. A quantitative evaluation of the amount of transcripts were obtained by densiometric scanning of autoradiograms. Δ, actin mRNA. The value of induced I-73 cells were normalized to 1.
●, µs mRNA; ○, µm mRNA. The value of total µ-chain mRNA of uninduced I-73 cells was set to 100 %.

The kinetics and the level of c-myc mRNA expression in the I-73 cells are similar to what has been reported for normal B-cells, activated to proliferation by anti-µ antibodies and BCGF (Smeland et al. 1985). A difference, however, is that in normal B-cells a decrease in c-myc mRNA to control levels was observed after 21 hours.

The level of c-myc protein

The finding that differentiation may occur in B-CLL cells without concomitant downregulation of the c-myc gene expression conflicts with the hypothesis that the c-myc product might prevent differentiation of several types of hematopoietic cells as suggested from the studies with the HL-60 and U-937 cell lines, and by the deregulation of c-myc expression noticed in BL. We therefore tested the possibility that a translation defect of the c-myc mRNA had occurred in the I-73 cells. However, as clearly demonstrated by the immunoprecipitation data using a c-myc protein specific antibody the c-myc mRNA was transcribed (Fig. 3). Apparently, thus the conclusion that B-cell differentiation may indeed proceed without downregulation of c-myc stands firmly after the protein studies. These results may also be useful to extend the results of Smeland et al. (1985) in that they show that the c-myc protein is a prerequisite but not sufficient in itself to make the cells enter the S-phase.

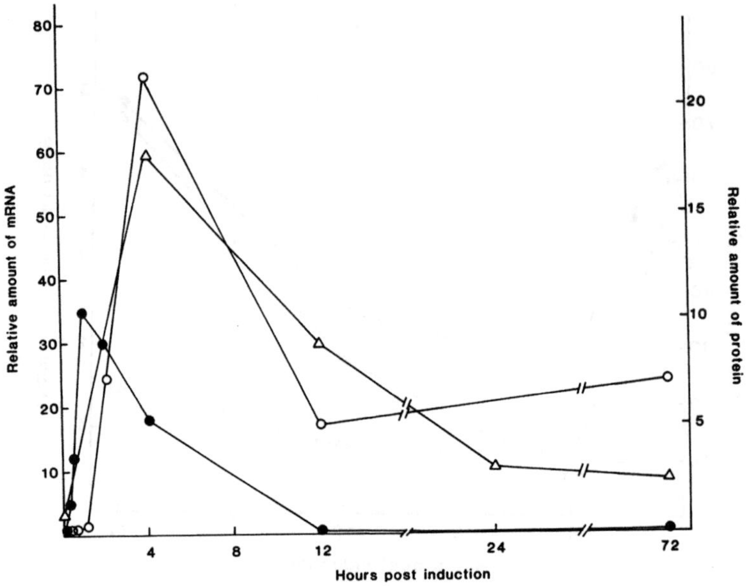

Fig. 3. Northern blot analysis of c-*myc* and c-*fos* expression and immunoprecipitation of c-*myc* protein. The autoradiograms were scanned as above. The value of uninduced I-73 cells were normalized to 1. ●, c-*fos* mRNA; ○, c-*myc* mRNA; △, p64 c-*myc*.

One may speculate why the I-73 cells become blocked in G1A, to express c-*myc* protein and simultaneously differentiate into Ig secretory cells. Obviously the findings may be artefactual in that the tissue culture conditions are deficient with respect to proper growth factors (e.g. BCGF) or that TPA would prevent proliferation of CLL cells. However, using TPA and the same culture conditions, we have identified some CLL tumor populations in which proliferation and differentiation into plasmablasts occur simultaneously.

The G1A block may also reflect a malignancy associated defect in the general control of gene expression in the I-73 cells. However, the G1 to G1 transition is similar to that of normal B-cells as are the phenotypic changes during the induced differentiation. This suggests that at least the set of genes involved in the differentiation process is orderly expressed and regulated in I-73 cells. Two other explanations may therefore be put forward. The first is that I-73 cells may be the malignant counterpart to B-cells programmed to rapidly convert into Ig secretory cells without proliferation (memory cells?). The second, and even more speculative explanation would be that I-73 cells represent aged B-cells unable to divide but inducible to c-*myc* mRNA expression similar to what has recently been observed in senescent fibroblasts when such cells are stimulated by platelet derived growth factor (Paulsson, personal communication). The I-73 CLL would according to this view represent a tumor clone with its proliferative (and immortal?) compartment present elsewhere (bone marrow, spleen) than in the peripheral blood. Such a CLL would become arrested, perhaps irreversibly in G0 after a certain number of cell divisions. They would then dislocate to peripheral blood where they remain unproliferative during the rest of their life span. Comparative studies on CLL populations isolated from spleen, bone-marrow and lymph nodes may help in elucidating further on this point.

The expression of c-fos

c-*fos* mRNA was detectable by northern blot analysis in uninduced cells at a level 2-fold that of TPA induced HL-60 cells. This significant level of c-*fos* mRNA increased rapidly after TPA-treatment (within 15 min.). The maximum level was reached after 1 hour (Fig. 3). The c-*fos* mRNA expression decreased to barely detectable levels at 12 hours. These results agree with previous data that c-*fos* is rapidly and transiently induced during the G0 to G1 transition in TPA-treated cells. Strikingly, however, is the finding that c-*fos* is detectable at comparatively high levels also in uninduced I-73 cells. If this is not an *in vitro* artefact constitutive expression of c-*fos* appears therefore not to be restricted to previously described cell types (e.g. macrophages, amnion cells).

SUMMARY AND CONCLUSIONS

Uninduced I-73 cells, like normal PBLs, appear to be arrested in the G0 phase of the cell cycle. When exposed to TPA they become activated and traverse synchronously into G1 where they once again become arrested. RNA/DNA quantitations and analyses of the expression of activation- and differentiation-associated surface antigens suggest that the majority of the cells become blocked in early-middle G1 (G1A), and a minority traverse to a late part of G1 before they arrest.

A switch in the ratio of μs/μm mRNA (from 1:1 to 4:1) occurs rapidly after TPA induction. This early increase in μs mRNA may be relatively selective as the increase in actin mRNA is noted somewhat later. Secretory IgM becomes detectable only at 24 hours.

c-*myc* mRNA expression increases drastically during the early period of activation, peaks at 4 hours and then decreases to reach a lower, but still high level at 12 hours. The c-*myc* mRNA expression then remains constant throughout the entire differentiation process of 72 hours.

c-*myc* mRNA is translated in amounts relative to the c-*myc* mRNA expression.

c-*fos* mRNA is detectable already in non-induced I-73 cells. Its level increases earlier than that of the c-*myc* mRNA, peaks at 1 hour and then decreases gradually to barely detectable levels at 12 hours post TPA induction.

The I-73 B-CLL clone thus appears to represent an interesting model both for studies of the nature of malignancy associated genetic changes and as a model for normal B-cell differentiation.

ACKNOWLEDGEMENTS

The studies summarized in this paper was supported by grants from the Swedish Cancer Society and by STU. We thank Mrs Eva Harryson for excellent assistance in the preparation of this paper.

REFERENCES

Benjamin D, Magrath JT, Triche TJ, Schroff RW, Jensen JP, Korsmeyer SJ (1984) Induction of plasmacytoid differentiation by phorbol ester in B-cell lymphoma cell lines bearing 8;14 translocations. Proc Natl Acad Sci USA 81:3547-3551

Bishop JM (1985) Viral oncogenes. Cell 42:23-38.

Carlsson M, Tötterman TH, Matsson P, Nilsson K (1986) Cell cycle progression of B-chronic lymphocytic leukemia cells induced to differentiate by TPA. To be published.

Crossman J, Neckers LM, Braziel RM, Trepel JB, Korsmeyer SJ, Bakhshi A (1984) In vitro enhancement of immunoglobulin gene expression in chronic lymphocytic leukemia. J Clin Invest 73:587-592.

Danersund A, Tötterman TH, Nilsson K, Egle-Jansson I, Kabelitz D, Sjöberg O (1985) Phorbol ester-induced differentiation of chronic B lymphocytic leukaemia cells - regulatory impact of autologous and allogeneic accessory cells. Clin exp Immunol 59:644-652.

Forsbeck K, Hellman L, Danersund A, Tötterman TH, Pettersson U, Nilsson K (1986) TPA-induced differentiation of chronic lymphocytic lèukaemia cells: Studies on chain expression. To be published.

Greaves MF (1979) Tumour markers, phenotypes, and maturation arrest in malignancy: A cell selection hypothesis. In: Boelsma E, Rumke P (eds) Tumour markers. Elsevier, Amsterdam p 201.

Huberman E, Callaham MF (1979) Induction of terminal differention in human promyelocytic leukemia cells by tumor-promoting agents. Proc Natl Acad Sci 76:1293-1297.

Kelly K, Cochran BH, Stiles CD, Leder P (1983) Cell-specific regulation of the c-myc gene by lymphocyte mitogens and platelet-derived growth factor. Cell 35:603-610.

Klein G, Klein E (1985) Evolution of tumours and the impact of molecular oncology. Nature 315:190-195.

Larsson L-G, Gray HE, Tötterman T, Pettersson U, Nilsson K (1986) Drastically increased expression of c-myc and c-fos oncogenes during in vitro differentiation of chronic lymphocytic leukemia (CLL) cells. To be published.

Mak TW, McCulloch (eds) (1982) Cellular and molecular biology of hemopoietic stem cell differentiation. J Cell Physiol, suppl 1.

Nilsson K, Andersson LC, Gahmberg CG, Forsbeck K (1980) Differentiation in vitro of human leukemia and lymphoma cell lines.In: Serrou B, Rosenfeld C (eds) International symposium on new trends in human immunology and cancer immuno-therapy. Doin Editeurs, Paris p 271.

Nilsson K, Ivhed I, Forsbeck K (1985) Induced differentiation in human malignant hematopoietic cell lines. In: Andersson LC, Gahmberg CG, Ekblom P (eds). Academic Press, London p 57.

Nilsson K, Tötterman T, Danersund A, Forsbeck K, Hellman L, Pettersson U (1985b) Phorbol ester (TPA)-induced differention of B-type chronic lymphocytic leukemia cells. In: Wahren B et al (eds) Molecular Biology of Tumor Cells. Raven Press, New York p 233.

Sachs L (1980) Constitutive uncoupling of pathways of gene expression that control growth differentiation in myeloid leukemia: A model for the origin and progression of malignancy. Proc Natl Acad Sci USA 77:6152-6156.
Smeland E, Godal T, Ruud E, Beiske K, Funderud S, Clark EA, Pfeifer-Ohlsson S, Ohlsson R (1985) The specific induction of myc proto-oncogene expression in normal human B cells is not a sufficient event for acquisition of competence to proliferate. Proc Natl Acad Sci USA 82:6255-6259.

Regulation of c-*myc* mRNA and Protein Levels During Activation of Normal Human B Cells

Erlend B. Smeland[1], Tore Godal[1], Klaus Beiske[1], Rosemary Watt[2], Susan Pfeifer-Ohlsson[1,3], and Rolf Ohlsson[1,3].

1) Laboratory of Immunology, Department of Pathology and the Norwegian Cancer Society, The Norwegian Radium Hospital, Montebello, N-0310 Oslo 3, NORWAY.
2) Molecular Oncology Group, Smith Kline and French Laboratories, Philadelphia, Pennsylvania 19101, USA.
3) Department of Oncology, University of Umeå, S-901 87 Umeå, SWEDEN.

INTRODUCTION

The myc oncogene has been implicated in the control of cellular proliferation in both normal and neoplastic cells. Recently, several cell lines have been shown to express c-myc mRNA and protein throughout the cell cycle (Thompson et al 1985; Hann et al 1985; Rabbitts et al 1985). However, in several cell systems triggering of quiescent cells into G_1 is accompanied by a marked burst of c-myc mRNA, peaking a few hours after stimulation (Kelly et al 1983; Goustin et al 1985; Smeland et al 1985a). This has focused on a possible function for the c-myc product during the induction of competence to respond to progression growth factors acting in G_1. This theory finds support in studies on fibroblast cell lines, where experimental manipulation of c-myc levels was related to cell cycle progression (Armelin et al 1984; Kaczmarek et al 1985). In both cases the increased myc levels provoked an increased sensitivity to the action of progression factors.
It is well established that B cell stimulation from a resting state into proliferation can be divided into at least two distinct steps (Howard et al 1984; Kehrl et al 1984; Melchers and Andersson 1984). Normal human peripheral blood B cells can thus be initially activated from G_0 to G_1 by polyclonal anti-immunoglobulins (anti-Ig). Using selected concentrations, little S phase entry is observed unless B cell growth factor (BCGF) is added (table 1). The monoclonal antibody 1F5, which reacts with the CD20 pan B cell antigen (Clark et al 1985), and a monoclonal anti-μ, AF6, are also both able to activate the cells into G_1 (Smeland et al, in preparation). However, both of them only weakly synergizes with BCGF (table 1). We have used these experimental approaches to explore the c-myc mRNA and protein levels under different triggering conditions.

Table 1. DNA synthesis in human B cells stimulated with anti-immunoglobulins and BCGF[a].

Treatment	Thymidine incorporation,cpm Withouth BCGF	Thymidine incorporation,cpm With BCGF
Control(medium only)	927 ± 194	2,261 ± 475
Sepharose anti-μ	2,490 ± 416	47,760 ± 4,777
Anti-μ (F(ab')$_2$-fragments)	4,526 ± 872	30,734 ± 4,102
AF6	858 ± 227	6,387 ± 1,321
1F5	2,245 ± 486	4,530 ± 692

a) Purified B cells (7.5x10^4 cells/well) were pulse labeled with (methyl-^{3}H)thymidine for the last 16 hours of a 64 hour incubation. Data are given as means ± SEM of 6 different experiments. The monoclonal anti-CD20 antibody, 1F5, and the monoclonal anti-μ, AF6, were kindly provided by Dr. E. A. Clark (Seattle, USA) and Dr. R. Jefferis (Birmingham, UK), respectively.

Current Topics in Microbiology and Immunology, Vol. 132

RESULTS AND DISCUSSION

G_1 Entry After Treatment With Anti-Immunoglobulins or 1F5.

The activation of resting cells into the G_1 phase of the cell cycle is accompanied by an increase in cellular volumes, RNA content, and in the expression of various activation antigens like the 4F2 antigen (DeFranco et al 1982; Darzynkiewicz et al 1980; Kehrl et al 1984). The volume responses after treatment of these B cells with anti-immunoglobulins and 1F5 is shown in Fig. 1.

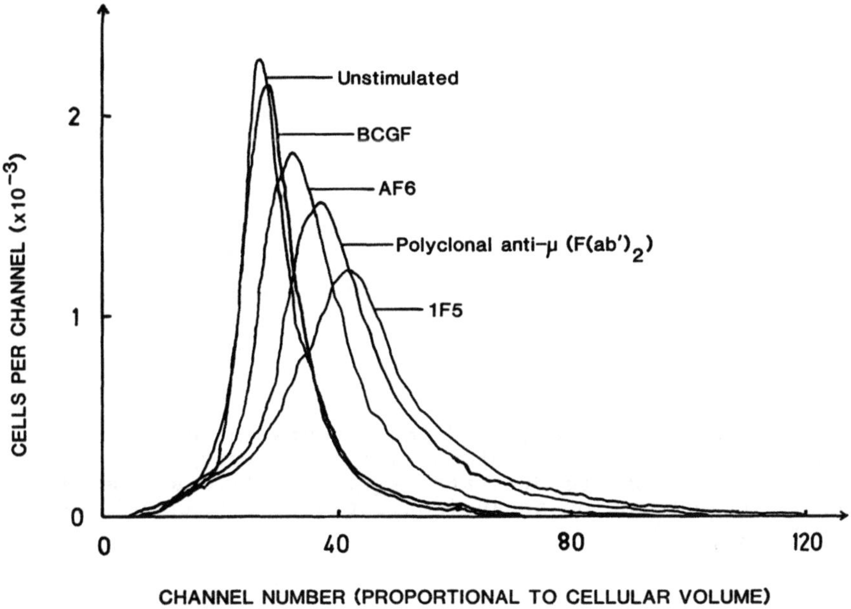

Fig. 1. Cellular volume distributions of human B cells cultured for 24 hours with the indicated stimuli.

In line with the volume responses, 1F5 and polyclonal anti-μ (F(ab')-fragments) have been found to induce a major increase in RNA synthesis, as determined by ^{3}H-uridine incorporation from 20 to 28 hours after stimulation, as well as a clear increase in 4F2 expression (Smeland et al 1985a, Smeland et al, in preparation). The changes were clearly smaller after AF6 treatment. Priming experiments confirmed the notion that polyclonal anti-μ and 1F5 trigger the cells into late G_1, while AF6 only activates the cells into early G_1 (Smeland et al, in preparation).

The Specific Induction of C-myc mRNA Expression in Normal B Cells is Mainly Due to an Increased Rate of Transcription.

The activation of peripheral blood B cells is accompanied by a specific 10-50 fold transient increase in c-myc mRNA levels, peaking at 2-4 hours after stimulation (Smeland et al 1985a). As can be seen from the Northern blot analysis in Fig. 2a, both polyclonal anti-µ, 1F5 and AF6 induced a marked increase in the c-myc mRNA levels, while there were virtually no changes in the levels of ß-actin mRNA.

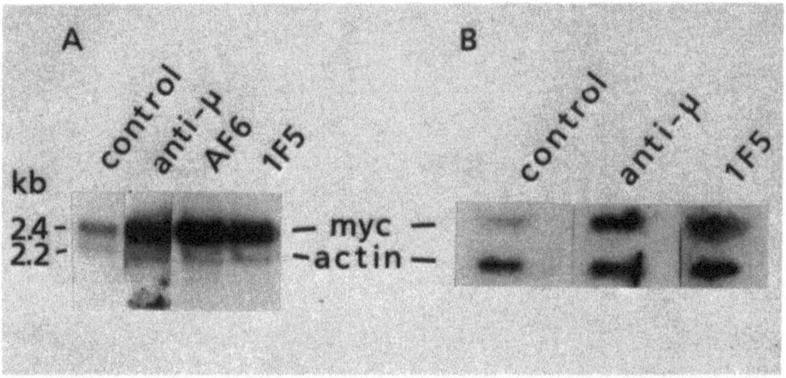

Fig 2. Purified B cells were cultured for 3 hours in medium only (controls) or with the indicated stimuli, and then subjected to A) Northern blot analysis of steady state c-myc mRNA levels, and (B) nuclear run-off transcription assay (reflecting the transcriptional rate of the c-myc gene).

Recently, it has been suggested that post-transcriptional regulation of c-myc mRNA stability might be the dominant mechanism underlying fluctuations in the steady-state levels of c-myc mRNA. Thus, in serum-starved fibroblast cells the c-myc gene is actively transcribed in G_0 cells without concomitant appearance of c-myc mRNA in the cytoplasm (Blanchard et al 1985). During activation posttranscriptional events operate to increase the cytoplasmic c-myc mRNA levels. In contrast, our nuclear run-off transcription experiments showed that the c-myc gene was transcribed at a low rate in unstimulated normal B cells (Fig. 2b). Stimulation with either polyclonal anti-µ or 1F5 led to a 5-10 fold increase in the transcriptional rate of the c-myc gene in relation to the ß-actin gene. Similar data has been reported for the T cell system (Krönke et al 1985). It is therefore conceivable that the operationally defined quiescence of in vitro maintained cell lines mechanistically differs from in vivo resting states of B and T cells, thereby confusing our understanding of the control of c-myc mRNA expression.

Induction of C-myc Protein During B Cell Activation.

The increase in c-myc mRNA levels following induction with either anti-μ or 1F5 was accompanied by a corresponding increase in $p65^{c\text{-}myc}$ levels, as demonstrated by Western blot analysis (Fig. 3). This implies the absence of important regulation of c-myc expression at the translational/posttranslational level.

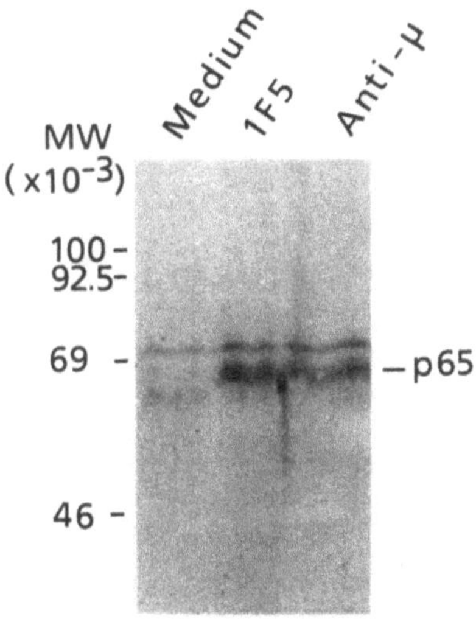

Fig. 3. Immunoblot analysis of c-myc protein in unstimulated and activated B cells.

To rule out a major heterogeneity of the c-myc signal in subpopulations of activated B cells, we performed immunocytochemistry on cytospin specimens (Fig. 4). Approximately 85% of the cells displayed a specific myc signal after stimulation with any of the inducing agens. These results imply that the expression of abundant levels of c-myc protein in B cells does not per se render the cells responsive to progression growth factors like BCGF. This contrasts the concept of c-myc as a dominant competence factor (Armelin et al 1984; Kaczmarek et al 1985). This discrepancy might reflect differences in the resting state of growth arrested in vitro maintained cell lines as opposed to the in vivo quiescence of peripheral blood B cells. In order to acquire competence to respond to BCGF, the B cells might require additional features, which are expressed, or indeed repressed, in quiescent Swiss 3T3 cells.

We can based on these results formulate two alternative models to explore the action of the c-myc protein. Firstly, the myc function could be independent of additional functions involved in the B cell cycle progression. Thus, whenever the c-myc protein is expressed, the myc specific function is exercised. The events complementing the myc activity in a positive or negative fashion to render the B cells competent, could be independantly expressed. This would suggest that the c-myc protein is a dominant feature of proliferating B cells. The putative presence of cis-acting elements acting on the c-myc promotor, analogously with the situation described for the c-fos gene (Treisman et al 1985), might allow myc to be expressed primarily in the G_1 phase of the cell cycle.

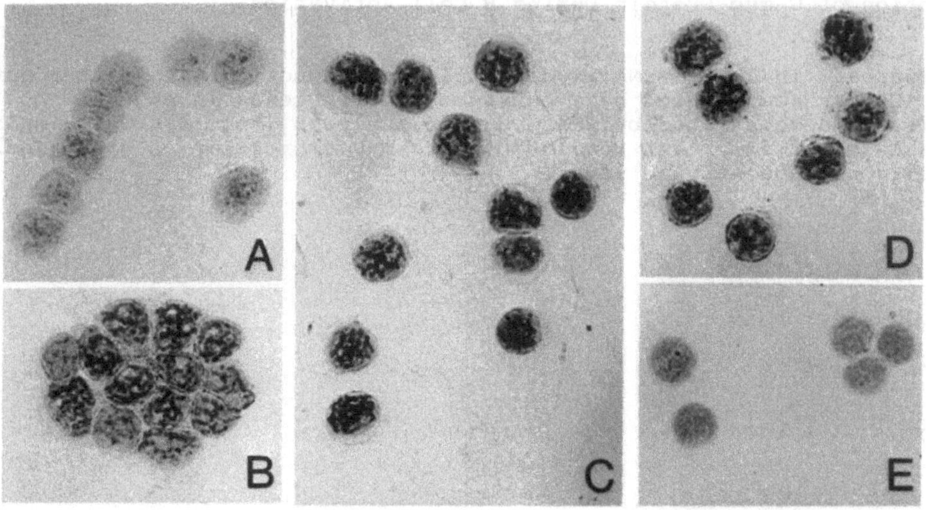

Fig 4. Immunocytochemical stainings of c-myc protein in unstimulated and activated B cells. The cells were incubated for 4 hours in medium only (A), or with 1F5 (B), AF6 (C), or polyclonal anti-μ (D). Cytospin specimens were prepared, and the cells were stained with a polyclonal rabbit anti-myc antiserum (Watt et al 1985) and Vectastain peroxidase ABC reagents. Pretreatment of the anti-myc antiserum with recombinant human myc protein blocked the signal in AF6 stimulated cells (E).

During tumor development, the c-myc gene could be expressed in a non-permissive part of the cell cycle through for example a genotypic change. Thereby it could modulate cell cycle specific repression and/or activation of other important genes.

The second model ascribes a less dominant role for the c-myc function, which would then not always operate whenever the myc protein is expressed. Instead it would depend on additional and simultaneously expressed features to promote optimal effects. In line with this concept, v-myc carrying retroviruses are only able to transform a fraction of hematopoietic cells, primarily of the myeloid lineage, although it can infect and replicate within all hematopoietic cell lineages. (Graf and Beug 1978). Thus the transforming properties associated with the c-myc oncogene depends on the host phenotype.

Our results do not at present distinguish between these two models. However, the recent results on c-myc subnuclear localization favors the second model (Evan and Hancock 1985). It was found that the bulk of c-myc protein is not tightly associated with any structural components. The authors interpret this finding to suggest that the c-myc function may operate only transiently, although the c-myc protein may be abundantly expressed.

CONCLUSIONS

We have shown that antibodies to surface IgM or to the CD20 antigen can induce c-myc mRNA and protein expression during the initial activation of human B cells. Yet, only the polyclonal anti-μ promotes competence to respond to BCGF. The observed lack of cooperativity between c-myc expression and BCGF is relevant when assessing the development of B cell neoplasias. Our data suggest that in addition to an abberant c-myc expression through a gene rearrangement, complementing functions are likely to be deregulated during tumor progression. An autocrine production of BCGF in B cell tumors (Gordon et al 1985), could then come into full operation and promote uncontrolled growth.

REFERENCES

Armelin HA, Armelin MCS, Kelly K, Stewart T, Leder P, Cochran BH, Stiles CD (1984) Functional role for c-myc in mitogenic response to platelet-derived growth factor. Nature 310: 655-660

Blanchard JM, Piechaczyk M, Dani C, Chambard JC, Franchi A, Pouyssegur J, Jeanteur P (1985) C-myc gene is transcribed at high rate in G_0 arrested fibroblasts and is post-transcriptionally regulated in response to growth factors. Nature 317: 443-445

Clark EA, Shu G, Ledbetter J (1985) Role of the Bp35 cell surface polypeptide in human B cell activation. Proc Natl Acad Sci USA 82: 1766-1770

Darzynkiewicz Z, Sharpless T, Staiano-Coico L, Melamed MR (1980) Subcompartments of the G_1 phase of cell cycle detected by flow cytometry. Proc Natl Acad Sci USA 11: 6696-6699

DeFranco AL, Kung JT, Paul WE (1982) Regulation of growth and proliferation in B cell subpopulations. Immunol Rev 64: 161-182

Evan GI, Hancock DC (1985) Studies on the interaction of the human c-myc protein with cell nuclei. Cell 43: 253-261

Gordon J, Ley SC, Melamed MD, English LS, Hughes-Jones NC (1984) Immortalized B lymphocytes produce B cell growth factor. Nature 310: 145-147

Graf T, Beug H (1978) Avian leukemia viruses. Interaction with their target cells in vivo and in vitro. Biochim Biophys Acta 516: 269-299

Goustin AS, Betsholtz C, Pfeifer-Ohlsson S, Persson H, Rydnert J, Bywater M, Holmgren G, Heldin C-H, Westermark B, Ohlsson R (1985) Coexpression of the sis and myc protooncogenes in developing human placenta suggests autocrine control of trophoblast growth. Cell 41: 301-312

Hann SR, Thompson CB, Eisenman RN (1985) C-myc oncogene protein synthesis is independent of the cell cycle in human and avian cells. Nature 314: 366-369

Howard M, Nakanishi K, Paul WE (1984) B cell growth and differentiation factors. Immunol Rev 78: 185-210

Kaczmarek L, Hyland JK, Watt R, Rosenberg M, Baserga R (1985) Microinjected c-myc as a competence factor. Science 228: 1313-1315

Krönke M, Leonard WJ, Depper JM, Greene WC (1985) Sequential expression of genes involved in human T lymphocyte growth and differentiation. J exp Med 161: 1593-1598

Kehrl JH, Muraguchi A, Butler JL, Falkoff RJM, Fauci AS (1984) Human B cell activation, proliferation and differentiation. Immunol Rev 78: 75-96

Kelly K, Cochran BH, Stiles CH, Leder P (1983) Cell specific regulation of the c-myc gene by lymphocyte mitogens and platelet-derived growth factor. Cell: 35: 603-610

Melchers F, Andersson J (1984) B cell activation: three steps and their variations. Cell 37: 715-720

Rabbitts PH, Watson JV, Lamond A, Forster A; Stinson MA, Evan G, Fisher W, Atherton E, Sheppard R, Rabbitts TH (1985) Metabolism of c-myc gene products: c-myc mRNA and protein expression in the cell cycle. EMBO J 4: 2009-2015

Smeland E, Godal T, Ruud E, Beiske K, Funderud S, Clark EA, Pfeifer-Ohlsson S, Ohlsson R (1985) The specific induction of myc proto-oncogene expression in normal human B cells is not a sufficient event

for acquisition of competence to proliferate. Proc Natl Acad Sci USA 82: 6255-6259
Smeland E, Funderud S, Ruud E, Blomhoff HK, Godal T (1985) Characterization of two murine monoclonal antibodies reactive with human B cells. Scand J Immunol 21: 205-214
Thompson CB, Challoner PB, Neiman PE, Groudine M (1985) Levels of c-myc oncogene mRNA are invariant throughout the cell cycle. Nature 314: 363-366
Treisman R (1985) Transient accumulation of c-fos RNA following serum stimulation requires a conserved 5' element and c-fos 3' sequences. Cell 42: 889-902
Watt RA, Shatzman AR, Rosenberg M (1985) Expression and characterization of the human c-myc DNA-binding protein. Mol Cell Biol 5: 448-456

Differential Expression of N-myc, c-myc and c-src Proto-oncogenes During the Course of Induced Differentiation of Murine Embryonal Carcinoma Cells

J.Sumegi* T.Sejersen** H.Björklund*** G.Klein* and N.R.Ringertz**

*Department of Tumor Biology, **Department of Medical Cell Genetics, Medical Nobel Institute and ***Department of Histology, Karolinska Institute, Box 60400, S-104 01 Stockholm, Sweden

INTRODUCTION

Proto-oncogenes the cellular homologues of retroviral oncogenes, appear to be normal cellular genes presumed to play a role in normal cellular processes like growth control and cellular differentiation. Their role in controlling cellular growth is strongly supported by the findings that several proto-oncogenes code for proteins closely related or identical to growth factors or growth factor receptors. It has been also found that the expression of proto-oncogenes c-myc and c-myb is diminished and the expression of c-fos is induced during differentiation of HL60 and U-937 cells (Mitchell 1985).

We describe here the results of a study on the expression of N-myc, c-myc and c-src proto-oncogenes in teratoma derived embryonal carcinoma cells. Murine teratocarcinoma are transplantable tumors that contain malignant stem cells; embryonal carcinoma cells and a variety of non-malignant differentiated cells believed to be derived from the embryonal carcinoma cells corresponding to derivatives of the three germ layers. Because of their potential to differentiate into a wide variety of cells, the embryonal carcinoma cells represent an interesting system to examine the regulation of proto-oncogene expression during terminal differentiation.

In this report we present evidence that the c-myc and N-myc proto-oncogenes are expressed at high levels in four murine teratocarcinoma stem cell lines; PCC3, PCC4, PCC7 and F9. We also report that in the case of retinoic acid and cAMP induced differentiation a decreased level of expression of N-myc and c-myc is detected in PCC7 and F9 cells. The down-regulation in the expression of both proto-oncogenes occurs at the post-transcriptional level. The decreased N-myc expression in the differentiated, neurofilament positive PCC7 cells is parallelled by a five fold increase in the expression of c.src gene.

MATERIAL AND METHODS

Cell Cultures and Induction.

PCC3 A/1, PCC4 azal (Jakob 1973) and PCC7 (Pfeiffer 1981) embryonal carcinoma cell lines were from Drs. H.Jakob and J-F. Nicholas. The F9 (Bernstine 1973) embryonal carcinoma cell line was provided by Dr.S.Grandchamp. NA is a hypoxanthine phosphorybosyl transferase deficient subline of mouse C1300 neuroblastoma (Augusti-Tocco 1969) was obtained from Dr.P.Nelson. Embryonal carcinoma cells were maintained in DMEM supplemented with 10% fetal calf serum, non-essential aminoacids and 0.12% (W/v) NaHCO3, 12 mM pyruvic acid and antibiotics. Balb/c 3T3 and NA cells were maintained in DMEM supplemented with 5% fetal calf serum. For induction of in vitro differentiation, PCC7 cells were treated for 3 days with 0.01 uM retinoic acid and for additional 3 days with 0.01 uM retinoic acid and 1.0 mM cAMP in DMEM supplemented with 2% fetal calf serum. F9 cells were induced fo form parietal or visceral endoderm as described previously (Sejersen 1985).

Isolation of RNA and DNA, Northern- and Southern-blot Analysis.

Current Topics in Microbiology and Immunology, Vol. 132

Total RNA was isolated by hot phenol extraction (Edmonds 1969), poly(A)+RNA was selected by oligo(dT)-cellulose chromatography (Aviv 1972). RNAs were analyzed by electrophoresis of 10-20 ug of total or 5 ug of poly(A)+ RNA through 1.5% agarose/formaldehyde gels followed by transfer to nitrocellulose and hybridization to radiolebeled DNA probes (Thomas 1980). The following cloned DNA fragments were used as hybridization probes; pNb1 (Schwab 1983), pMC-54 (Stanton 1983), a PvuII E fragment of the v-src oncogene (deLorbe 1980), AFP1 (Tilgham 1979), pAM91 (Minty 1981) and pCH3-3E (Harvey 1981). The isolation of high molecular weight DNA and Southern-blot analysis were done as described earlier (Sumegi 1983).

Nuclear Run-on Transcription Assay.

For the nuclear run-on transcription assay the nuclei were isolated as described by Schibler (1983). The nuclei were stored in nuclei storage buffer at -70C° until use. Nuclei were thawed for the run-on transcription assay and incubated for 30 min at 26C° in 2 ml of 70 mM KCl, 5 mM MgCl2, 2.5 mM dithiotreitol, 0.1 mM EDTA, 0.4 mM each of ATP, GTP, CTP and 250 uCi 32P-UTP (Amersham). 5x10 cpm of labeled and purified RNA was hybridized for 4 days to cDNA clones immobilized on nitrocellulose filters (5 ug DNA per slot).

RESULTS

Structure and Expression of c-myc and N-myc genes.

The restriction enzyme map of the murine c-myc and N-myc loci is shown in the Fig. 1. The mouse N-myc locus is organized into three exons and two introns likewise the c-myc gene. To better understand the structural relationship of the N-myc gene to the c-myc gene the regions of homology in N-myc was mapped and related to that of the c-myc gene.

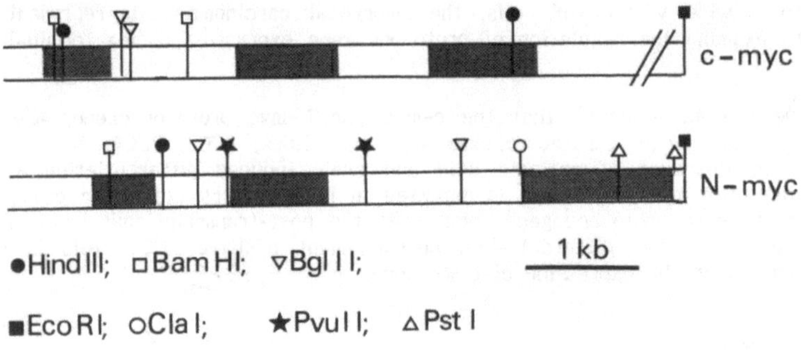

Fig.1. Restriction enzyme map of the murine c-myc and N-myc genes.Regions with high degree of homology are underlined.

Four mouse teratocarcinoma stem cell lines; PCC3, PCC4, PCC7, F9 and mouse Balb/c 3T3 fibroblast and NA neuroblastoma cell lines were tested for the expression of c-myc and N-myc genes. The PCC3 and to a lesser extent PCC4 represent multipotent embryonal carcinoma lines, their differentiation both in vivo and in vitro give rise to a great variety of differentiated tissues. The PCC7 and F9 cells have very limited differentiative capacity. All four embryonal carcinoma cell lines but NA and Balb/c 3T3 were found to express a 3.0 kb N-myc transcript (Fig. 2). We have also found that PCC3, PCC4, F9, NA, and Balb/c 3T3 cells abundantly express the c-myc mRNA whereas the PCC7 shows no detectable c-myc expression. To determine whether the abundant expression of the N-myc gene in the murine embryonal carcinoma lines is due to geneamplification, we performed quantitative Southern-blot analysis of the genomic DNA of PCC3, PCC4, PCC7, F9 in which the N-myc was expressed at relatively high level.

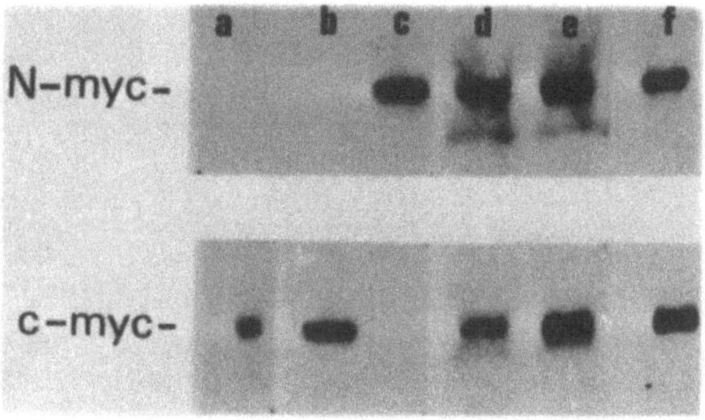

Fig.2. N-myc and c-myc expression in mouse teratocarcinoma stem cells. The cells were cultured and the RNAs were isolated, purified, separated in agarose/formaldehyde gel and transferred to nitrocellulose filter as described in Materials and Methods. Hybridization was as described earlier (Sejersen 1985). Lane a: 15 ug of Balb/c 3T3 poly(A)+RNA, lanes b-f 40 ug of total RNA of NA (b); PCC7 (c); PCC3 (d); PCC4 (e) and F9 (f).

Southern-blot analysis revealed the presence of a single-copy of the N-myc gene per haploid genome in all the four EC lines studied (Fig.3). Therefore the abundant expression of N-myc in these embryonal carcinoma cell lines is not the consequence of gene amplification.

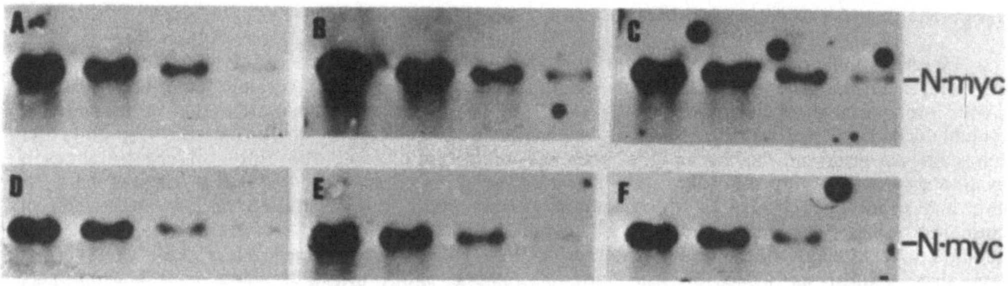

Fig.3. Southern-blot analysis of N-myc in genomic DNA from mouse cells. High molecular weight DNAs were isolated from Balb/c 3T3 mouse fibroblast (A), NA mouse neuroblastoma (B), PCC7 (C), PCC3 (D), PCC4 (E) and F9 (F) mouse embryonal carcinoma cells as described earlier (Sumegi 1983). 10 ug, 5 ug, 2.5 ug and 1.25 ug of each was digested to completion with EcoRI. The restriction fragments were separated on a agarose gel (0.7%) and transferred to nitrocellulose filter, then hybridized with nick-translated 32P-labelled pNb-1 DNA as described previously (Sumegi 1983).

The Level of N-myc Transcript in Differentiated PCC7 Cells.

In a recent study it was observed that when human neuroblastoma cells were induced to differentiate in vitro the N-myc expression rapidly decreased (Thiele 1985). In order to see whether the PCC7 mouse teratocarcinoma stem cells show a similar down-regulation of the N-myc expression upon differentiation we have measuered the levels of N-myc RNA in proliferating and differentiated cells. Although the PCC7 cells differentiate spontaneously into cholinergic neurons (Pfeiffer 1981), we induced the terminal differentiation by the addition of retinoic acid and cAMP (see Materials and Methods) in order to induce more pronounced and homogeneous formation of nerve cells. This differentiation process results in gross changes in cell morphology. After a lag of about 2-3 days after induction, the cells started to undergo a marked phenotypic conversion, as assessed by the characteristic neurite outgrowth (Fig.4) and by the marked decrease in DNA synthesis (data not shown). Immune-fluorescence staining with anti-neurofilament anti-serum showed a strong fibrillar fluorescence in the differentiated PCC7 cells (Fig.4).

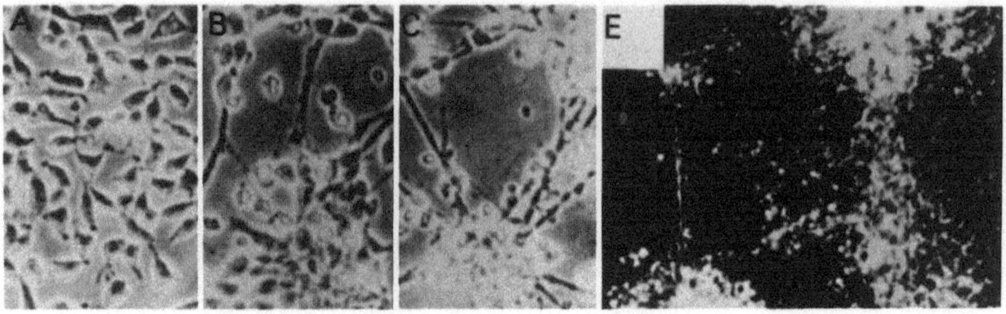

Fig.4.Morphological changes of PCC7 cells during retinoic acid and cAMP induced differentiation. PCC7 cells were cultured and induced to differentiate as described in Materials and Methods. Cells before (A), 4 (B) and 6(C) days after induction. Immunfluorescence staining of PCC7 cells with anti-neurofilament anti-serum at the sixth day of the induction (E).

N-myc expression was assessed by Northern-blot analysis of total RNA from retinoic acid/cAMP induced or control cultures. The densitometric analysis of Northern-blots revealed an 83% decrease in the level of N-myc expression in retinoic acid/cAMP treated cultures compared with control cultures (Fig.5). A detectable decrease in the level of RNA hybridizing to the pNb-1 probe was already observed by 6 hours after treatment in differentiating cells (data not shown).

N-myc and c-myc expression in differentiating F9 cells.

The F9 embryonal carcinoma cell line provides us with another model system for the study of differentiation. The F9 cells differentiate after treatment with retinoic acid and dibutyryl cAMP into parietal endoderm (Strickland 1978). Ten days after induction the cells were of typical endoderm morphology. Visceral endoderm was induced by culturing the F9 cells for ten days as embryoid bodies in the presence of retinoic acid. The fully differentiated cells expressed alpha-fetoprotein (data not shown). The F9 unlike the PCC7 cells express both N-myc and c-myc mRNA (Fig.2) which enabled us to study the regulation of the expression of both proto-oncogenes in the same cell type. By Northern-blot hybridization we found that 10 days after induction the N-myc expression was maximally depressed (Fig.5) cell cycle arrest was also maximal as judged by the lack of histone mRNA synthesis (data not shown). There was an 85% decrease in the level of N-myc expression at ten days after the induction in both parietal and visceral endoderm cells (Fig.5). The rehybridization of the blots with a c-myc specific DNA probe showed a similar pattern of down-regulation of c-myc gene. The blots were also hybridized with actin probe in order to verify that equal amounts of RNA were loaded in each lane (data not shown).

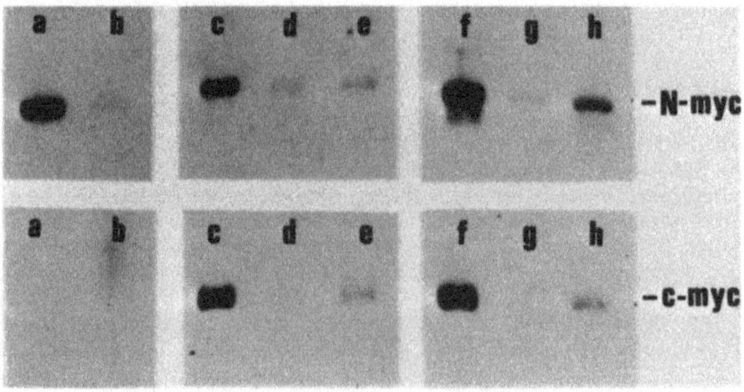

Fig.5. The effect of terminal differentiation on steady-state N-myc and c-myc mRNA levels in PCC7 and F9 embryonal carcinoma cells. The cells were cultured, induced and the RNA was

isolated and Northern-blots prepared and hybridized as described in Materials and Methods. RNAs isolated from control PCC7 (a); PCC7 at sixth day after induction (b); control F9 (c and f) and F9 at tenth day after induction to parietal (d) and visceral (g) endoderm were hybridized to N-myc and c-myc specific DNA probes (see Materials and Methods).

Induction of c-src Expression in Differentiated PCC7 Cells.

Addition of retinoic acid and cAMP is sufficient to commit the PCC7 cells to a cholinergic differentiation pathway. The implication of pp60-src in the neuronal differentiation (Brugge 1985) led us to analyze the expression of c-src gene in the course of terminal differentiation of PCC7 cells. As the Fig.6. shows the formation of nerve-like cells from PCC7 undifferentiated embryonal carcinoma cells has resulted in altered expression of the proto-oncogene c-src The 4.0kb src-specific mRNA is hardly detectable in proliferating PCC7 stem cells (Fig.6.).The level of c-src transcript in the terminally differentiated PCC7 cells appears to be five fold higher than prior to induction. The elevated level of c-src mRNA in the differentiated PCC7 cells is due to transcriptional activation of the gene as judged by the results obtained by the in vitro nuclear "run-on" transcription assay (Fig.7).

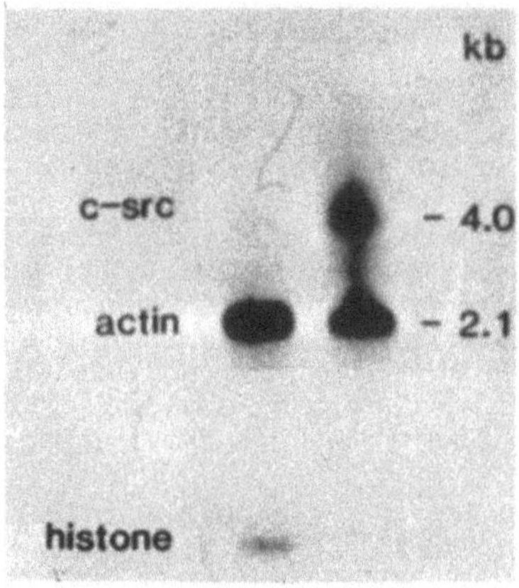

Fig.6. Steady-state level of c-src mRNA in control and differentiated PCC7 cells.
RNA from control (a) and from differentiated (b) PCC7 cells was analyzed as described in Fig.1.

Post-transcriptional Control of the N-myc and c-myc Expression in Differentiating PCC7 and F9 Cells.

In order to analyse whether control is exerted at the transcriptional level during PCC7 and F9 differentiation, we measuered the transcription rate of N-myc and c-myc in isolated nuclei at various times after retinoic acid and cAMP addition by the nuclear run-on transcription assay. In vitro transcripts were generated by elongation of previously initiated RNA chains during incubation of nuclei isolated from cells at various stages of differentiation in the presence of (alpha-32P)-UTP as described by Schibler (1983). In this in vitro nuclei transcription assay the initiation of new transcript is prevented by the high salt concentration and by the presence of heparin. Therefore this assay provides a reasonable measurement of the number of polymerase molecules actively engaged in transcription before the cell lysis. The Fig.7. shows that the rate of transcription of N-myc and c-myc does not change during differentiation of PCC7 and F9 cells.

DISCUSSION

The myc family of proto-oncogenes comprises three known members (Zimmerman 1986). The L-myc is the least known of the three and has been found amplified/expressed in human small cell lung cancer (Nau 1986). The other two members, c-myc and N-myc show remarkable homology in their coding exons (Colby 1983). In recent reports it has been shown that on co-transfection with the c-Ha-ras oncogene both c-myc and N-myc can induce the neoplastic transformation of rat embryo fibroblasts (Schwab 1985, Yancopoulos 1985). The c-myc oncogene has been found rearranged or amplified and activated in various animal tumors. It is also expressed in most divinding cells. In contrast, the expression of N-myc appears to be restricted to a certain

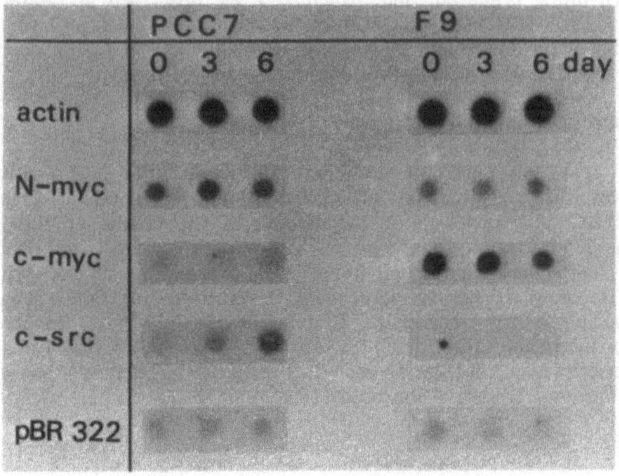

Fig.7. Transcriptional analysis of N-myc, c-myc and c-src during the differentiation of PCC7 and F9 cells. The experimental condition was as described in Materials and Methods.

set of tumors with neuroectoderm origin (Schwab 1985). Several observations implicate the N-myc gene in the development and/or progression of human neuroblastoma, retinoblastoma and small cell lung cancer. Based on these findings it has been suggested that the N-myc is expressed early in the development of neuroectodermal tissues (Thiele 1985). The finding of high level of N-myc expression without gene amplification in PCC7 cells seems to support this suggestion. However, the detection of N-myc expression in F9, an embryonal carcinoma cell line committed to differentiate into extra-enbryonal endoderm and in two multipotent stem cell lines (PCC3 and PCC4) suggests that the N-myc is not simply a neuroectoderm specific gene.

It is remarkable that the proliferating PCC7 cells do not show c-myc expression suggesting that the cell proliferation, at least in certain types of cells, does not have the c-myc expression as a mandatory requirement.

The expression of N-myc was down-regulated in the course of in vitro differentiation of PCC7 cells. The reduction of N-myc mRNA level in PCC7 cells occured gradually and in parallel with diminishing of the cell proliferation. However, the rate of reduction in the N-myc expression in differentiating PCC7 cells appears to be slower process than that reported in differentiating human neuroblastoma cells. The expression of both N-myc and c-myc was down-regulated in induced F9 cells. This differentiation-associated down-regulation of N-myc and c-myc follows different kinetics (Sejersen unpublished). The reduction of c-myc expression is an early event in the differentiation process. The reduction of N-myc expression can be detected only at the later stage of differentiation of the F9 cells. This suggests that in contrast to the similarities in structure and function of the c-myc and N-myc genes, their expression may be differently regulated.

Our data obtained by Northern analysis and in vitro transcription assay indicate that the c-myc and N-myc expression is not regulated at the level of transcription, at least in the course of cellular differentiation, but rather by a post-transcriptional mechanism, which may affect the half-life of the transcripts. It is noteworthy that the half-life of the c-myc and N-myc mRNAs is different. We have found that the half life of the myc RNA is 30 min (Sejersen unpublished). In contrast the N-myc mRNA seems to have 2-3 times longer half-life than the c-myc RNA.

The cellular protein encoded by the c-src gene is abundantly expressed during development of neural tissues of chicken and rat (Brugge 1985) The pp60-c-src is particularly abundant in brain, retina and spinal ganglia. The tissue specific expression of the c-src gene strongly suggests that the product of this proto-oncogene plays role in terminally differentiated neurons.

In accordance with these findings the c-src gene expression is induced in the differentiated PCC7 cells. By run-on nuclear transcription assay it is shown that the enhanced level of c-src specific mRNA is due to a transcriptional activation of the gene. The highest level of c-src RNA transcription was detected at the stage when the cell proliferation ceased. This suggests that the induction of the c-src expression in the PCC7 cells is more likely to be a consequence than a cause of the cellular differentiation.

REFERENCES

Augusti-Tocco,G. and Sato,G. (1969) Establishment of functional clonal lines of neurons from mouse neuroblastoma. Proc.Natl.Acad.Sci. USA 64;311-315

Aviv,H. and Leder,P. (1972) Purification of biologically active globin messenger RNA by chromatography on oligothymidylic acid-cellulose. Proc.Natl.Acad.Sci. USA 69;1408-1412

Bernstine,E.G., Hooper,M.L., Grandchamp,S. and Ephrussi,B. (1973) Alkaline phosphatase activity in mouse teratoma. Proc.Natl.Acad.Sci. USA 70;3899-3903

Brugge,J.S., Cotton,P.C., Queral,A.E., Barrett,J.N., Nonner,D. and Keane,R.W. (1985) Neurones express high levels of a structurally modified, activated form of pp60-c-src. Nature (London) 316;554-557

deLorbe,W.J., Luciv,P.A., Godman,H.M., Varmus,H.E. and Bishop,J.M. (1980) Molecular cloning and characterization of avian sarcoma virus circular DNA molecules. J.Virol. 36;50-61

Harvey,R.P., Krieg,P.A., Robins,A.J., Coles,L.S. and Well,J.R.E. (1981) Non-tandem arrangement and divergent transcription of chicken histone genes. Nature (London) 294;49-53

Jakob,H., Bonn,T., Gaillard,J., Nicolas,J-F. and Jacob, F. (1973) Teratocarcinome de la Souris, Isolement, Culture et Proprietes de Cellules a Potentialites Multiples. Ann. Microbiol. Inst. Pasteur 124B;269-282

Minty,A.J., Caravatti,M., Robert,B., Cohen,A., Daubas,P., Weydert,A., Gros,F. and Buckingham,M.E. Mouse actin messenger RNAs. J.Biol.Chem. 256;1008-1014

Mitchell,L.R., Zokas,L., Schreiber,R.D. and Verma,I.M. (1985) Rapid induction of the expression of proto-oncogene fos during human monocytic differentiation Cell 40;209-217

Nau,M.M., Brooks,J.B., Battey,J., Sausville,E., Gazdar,A.F., Kirsch,I.R., McBride, O.W., Bertness,V., Hollis,G.F. and Minna,J.D. (1985) L-myc, a new myc related gene amplified and expressed in human small cell lung cancer Nature 318;69-73

Pfeiffer,S.E., Jakob,H., Mikoshiba,K., Dubois,P., Guenet,J.L., Nicolas,J-F. Gaillard,J., Chevance, G. and Jacob,F. (1981) Differentiation of a teratocarcinoma line: preferential development of cholinergic neurons. J.Cell.Biol. 88;57-66

Schibler,U., Hagenbüchle,O., Wellauer,P.K. and Pittet,A.C. (1983) Cell 33;501-508

Schwab,M., Varmus,H.E. and Bishop,J.M. (1985) Nature 316;160-162

Sejersen,T., Sumegi,J. and Ringertz,N.R. (1985) Expression of cellular oncogenes in teratoma derived cell lines. Exptl.Cell.Res.160;19-30

Stanton,L.W., Watt,R. and Marcu,K.B. (1983) Translocation, breakage and truncated transcripts of c-myc oncogene in murine plasmacytomas. Nature (London) 303;401-406

Strickland,S. and Madhavi,V. (1978) The induction of differentiation in teratocarcinoma stem cells by retinoic acid. Cell 15;393-403

Sumegi,J., Spira,J., Bazin,H., Szpirer,J., Levan,G. Klein,G. (1983) Rat c-myc oncogene is located on chromosome 7 and rearranges in immunocytomas with t(6:7) chromosomal translocation. Nature 306;497-499

Thiele,C.J., Reynolds,C.P. and Israel,M.A. (1985) Decreased expression of N-myc precedes retinoic acid induced morphological differentiation of human neuroblastoma. Nature 313;404-406

Thomas,P.S. (1980) Hybridization of denatured RNA and small DNA fragments transferred to nitrocellulose Proc.Natl.Acad.Sci. USA 77;5201-5205

Zimmerman,K.A., Yancopoulus, G.D., Collum,R.G. Smith,R.K. Kohl,N.E. Denis,K.A., Nau,M.M., Witte, O.N., Toran-Allerand,D., Gee,C.E., Minna,J.D. and Alt,F.W. (1986) Differential expression of myc family genes during murine development. Nature 319;780-783

Tilgham, S.M., Juiyssus,D., Gorin,M.B., Ruiz,J.P.G. and Ingram, R.S. (1979) The presence of intervening sequences in the alpha-fetoprotein gene of the mouse J.Biol.Chem. 254;7393-7399

Complex Regulation of c-myc Gene Expression in a Murine B Cell Lymphoma

R.A. Levine, J.E. McCormack, A. Buckler and G.E. Sonenshein

Department of Biochemistry, Boston University Medical School, Boston, MA 02118, USA

INTRODUCTION

Alterations in the structure of the c-myc gene have implicated this oncogene in many types of B cell neoplasias. Changes include chromosomal translocation to an immunoglobulin gene locus, retroviral insertion into the c-myc promoter, and gene amplification. While in most cases the change in c-myc gene structure leaves the protein product unaffected, the regulation of expression of the gene may be altered. In many cell systems, e.g. splenic lymphocytes, untransformed fibroblast lines, and rat liver (Kelly et al., 1983, Campisi et al., 1984, Goyette et al., 1984), expression of c-myc mRNA is low in quiescence and increases rapidly upon exit from the G0 state. Quiescent B lymphocytes contain barely detectable levels of c-myc mRNA. Upon stimulation with the mitogen LPS, c-myc mRNA levels increase 20 to 30 fold within 2-3 hours (Kelly et al., 1983). Terminal differentiation is accompanied by a decrease in expression of c-myc mRNA (Campisi et al., 1984, Grosso and Pitot 1985, Lachman and Skoultchi, 1984). These results suggest a role for the c-myc gene in the control of proliferation and differentiation. Since maturation of B cells involves several stages of differentiation, including terminal differentiation to nonproliferating plasma cells, it seemed likely that alterations in c-myc gene regulation might lead to aberrant B cell growth and differentiation.

The murine lymphoma WEHI 231 cell line has been characterized as an early B cell on the basis of surface markers and biological properties (Boyd and Schrader 1981). We have employed WEHI 231 as a model system to study changes in c-myc gene expression accompanying cessation of B cell proliferation (McCormack et al., 1984). The c-myc genes in this line are unrearranged. Incubation of exponentially growing cultures of WEHI 231 cells with goat anti-(mouse Ig) antiserum (GaMIg) resulted in a rapid increase in the amount of c-myc mRNA within the first 2 hours. Then, the level dropped precipitously, such that it was 5-10 fold lower than control values after 6 hours. In contrast, the amounts of most major mRNAs, as judged by translation in a cell-free system, were only slightly affected. In the period between 2 and 4 hours after treatment, c-myc mRNA decayed with a half-time of 20-30 minutes. We have now examined the effect of GaMIg treatment on the regulation of c-myc gene expression and find evidence for control at multiple sites, including post-transcriptional and transcriptional levels.

Current Topics in Microbiology and Immunology, Vol. 132

RESULTS

Induction of c-myc mRNA by GaMIg Treatment

Previously we reported that treatment of WEHI 231 cells with GaMIg dramatically altered the levels of c-myc cytoplasmic mRNA within 2 hours (McCormack et al., 1984). We have now extended these studies by examining earlier time points. Cytoplasmic RNA was isolated from control cells and from cells treated with anti-Ig for 15, 30, 60, and 120 minutes, or in a separate experiment at 2, 4, 8, and 24 hours. Levels of c-myc mRNA in these samples were assessed by densitometric scanning of autoradiograms produced by Northern blot analysis using a murine c-myc genomic probe (Fig. 1). An increase in c-myc message is noticed within 30 minutes of treatment, reaching a level approximately 20 fold greater than that of control cells by 1 hour; after this time, the levels drop rapidly below the control value. As we have shown previously (McCormack et al., 1984), this is not the result of a general increase in cytoplasmic mRNA, but instead reflects a selective regulation of the expression of the c-myc gene.

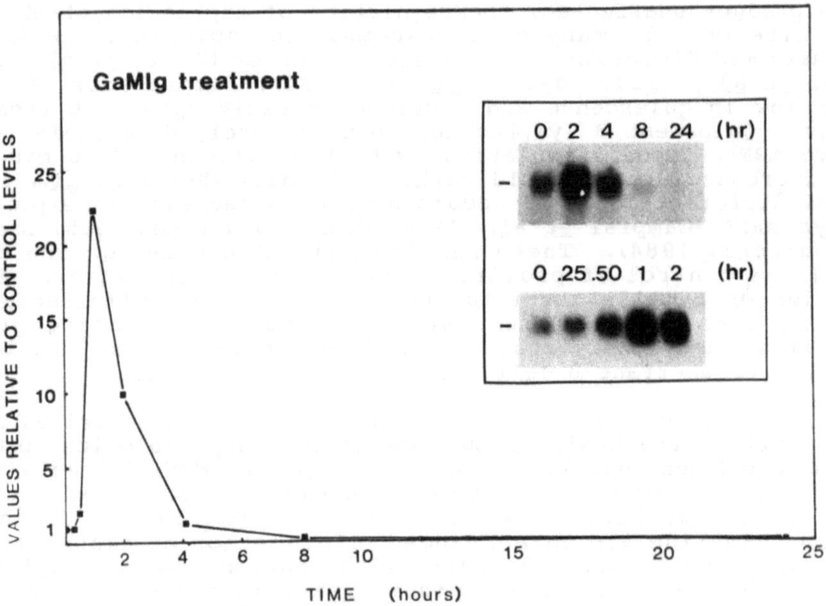

Fig. 1. Effects of GaMIg treatment on cytoplasmic levels of c-myc mRNA.

In order to determine whether the change in c-myc mRNA levels were due to alteration in the synthesis of the message, we examined the effect of GaMIg treatment on transcription of the c-myc gene. Nuclei were isolated from cells treated for varying lengths of time; these nuclei were then incubated with ^{32}P-labelled ribonucleotides under conditions permitting the elongation of nascent transcripts present at the time the nuclei were isolated (Greenberg and Ziff 1984). These "run-on" transcripts were then hybridized to nitrocellulose filters to which an excess of plasmid containing a c-myc cDNA clone (Stanton et al., 1983) had been bound; pUC19 vector DNA served as background control. As can be seen in Fig. 2, transcription of c-myc began to increase between 15 and 30 minutes, peaking

7-12 fold above the control value after approximately 1 hour of treatment. After this time c-myc transcription declined rapidly and was barely detectable after 8 hours of treatment.

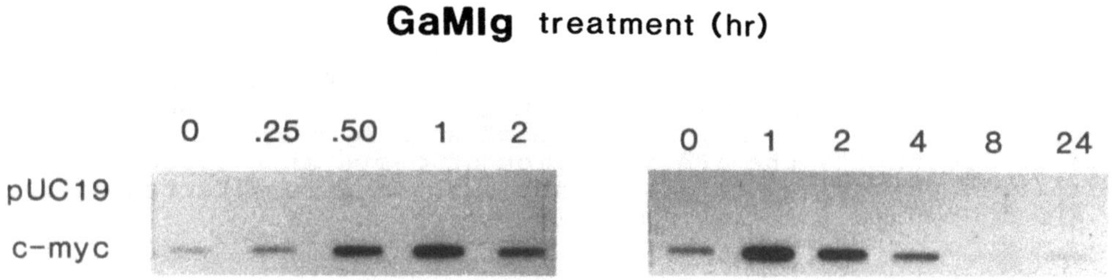

Fig. 2. Transcriptional "run-on" analysis of changes in c-myc gene expression following GaMIg treatment.

As we noted previously, the c-myc message displays a very short half-life during the period following anti-Ig treatment (McCormack et al., 1984). Jeanteur and coworkers have determined a half-life of approximately 15 minutes for the c-myc message in human lymphoblastoid lines (Dani et al., 1984). In order to determine whether changes in mRNA stability play a role in regulating c-myc message levels following GaMIg treatment, cells were treated with anti-Ig for either 10 minutes or 2 hours; then further RNA synthesis was inhibited by treatment with actinomycin D. Cytoplasmic RNA was extracted from aliquots of cells at various times after addition of actinomycin D, and levels of c-myc mRNA were quantitated as above. When the Northern blots were scanned, a $t_{1/2}$ for the decay of c-myc message of 10-12 minutes was obtained after 2 hours of anti-Ig treatment; the same value was obtained for exponentially growing WEHI 231 cells in the absence of GaMIg. In contrast, cells treated with GaMIg for only 10 minutes displayed a significantly slower rate of turnover; the $t_{1/2}$ of decay of c-myc mRNA was approximately 25 minutes in these cells (data not shown). Thus the changes in c-myc mRNA levels following treatment with GaMIg appear to be the result of alterations in the rate of synthesis of the mRNA in the nucleus and the rate of its turnover in the cytoplasm.

Phorbol Esters Induce c-myc mRNA

Regulatory molecules, such as hormones and growth factors, which bind to cell-surface receptors generally exert their effects by activating intracellular "second messenger" systems. The polyphosphoinositol phosphate/protein kinase C pathway has been implicated in the transduction of growth regulatory signals in many cell types, including B cells. In order to determine whether this pathway might play a role in the response of WEHI 231 cells to anti-Ig, we treated these cells with the phorbol ester TPA (12-0-tetradecanoyl phorbol 13-acetate), a potent activator of protein kinase C (Nishizuka, 1985). Initial studies indicated that incubation in the presence of 5×10^{-8}M TPA inhibited DNA synthesis and WEHI 231 cell growth within 24-48 hours; this is similar to the kinetics of GaMIg-induced growth arrest of these cells. We next examined levels of cytoplasmic c-myc mRNA in WEHI 231 cells following treatment with TPA for various periods of time, using the same methods employed above; the results are summarized in Fig. 3. As in anti-Ig treated cells, there is an early and rapid increase in cytoplasmic c-myc mRNA levels, peaking approximately 1 hour after treatment. The kinetics of the subsequent decline, however, were different for the two treatments. Following an initial rapid decrease in c-myc mRNA concentration, which results in a return to the level seen in exponentially growing cells by 4 hours, no further decline is seen during the next 4 hours. Thus after 8 hours of TPA treatment, c-myc message had only declined to control levels, whereas the mRNA was virtually undetectable after 8 hours of anti-Ig treatment. As with anti-Ig treatment, the TPA induction of c-myc mRNA appears to be relatively selective, as only minor changes were detected in the levels of control RNAs (as discussed above).

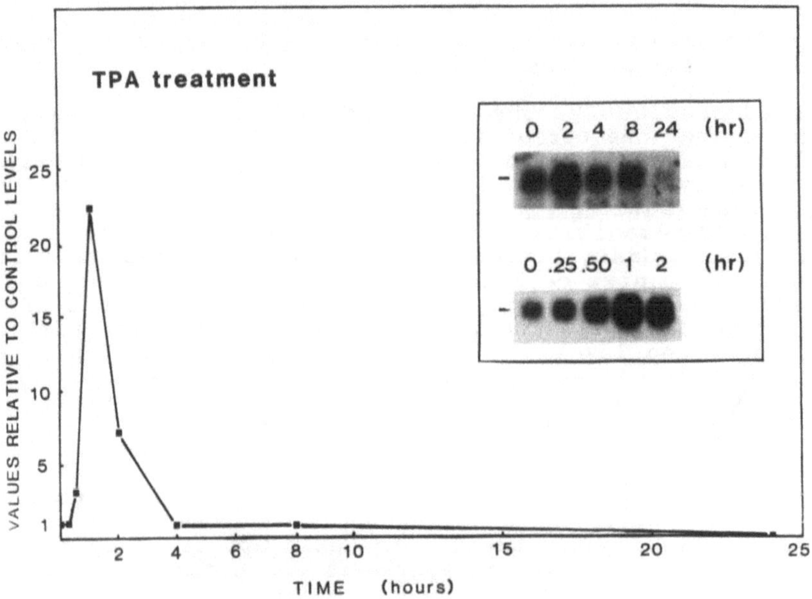

Fig. 3. Effects of TPA treatment on cytoplasmic levels of c-myc mRNA.

In order to determine whether the difference in c-myc induction by anti-Ig and TPA might be accounted for at the transcriptional level, nuclear "run-on" assays were performed on TPA-treated cells (Fig. 4). TPA induced a rapid (15-30 minute) increase in c-myc transcription, peaking at about 1 hour of treatment. Following a decline between 1 and 4 hours, transcription remained at a level comparable to that in untreated, control cells through the 8th hour, but declined further by 24 hours. These kinetics parallel the changes in cytoplasmic mRNA levels.

Sense vs Anti-sense Transcription

Marcu and coworkers have observed in nuclear "run-on" assays that both strands of an unrearranged c-myc gene are transcribed (see this volume). The transcriptional analyses described above employed a double-stranded cDNA clone, which would detect both coding , sense transcripts as well as non-coding, anti-sense transcripts. In order

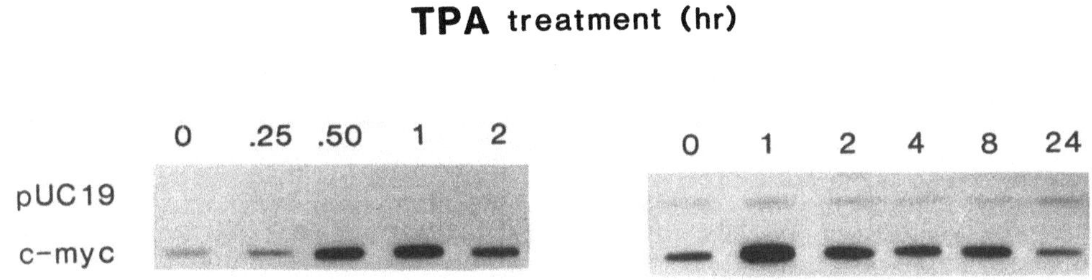

Fig. 4. Transcriptional "run-on" analysis of changes in c-myc gene expression following TPA treatment.

to determine whether transcription in both directions was coordinately or individually regulated in this system, nuclear "run-on" experiments were repeated using single-stranded DNA probes to detect sense and anti-sense transcripts separately. A Bam HI-Hind III genomic DNA fragment encompassing exons 2 and 3 of c-myc was cloned in both orientations in M13 vectors; single-stranded DNA was prepared from each construct. Radiolabelled nuclear RNA was prepared from control cells and from cells treated with either GaMIg or TPA for 1 or 24 hours; these RNAs were hybridized to filters bearing sense specific, anti-sense specific, and double stranded cDNA probes (Fig. 5). The results show that there is no detectable change in net anti-sense transcription with either treatment. All of the previously noted changes in transcription of the c-myc gene can be accounted for by fluctuations in the rate of sense strand transcription.

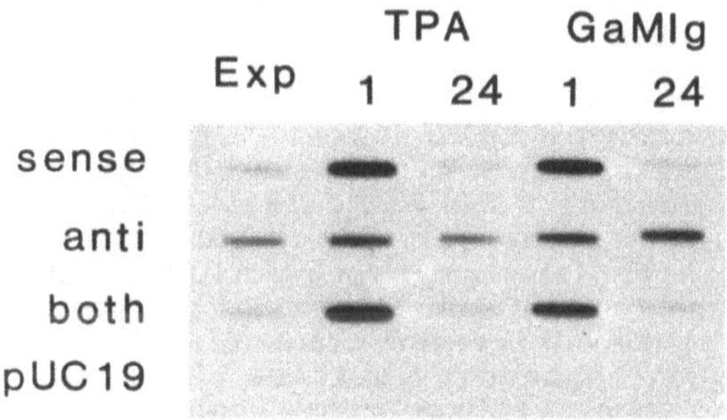

Fig. 5. Effects of GaMIg and TPA treatments on transcription of c-myc mRNA coding and non-coding strands.

DISCUSSION

The dramatic changes in cytoplasmic c-myc mRNA levels induced during growth arrest of WEHI 231 cells result from regulation at several steps in gene expression. The major regulation appears to be at the level of transcription. When exponentially growing cells are treated with either GaMIg or TPA, the rate of transcription from the c-myc locus changes markedly, preceding fluctuations in cytoplasmic mRNA. Transcriptional control of c-myc has been noted in several other systems. Greenberg and Ziff (1984) have demonstrated changes in c-myc transcription accompanying the large changes in c-myc mRNA levels following addition of serum to quiescent 3T3 fibroblasts. The terminal differentiation of the human promyelocytic leukemia line HL60 induced by TPA or DMSO is accompanied by a drop in the level of c-myc mRNA, the result of a decrease in transcription of this gene (Grosso and Pitot 1985).

In addition to this transcriptional regulation, the c-myc gene in WEHI 231 appears to be subject to post-transcriptional regulation, as well. A transient stabilization of c-myc mRNA is observed shortly after GaMIg treatment is initiated. The rate of decay of cytoplasmic c-myc mRNA is slower 10 minutes post treatment than in exponentially growing cells or at a later time (2 hours) during the course of the GaMIg treatment, when c-myc mRNA levels are dropping. (Work is in progress to determine whether a similar regulation of message stability occurs during TPA treatment.) Although the transcriptional rate appears to be the major determinant of c-myc mRNA levels in this system, this coordination of transcription and decay rates serves not only to increase the maximum attainable level of cytoplasmic message, but also shortens the time needed to achieve this maximum. Changes in c-myc message stability have also been observed in lymphoblastoid Daudi cells following interferon treatment (Dani et al., 1985). Altered message stability may also help explain changes in c-myc message levels which are not accompanied by transcriptional changes, such as those seen in F9 teratocarcinoma cells undergoing terminal differentiation (Dony et al., 1985, Dean et al., 1986), and Chinese hamster lung fibroblasts treated with thrombin and insulin (Blanchard et al., 1985). The mechanism of stabilization of c-myc mRNA is not known at present; we hypothesize a selective ribonuclease activity which may be transiently inactivated.

A third possible regulatory mechanism, which must be further explored, is suggested by the presence of anti-sense (non-coding strand) transcription of the c-myc gene. During the time course of GaMIg or TPA treatment of WEHI 231 cells, little change is seen in the levels of anti-sense strand transcription; the overall transcriptional changes detected using double-stranded probes can be accounted for by changes in sense-strand transcription. This means that the ratio of sense/anti-sense transcription fluctuates in these cells, and appears to be lowest in those cells which have entered a quiescent state. These data are consistent with a model in which anti-sense transcription of RNA plays a regulatory role in the nucleus, setting a threshold level which must be exceeded by sense transcription before significant amounts of mRNA are exported to the cytoplasm. This might allow for more rapid changes in the expression of c-myc mRNA levels than an on-off mechanism. Much more work, however, must be done before the meaning of the observed anti-sense transcription of c-myc is understood. These findings and the previous observations by Marcu and colleagues indicate that strand-specific probes must be employed in future measurements of c-myc gene transcription.

It is clear that the frequently observed chromosomal translocations involving the c-myc locus (Adams et al., 1982, Shen-Ong et al., 1982, Taub et al., 1982) would be expected to have dramatic effects on the regulation of expression of this gene. In most murine plasmacytomas, such translocations remove the normal c-myc promoter(s) and presumptive 5' regulatory regions from the protein-coding portion of the gene (Stanton et al., 1983, Marcu and coworkers, this volume). This alteration in structure would presumably release the c-myc gene from the normal transcriptional regulation observed in these and other studies mentioned above. Our finding of regulation of message stability raises the further possibility that the aberrant transcripts produced by translocated genes might escape normal turnover regulation. Studies of turnover rates in lymphoid cell lines bearing translocated c-myc genes indicate that aberrant transcripts from such alleles are indeed more stable (by a factor of 2-4) than are c-myc transcripts in lines without translocations (Piechaczyk et al., 1985, our unpublished observations). Work is in progress to determine whether this is indeed the result of altered message structure, as has been postulated, and whether these messages display equal sensitivity to the putative selective ribonuclease activity in these cells.

A further intriguing possibility is that translocations of c-myc affect not only the 5' end of the sense transcripts (mRNA), but also the 3' end of anti-sense transcripts. We have previously described anti-sense c-myc transcripts arising from translocated c-myc alleles in two murine plasmacytomas, MOPC 315 and HOPC 1 (Ponte et al., 1981, Dean et al., 1983). These transcripts begin within the c-myc locus, in an anti-sense direction, and cross the recombination junction into the translocated heavy chain constant region domain; they are thus transcribed in the sense direction for the heavy chain constant region domain. The immunoglobulin portion of these aberrant transcripts is properly spliced and polyadenylated and the processed transcripts are transported to the cytoplasm (manuscript in preparation). If anti-sense transcription of an unrearranged c-myc gene normally plays a regulatory role, it is possible that the processing of these aberrant transcripts results in further deregulation of the translocated c-myc gene.

REFERENCES

Adams, J, Gerondakis, S, Webb, E, Mitchell, J, Bernard, O and Cory, S (1982) Transcriptionally active DNA region that rearranges frequently in murine lymphoid tumors. Proc Natl Acad Sci USA 79:6996-6970

Blanchard, JM, Piechaczyk, M, Dani, Ch, Chambard, JC, Franchi, A, Pouyssegur, J, and Jeanteur, Ph (1985) c-myc gene is transcribed at high rate in G_o-arrested fibroblasts and is post-transcriptionally regulated in response to growth factors. Nature 317:443-445

Boyd, A and Schrader, JW (1981) The regulation of growth and differentiation of a murine B-cell lymphoma: II. The inhibition of WEHI 231 by anti-immunoglobulin antibodies. J Immunol 126:2466-2469

Campisi, J, Gray, H, Pardee, AB, Dean, M, Sonenshein, GE (1984) Cell-cycle control of c-myc but not c-ras expression is lost following chemical transformation. Cell 36:241-247.

Dani, Ch, Blancard, J M, Piechaczyk, M, El Sabouty, S, Marty, L, Jeanteur, Ph (1984) Extreme instability of myc mRNA in normal and transformed human cells. Proc Natl Acad Sci USA 81:7046-7050

Dani, Ch, Mechti, N, Piechaczyk, M, Lebleu, B, Jeanteur, Ph, Blancard, JM (1985) Increased rate of degradation of c-myc mRNA in interferon-treated Daudi cells. Proc Natl Acad Sci USA 82:4896-4899

Dean, M, Kent, RB, Sonenshein, GE (1983) Transcriptional activation of immunoglobulin α heavy-chain genes by translocation of the c-myc oncogene. Nature (London) 305:443-446

Dean, M, Levine, RA, and Campisi, J (1986) c-myc regulation during retinoic acid-induced differentiation of F9 cells is post-transcriptional and associated with growth arrest. Molec Cell Biol 6:518-524

Dony, L, Kessel, M, and Gruss, P (1985) Post-transcriptional control of myc and p53 expression during differentiation of the embryonal carcinoma cell line F9. Nature 317:636-639

Goyette, M, Petropoulos, C, Shank, P, Fausto, N (1984) Regulated transcription of c-Ki-ras and c-myc during compensatory growth of rat liver. Mol Cell Biol 4:1493-1498

Greenberg, ME and Ziff, EB (1984) Stimulation of 3T3 cells induces transcription of the c-fos proto-oncogene. Nature 311:433-438

Grosso, LE and Pitot, HC (1985) Transcriptional regulation of c-myc during chemically induced differentiation, Cancer Res 45:847-850

Kelly, K, Cochran, B, Stiles, C, Leder, P (1983) Cell-specific regulation of the c-myc gene by lymphocyte mitogens and platelet-derived growth factor. Cell 35:603-610

McCormack, JE, Pepe, VH, Kent, RB, Dean, M, Marshak-Rothstein, A, Sonenshein, GE (1984) Specific regulation of c-myc oncogene expression in a murine B-cell lymphoma. Proc Natl Acad Sci USA 81:5546-5550

Nishizuka, Y (1984) The role of protein kinase C in cell surface signal transduction and tumor promotion. Nature 308:693-698

Piechaczyk, M, Yang, J-Q, Blanchard, JM, Jeanteur, Ph, Marcu, KB (1985) Posttranscriptional mechanisms are responsible for accumulation of truncated c-myc RNAs in murine plasma cell tumors. Cell 42:589-597

Ponte P, Siekevitz, M, Schwartz, R, Gefter, M, and Sonenshein, GE (1981) Transcription of immunoglobulin heavy-chain sequences from the excluded allele. Nature 291:594-596

Shen-Ong, G, Keath, E, Piccoli, S and Cole, M (1982) Novel myc oncogene RNA from abortive immunoglobulin-gene recombination in mouse plasmacytomas. Cell 31:443-452

Stanton, LW, Watt, R, Marcu, KB (1983) Translocation, breakage and truncated transcripts of c-myc oncogene in murine plasmacytomas. Nature 303:401-406

Taub, R, Kirsch, I, Morton, C, Lenoir, G, Swan, D, Tronick, S, Aaronson, S, and Leder, P (1982) Translocation of the c-myc gene into the immunoglobulin heavy chain locus in human Burkitt lymphoma and murine plasmacytoma cells. Proc Natl Acad Sci USA 79:7837-7841

Activation of Proto-oncogene Expression by Growth Regulatory Signals

W. Ran, M. Dean*, R. A. Levine, J. Campisi

Department of Biochemistry, Boston University Medical School, 80 E. Concord St., Boston, MA 02118

*Frederick Cancer Research Facility, Frederick, MD 21701

INTRODUCTION

c-myc and c-fos are proto-oncogenes that encode unstable proteins localized in the cell nucleus (Curran et al. 1984; Kruijer et al. 1984; Muller er al. 1984; Eisenman et al. 1984; Rabbitts et al. 1985). Both proto-oncogenes, but especially c-myc, have been implicated in the establishment or progression of a variety of tumors. In many lymphoid tumors, the c-myc gene has undergone structural alterations in 5' noncoding sequences that are believed important for normal regulation (Stanton et al. 1983; Leder et al. 1983). By contrast, certain tumorigenic fibroblasts have lost the ability to regulate c-myc expression properly, apparently because of mutation(s) outside the c-myc gene (Campisi et al. 1984; Dean, Vande Woude, Campisi, in preparation).

We are particularly interested in the intracellular pathways that regulate c-myc and c-fos expression in normal and transformed cells. In normal mammalian fibroblasts in culture, the transcription, mRNA, and protein of both genes have been shown to increase many fold beginning 5 (c-fos) to 30 (c-myc) minutes after quiescent cells are stimulated to resume proliferation by addition of fresh serum or purified mitogens (Kelly et al. 1983; Greenberg et al. 1984; Kruijer et al. 1984; Muller et al. 1984). The mitogens that activate the expression of these proto-oncogenes include platelet-derived growth factor (PDGF), epidermal growth factor (EGF) and phorbol ester tumor promoters such as tetradecanoylphorbol acetate (TPA). Of these mitogens, PDGF and TPA share a common mechanism. Both activate protein kinase-C, a seryl-threonyl kinase important in several cell processes, including cell proliferation. PDGF activates this kinase indirectly by stimulating phosphatidylinositol hydrolysis, generating diacylglycerol. Diacylglycerol and TPA are direct activators of protein kinase-C (Nishizuka 1984; Hokin 1985). By contrast, EGF does not stimulate phosphatidylinositol hydrolysis nor does it activate protein kinase-C (Coughlin et al. 1985; Besterman et al. 1986). It is likely, therefore, that EGF activates proto-oncogene expression by a unique pathway, distinct from that utilized by PDGF.

In this study, we show that under certain culture conditions TPA does not activate proto-oncogene expression, although the activation of at least one other growth-regulated gene occurs normally. Thus, there may be selective regulation over the action of protein kinase-C towards the c-myc and c-fos proto-oncogenes. Moreover, we provide evidence that, under these same culture conditions, the second messengers that are utilized by EGF to activate c-myc and c-fos expression are cyclic-AMP and calcium.

REGULATION OF PROTO-ONCOGENE EXPRESSION BY PHORBOL ESTER

We used murine BALB/c 3T3 fibroblasts (clone A31) for our studies. These nontumorigenic cells become proliferatively quiescent when grown to confluence (density arrested) or when given a suboptimal serum

Current Topics in Microbiology and Immunology, Vol. 132

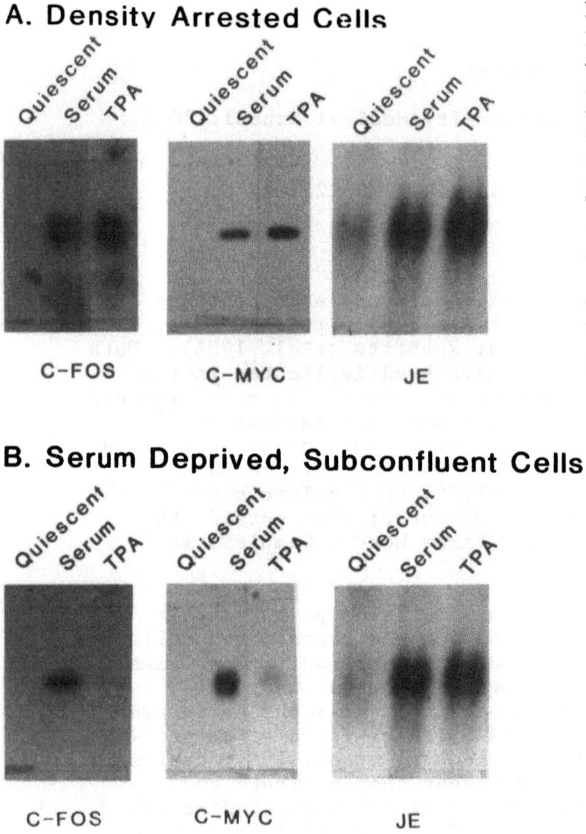

Fig. 1 Induction of proto-oncogene mRNA by TPA. A31 cells were growth arrested by growth to confluence (density arrested) or by serum deprivation at subconfluence (0.4% calf serum, 48 hours). The cells were stimulated by 15% serum or 100 nM TPA. Cytoplasmic RNA was isolated after 45 or 120 min. and analyzed for c-fos mRNA (45 min. samples) by Northern blot analysis, or for c-myc mRNA (120 min. samples) by S1 nuclease analysis, both as previously described (Dean et al. 1986).

concentration at subconfluence. Regardless of the method of growth arrest, A31 cells contained very little c-myc or c-fos cytoplasmic mRNA when quiescent (Fig. 1). When serum was added to these quiescent cells, c-fos and c-myc mRNA was induced 20-fold or more within 45 and 120 minutes respectively, again regardless of the method of growth arrest (Fig. 1). However, the method of growth arrest profoundly influenced the ability of TPA to induce proto-oncogene mRNA levels. TPA was a potent inducer of c-myc and c-fos mRNA in density arrested cells, whereas it was a poor inducer of these mRNAs in serum deprived, subconfluent cells (Fig. 1).

We found that the level of protein kinase-C in density arrested cells and serum deprived, subconfluent cells was similar, and that the ability of TPA to stimulate phosphorylation of the major 80 kDa protein kinase-C substrate was unimpaired in the serum deprived cells. In addition, TPA was fully able to induce the mRNA of JE, a PDGF-inducible gene (Cochran et al. 1983), regardless of the method of growth arrest (Fig. 1). Thus, in serum deprived cells proto-oncogene expression, but not JE expression, could not be activated by TPA.

To better understand the differential regulation of the proto-oncogenes and JE by TPA, we determined the level of c-myc and JE transcription in nuclei isolated from quiescent cells and from cells 1 hour after stimulation by serum or TPA (Fig. 2). Serum and TPA induced a 3- to 5-fold increase in the transcription of both c-myc and JE in density

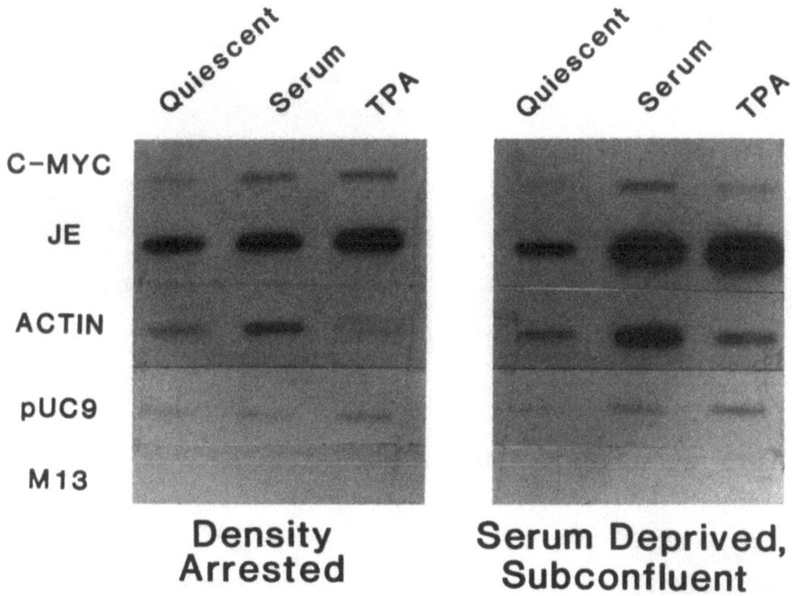

Fig. 2 Transcriptional regulation of c-myc and JE by TPA. A31 cells were made quiescent and stimulated as described in the legend to Fig. 1. After 1 hr, nuclei were isolated and run-off transcripts were analyzed for c-myc and JE sequences, as previously described (Dean et al. 1986).

arrested cells. In serum deprived cells, by contrast, serum and TPA induced JE transcription by about 10-fold; however, c-myc transcription was induced 3- to 5-fold by serum, but less than 2-fold by TPA. These results suggest that under certain conditions of growth arrest the action of protein kinase-C may be selectively regulated such that the transcription of some genes (JE) can be activated, whereas transcription of the c-myc and c-fos proto-oncogenes cannot be activated. We do not yet know whether this selectivity is achieved by regulation of some aspect of the kinase, for example its localization or accessibility to its substrates, or whether the selectivity is regulated at the level of the substrates.

REGULATION OF PROTO-ONCOGENE EXPRESSION BY EGF

Our finding that the expression of c-myc and c-fos is not activated by protein kinase-C in serum deprived cells suggested that EGF, which does not stimulate phosphatidylinositol turnover, may be an important activator of proto-oncogene expression in serum deprived cells. In contrast to TPA, we found that EGF was indeed a relatively good inducer of proto-oncogene mRNA in serum deprived cells, but that it was a poor inducer in density arrested cells (Fig. 3). This result is consistent with the idea that at least two pathways may lead to increased c-myc and c-fos expression: a TPA (protein kinase-C)-directed pathway that is most active in density arrested cells, and an EGF-directed pathway that is most active in serum deprived, subconfluent cells. Moreover, the differential response to EGF suggested that it might be possible to identify intracellular messengers that mediate EGF action.

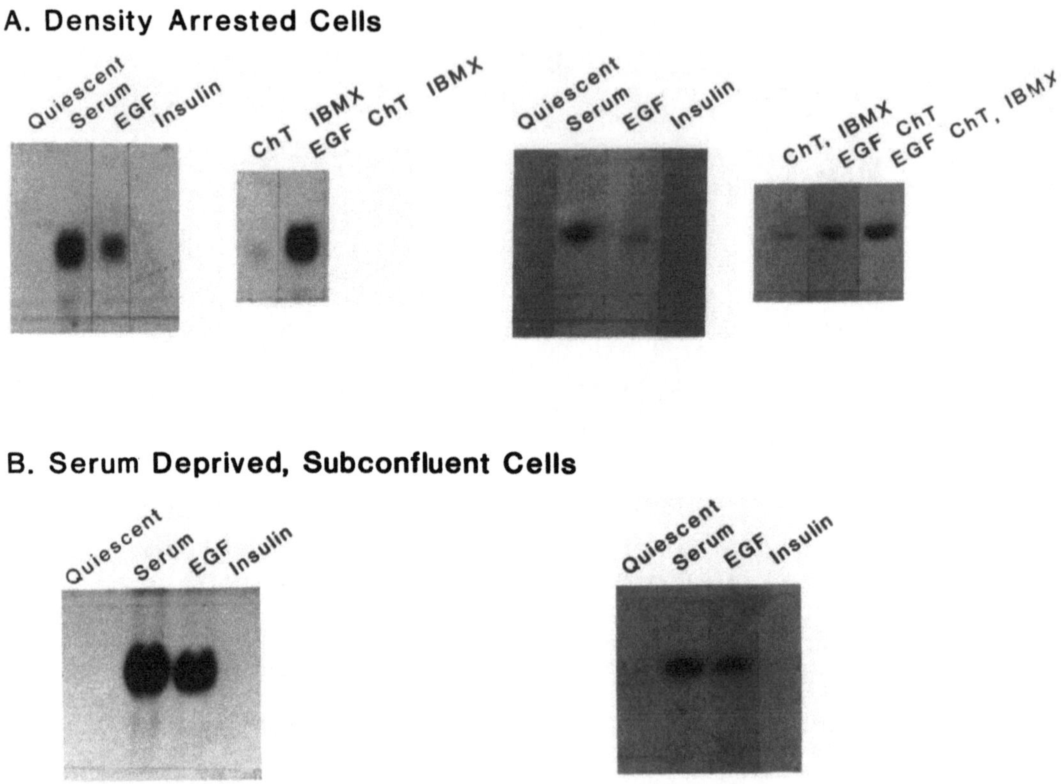

Fig. 3 Regulation of proto-oncogene mRNA by EGF and cyclic-AMP. Quiescent A31 cells were stimulated, and cytoplasmic RNA was extracted and analyzed as described in the legend to Fig. 1. Cholera toxin (ChT) was added at 1 ug/ml and isobutylmethylxanthine (IBMX) was added at 0.1 mM.

We have noted that serum deprived cells maintain intracellular cyclic-AMP at nearly twice the level maintained by density arrested cells, and several investigators have shown that the mitogenic potential of EGF can be increased by agents that elevate intracellular cyclic-AMP (Pruss et al. 1979; Olashaw et al. 1984). It is possible, therefore, that the ability to induce proto-oncogene mRNA by EGF in serum deprived, but not density arrested, cells is due in part to the intracellular cyclic-AMP level. To explore this idea, we treated density arrested cells with EGF and cholera toxin or isobutylmethylxanthine (Fig. 3). These drugs increase intracellular cyclic-AMP by activating adenylate cyclase, or inhibiting the phosphodiesterase responsible for degrading cyclic-AMP, respectively. Either cholera toxin or cholera toxin plus isobutylmethylxanthine substantially potentiated the ability of EGF to induce c-myc and c-fos mRNA in density arrested cells. However, these drugs did not potentiate the ability of TPA to induce proto-oncogene mRNA. This result suggests that cyclic-AMP cooperates with the EGF-directed pathway and not the TPA-directed pathway, and is consistent with the notion that these are independent pathways regulated by different intracellular messengers.

In addition to production of diacylglycerol, phosphatidylinositol hydrolysis also produces inositol triphosphate. This molecule releases calcium from an intracellular store. Thus, growth factors that stimulate phosphatidylinositol hydrolysis characteristically give rise to a large, transient increase in intracellular free calcium (Hokin 1985). Although EGF does not stimulate phosphatidylinositol hydrolysis, it has been shown in some (but not all) cell systems that EGF nonetheless causes an increase in intracellular free calcium; however, the source of the calcium appears to be extracellular (Hesketh et al. 1985). To explore the role of calcium influx in the activation of proto-oncogene expression, we treated density arrested cells with the calcium ionophore A23187. When used alone, this drug had no effect on c-myc or c-fos mRNA levels. However, when administered together with cholera toxin, both proto-oncogene mRNAs were induced to approximately the level induced by EGF and cholera toxin (data not shown). Taken together, our results suggest that cyclic-AMP is a positive regulator of c-myc and c-fos mRNA levels providing the cells receive a simultaneous signal, probably calcium influx, from EGF.

DISCUSSION

Our results suggest that at least two post-receptor pathways operate to activate c-myc and c-fos mRNA levels. We found that we could sensitize A31 cells to use a TPA (protein kinase-C)-directed pathway or an EGF-directed pathway by manipulating the culture conditions. In density arrested cells, the TPA-directed pathway was most active. This is not surprising since it is well-established that PDGF, which activates protein kinase-C, is a potent inducer of both gene expression and mitogenesis in density arrested cells (Greenberg et al. 1984; Kelly et al. 1983; Kruijer et al. 1984; Muller et al. 1984). The relative impotence of EGF in density arrested cells could be explained the relatively low level of intracellular cyclic-AMP in these cells. In serum deprived, subconfluent cells, the EGF-directed pathway was most active, possibly because these cells maintain a relatively high cyclic-AMP level. It is not clear why the TPA-directed pathway is blocked in serum deprived cells. However, it is noteworthy that not all actions of TPA are blocked in serum deprived cells. In particular, at least one other growth-regulated gene (JE) was inducible by TPA in serum deprived cells. Additional experiments are needed before we can understand the significance and mechanism(s) of the specificity of this block to proto-oncogene induction by TPA.

We are currently determining whether the expression of other growth-regulated genes is also enhanced by EGF, and whether EGF and cyclic-AMP act at transcriptional or post-transcriptional levels in A31 cells. At this time, it is not known whether TPA and EGF operate within pathways that remain distinct, or whether the pathways converge at one or more points to alter a unique regulator(s) of gene expression. Nonetheless, our finding that cyclic-AMP enhances the induction of c-myc and c-fos mRNA by EGF suggests a mechanism by which this cyclic nucleotide could act as a postive growth regulator in the proliferation of normal cells. Moreover, it is known that the ras oncogene family is related to a family of proteins (G proteins) that regulate adenylate cyclase (Gilman 1984; Hurley et al. 1984) and, therefore, our results further suggest a mechanism by which derangements in cyclic-AMP metabolism could lead to malignant transformation.

REFERENCES

Besterman JM, Watson SP, Cuatrecasas P (1986) Lack of association of epidermal growth factor-, insulin-, and serum-induced mitogenesis with stimulation of phosphatidylinositide degradation in BALB/c 3T3 fibroblasts. J Biol Chem 261:723-727

Campisi J, Gray HE, Pardee AB, Dean M, Sonenshein GE (1984) Cell-cycle control of c-myc but not c-ras expression is lost following chemical transformation. Cell 36:241-247

Cochran BH, Reffel AC, Stiles CD (1983) Molecular cloning of gene sequences regulated by platelet-derived growth factor. Cell 33:939-947

Coughlin SR, Lee WF, Williams PW, Giels GM, Williams LT (1985) c-myc gene expression is stimulated by agents that activate protein kinase-C and does not account for the mitogenic effect of PDGF. Cell 43:243-251

Curran T, Miller DA, Zokas L, Verma IM (1984) Viral and cellular fos proteins: A comparative analysis. Cell 36:259-268

Dean M, Levine RA, Campisi J (1986) c-myc regulation during retinoic acid-induced differentiation of F9 cells is posttranscriptional and associated with growth arrest. Molec Cell Biol 6:518-524

Eisenman RN, Hann SR (1984) myc-Encoded proteins of chickens and men. Curr Top in Microbiol and Immunol 113:192-197

Gilman AG (1984) G proteins and dual control of adenylate cyclase. Cell 36:577-579

Greenberg ME, Ziff EB (1984) Stimulation of 3T3 cells induces transcription of the c-fos proto-oncogene. Nature 311:433-437

Hesketh TR, Moore JP, Morris JDH, Taylor MV, Rogers J, Smith GA, Metcalfe JC (1985) A common sequence of calcium and pH signals in the mitogenic stimulation of eucaryotic cells. Nature 313:481-484

Hokin LE (1985) Receptors and phosphoinositide-generated second messengers. Ann Rev Biochem 54:205-235

Hurley JB, Simon MI, Teplow DB, Robishaw JD, Gilman AG (1984) Homologies between signal transducing G proteins and ras gene products. Science 226:860-862

Kelly K, Cochran BH, Stiles CD, Leder P (1983) Cell-specific regulation of the c-myc gene by lymphocyte mitogens and platelet-derived growth factor. Cell 35:603-610

Kruijer W, Cooper JA, Hunter T, Verma IM (1984) Platelet-derived growth factor induces rapid but transient expression of the c-fos gene and protein. Nature 312:711-715

Leder P, Battey J, Lenoir G, Moulding C, Murphy W, Potter H, Stewart T, Taub R (1983) Translocations among antibody genes in human cancer. Science 222:765-771

Muller R, Bravo R, Burckhardt J, Curran T (1984) Induction of c-fos gene and protein by growth factors precedes activation of c-myc. Nature 312:716-720

Nishizuka Y (1984) The role of protein kinase C in cell surface signal transduction and tumor promotion. Nature 308:693-698

Olashaw NE, Leof EB, O'Keefe EJ, Pledger WJ (1984) Differential sensitivity of fibroblasts to epidermal growth factor is related to cyclic-AMP concentration. J Cell Physiol 118:291-297

Pruss RM, Herschman HR (1979) Cholera toxin stimulates division of 3T3 cells. J Cell Physiol 98:469-474

Rabbitts PH, Watson JV, Lamond A, Forster A, Stinson MA, Evan G, Fischer W, Atherton E, Sheppard R, Rabbitts TH (1985) Metabolism of c-myc gene products: c-myc mRNA and protein expression in the cell cycle. EMBO J 4:2009-2015

Stanton LW, Watt R, Marcu KB (1983) Translocation, breakage and truncated transcripts of c-myc oncogene in murine plasmacytomas. Nature 303:401-406

ACKNOWLEDGEMENTS

This work was supported by grant #PCM8403268 from the National Science Foundation and a grant from the Life and Health Insurance Medical Research Fund to JC. MD is recipient of a postdoctoral fellowship and JC is recipient of a Cancer Research Scholar Award, both from the American Cancer Society. Additional support was provided by the National Cancer Institute under contract NO1-CO-23909 with Litton Bionetics Corporation.

Biological Effects of High Level c-myc Expression in FR3T3 Fibroblasts

M. Zerlin[1], M. A. Julius[1], C. Cerni[2] and K. B. Marcu[1]
[1]Biochemistry Department, SUNY at Stony Brook, Stony Brook, NY, 11794; [2]Tumor Biology Institute, Vienna, Austria

INTRODUCTION

The contribution(s) made by the c-*myc* proto-oncogene to cellular transformation remains obscure and controversial. Introduction of a c-*myc* gene into primary fibroblast cells facilitates continuous growth *in vitro* yet these cells retain a normal morphology, are unable to grow in soft agar and, are not tumorigenic in syngeneic hosts or athymic mice (Land et al. 1983; Mougneau et al. 1984; Connan et al. 1985). C-myc activity has also been associated with the competency of cells to enter and progress through the cell cycle (Thompson et al. 1985; Kaczmarek et al. 1985). This picture of c-*myc* gene function loses its apparent simplicity within the context of cell lines that have been established spontaneously in culture. An activated c-*myc* gene within certain immortalized cell lines such as Rat2 (Topp 1981) or NIH3T3 (Jainchill et al. 1969) for example, promotes growth in low serum and in soft agar at low efficiency and, converts cells to a tumorigenic phenotype (Keath et al. 1984; Kelekar and Cole 1986). By these latter criteria c-*myc* could be considered a transforming gene.

We have investigated the role of c-*myc* in cellular transformation by assessing the effects of an activated c-*myc* gene in a cell line established spontaneously in culture. The data suggest that high levels of c-*myc* are necessary but not sufficient for transformation and tumorigenicity.

Characterization of Late and Early Passage FR3T3 Cells Expressing High Levels of c-*myc* RNAs

The fibroblast clones described here are derived from the Fisher rat cell line FR3T3. This well-characterized line does not grow in soft agar or in low serum and, is not tumorigenic in syngeneic hosts (Seif and Cuzin 1977; Rassoulzadegan et al. 1982). It is therefore, an ideal cell line to measure various parameters of transformation or tumorigenicity. The activated c-*myc* gene in this study consists of the coding exons of a normal mouse c-*myc* cDNA clone, pMc-myc54 (Stanton et al. 1983), inserted into a derivative of the MoMuLV LTR-driven EVX retroviral vector, FVXM (Kriegler et al. 1984; M. Kriegler unpublished results).

Multiple stable transformants were derived from FR3T3 cells that were maintained in culture for about 60 generations (late passage) or 10 generations (early passage) prior to cotransfection with FVXMc-*myc* and the pSV2NEO selectable marker gene (Southern and Berg 1982). Late and early passage FR3T3 cells are indistinguishable morphologically but an activated c-*myc* gene has dramatically different affects on them. G418 resistant colonies were selected randomly and replated in order to facilitate the identification of those clones that might show an aberrant morphology possibly as a result of high c-*myc* levels. Among twelve late passage G418 resistant colonies replated four were found to share the same characteristics: high refractility, raised morphology and, slight disorganization in monolayer culture. A representative clone, FRFVXMc-*myc*-8 is shown in monolayer culture in Figure 1b. Its morphology is clearly distinguishable from the control, a pool of FR3T3 clones that contain the pSV2NEO construct only (Fig. 1a). Still greater disorganization is achieved by the introduction of a v-Ha-ras retroviral construct HrasNVX (Stanton and Marcu, unpublished) into FR3T3 late passage cells.

Current Topics in Microbiology and Immunology, Vol. 132

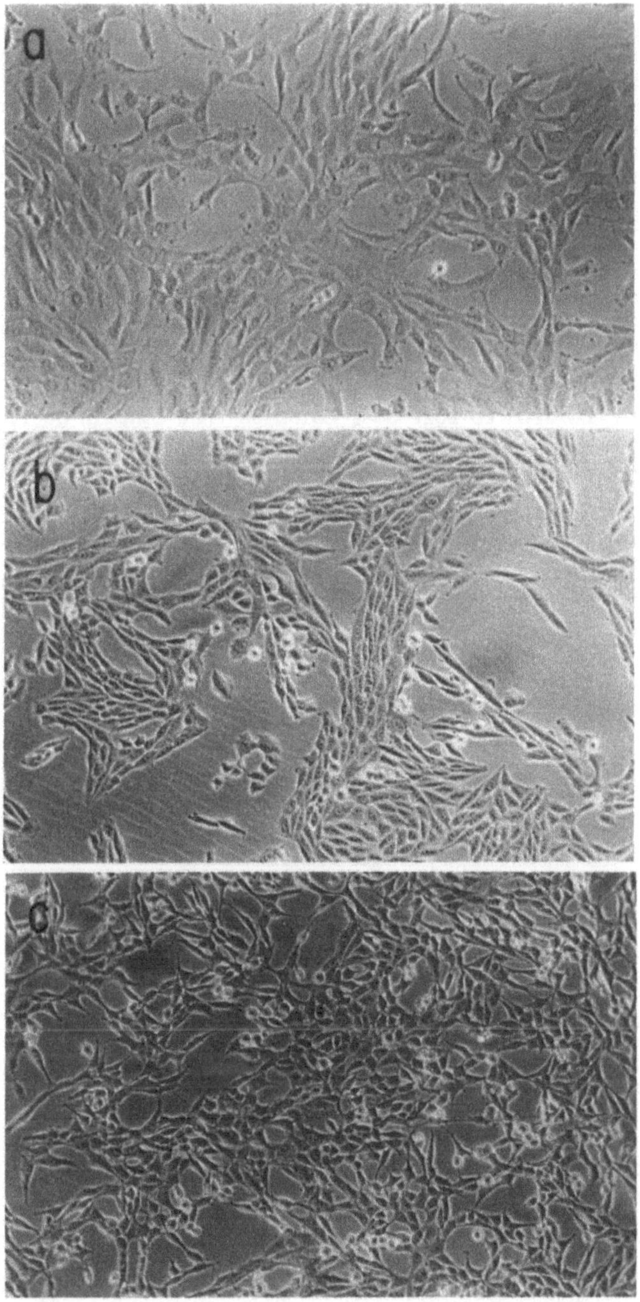

Fig. 1 Subconfluent monolayer cultures of (a) FR SV NEO pool, (b) FRFVXM c-myc-8 and, (c) FR V-RAS pool grown in DME containign 10% calf serum. Pools are comprised of approximately 100 clones (magnification 100X).

FR3T3 late passage cells that contain an activated c-myc gene typically grow to higher saturation densities than cells containing only the selectable marker. In Figure 2 for example, FRFVXMc-myc-8 and the FR SV NEO pool grow at approximately the same rate. However, at confluence FRFVXMc-myc-8 is five times more dense. Similar results have been obtained by others (Keath et al. 1984; Kelekar and Cole 1986). Although an activated c-myc gene appears to confer upon FR3T3 a growth advantage in 10% serum it is unable to do so in 0.5% serum (see Fig. 2). In fact, both FRFVXMc-myc-8 and the FR SV NEO pool remain essentially at stationary phase suggesting that FR3T3 clones that contain activated c-myc genes and control clones have the same serum requirements.

The ability of FR3T3 late passage clones to form colonies in soft agar in response to elevated levels of c-myc is perhaps the most striking affect of the c-myc gene described here. Table 1 shows that the cloning efficiencies of c-myc transfected clones are 30-45%. These values compare favorably with those obtained for rat fibroblast clones transfected by HrasNVX(60%). Without an activated c-myc gene however, the cloning efficiency of FR3T3 is less than 1%. Morphology that is typical of FRFVXMc-myc soft agar colonies is depicted in Figure 3a and is compared to soft agar colonies that contain activated v-Ha-ras genes in Figure 3b. FRFVXMc-myc colonies are smaller than ras colonies (see Table 1, as well) and are somewhat more compact. That FRFVXMc-myc late passage clones are indeed transformed is evident by their ability to form tumors having a latency period of 3-4 weeks (see Table 1). Again, without an activated c-myc gene FR3T3 late passage cells have not been observed to form tumors during 28 weeks of observation.

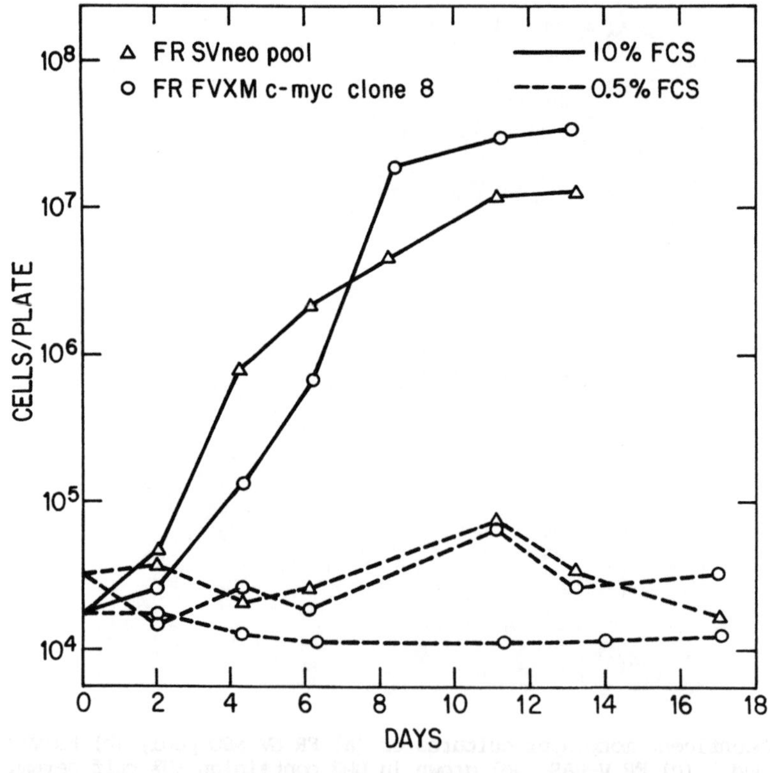

Fig. 2 Growth curves of FR SV NEO pool (triangles) and FRFVXM c-myc-8 (circles). Cells were seeded at densities of 2.5×10^4 or 5.10^4 cells per 60mm dish in DME and fetal calf serum and subsequently trypsinized for counting. Each point represents the mean value of at least two determinations.

Referring to Table 1, c-myc mRNA levels in FRFVXM c-myc late passage clones are 40-100 fold higher than the endogenous steady-state level in FR SV NEO control cells. Elevated c-myc levels in these clones cannot be attributed to the method by which they were selected because similarly high levels of c-myc also occurs in a pool of G418 resistant clones that were selected randomly and without regard to morphology (see Table 1 and Figure 4). We conclude that the characteristics of FRFVXMc-myc late passage clones correlate with, and are likely a response to elevated levels of c-myc mRNA.

Strikingly, this correlation does not extend to early passage clones despite the fact that c-myc mRNA levels are 5-30X above the endogenous level as determined by comparisons to FR SV NEO control cells (data not shown). In fact, thirty two early passage clones have been examined and none exhibit characteristics of c-myc late passage clones except for increased refractility and elevated c-myc mRNA. We conclude that the activated c-myc gene is cooperating with another gene(s) specific to FR3T3 late passage cells to create a transformed phenotype.

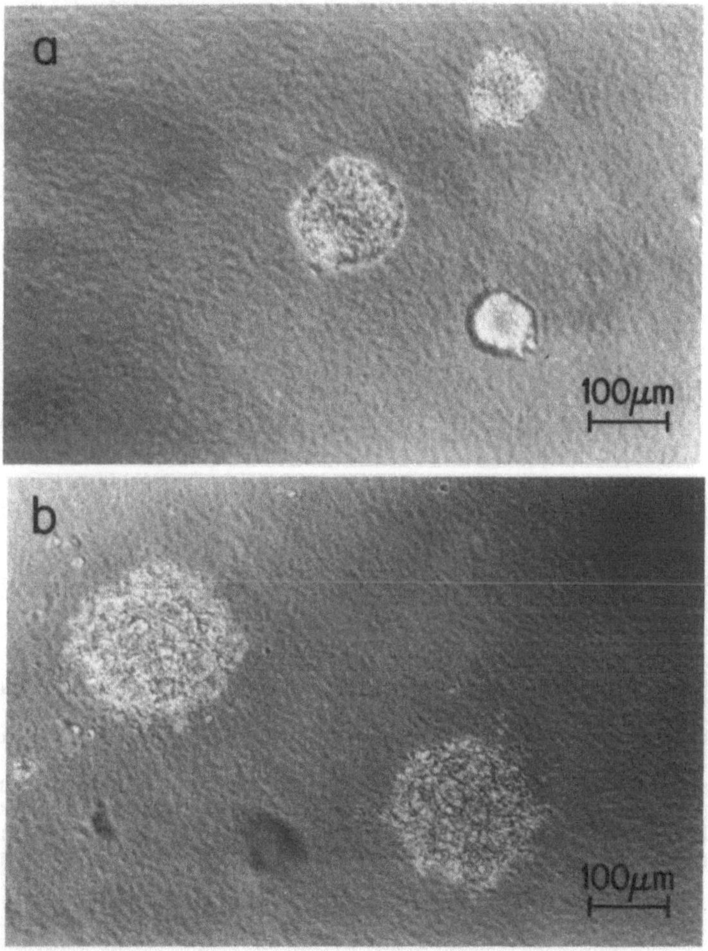

Fig. 3. Colony growth in soft agar of (a) FRFVXMc-myc-8 and (b) Rat-2 RAS-NEO-2. Cells were seeded at a density of 1×10^4 cells per 60mm dish in DME containing 10% calf serum and 0.25% agarose. Colonies were photographed about six weeks later at 100X magnification.

Recently, Stern et al. have shown that FR3T3 cells containing activated c-myc genes can grow in soft agar in response to epidermal growth factor (Stern et al. 1986). We have confirmed their observation by showing that our early passage FVXMc-myc clones can grow in soft agar only when stimulated by EGF. Late passage FRFVXMc-myc clones on the other hand, grow readily in soft agar in the absence of EGF. As expected, introduction of EGF into the medium does not enhance the ability of these late passage FRFVXMc-myc clones to grow in soft agar. Thus, growth factor independence of late passage cells is achieved by the introduction of an activated c-myc gene and the acquisition of a factor(s) by late passage cells.

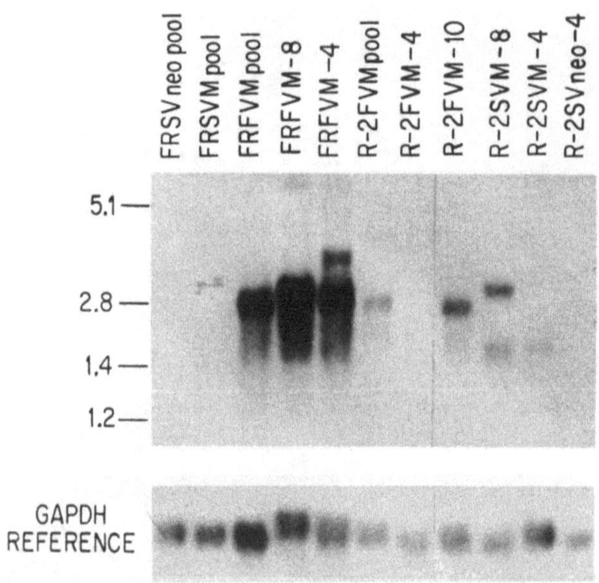

Fig. 4 Northern blots of c-myc transcripts in various fibroblast lines. About 2 ug poly(A)+ RNA was electrophoresed through formaldehyde-agarose gel (Zeevi et al. 1981), transferred to nitrocellulose (Thomas 1980) and, hybridized to a c-myc exon 2 probe (Stanton et al 1983) and, to a glyceraldehyde 3-phosphate dehydrogenase (GAPDH) cDNA clone (Fort et al, 1985). Clone designations are described in Table 1. SVM lines contain the pSVc-myc-1 expression vector (Land et al 1983). Predicted sizes of c-myc transcripts are 1.7 Kb for pSVc-myc-1 and, 2.8 Kb for FVXMcmyc. Endogenous c-myc RNAs (2.4 Kb) are not apparent in this exposure.

TABLE 1. PROPERTIES OF C-MYC TRANSFECTED FR3T3 CELL LINES

CELL LINE	C-MYC LEVEL	COLONY FORMATION IN SOFT AGAR		TUMORIGENICITY	
		CLONING EFFICIENCY (%)	MEAN COLONY SIZE (μM)	LAT. (W)	FREQUENCY
FRFVXM C-MYC-3	~40	32.5	87±33	3-4	5/5
FRFVXM C-MYC-4	~100	44.7	92±29	3	5/5
FRFVXM C-MYC-8	~100	26.4	131±39	3-4	5/5
FRFVXM C-MYC-12	~50	40.5	102±24	4	5/5
FRFVXM C-MYC POOL	~40	26.7	110±32	4	5/5
FR SV NEO POOL	1	0.7	≤40	-	0/5
FR V-RAS	ND	62.4	156±48	1-2	5/5
R-2 RAS-NEO-2	ND	59.3	220±112	ND	ND

Conclusions

There is abundant data in the literature to support the hypothesis that cellular transformation occurs as a step-wise process, presumably by the accumulation of genes that exert their effects collectively (for reviews see Cairns 1975; Klein and Klein 1985). Late and early passage FR3T3 cells appear to be indistinguishable. In the presence of an activated c-myc gene however, the phenotype of the late passage cell is altered dramatically whereas its early passage counterpart acquires only slight refractility. These results are concordant with the original observation that the c-myc gene is unable to transform primary embryo fibroblasts without the cooperative effect of a class 2 transforming gene (Land et al. 1983; Lee et al. 1985). These data also emphasize that interpretations of oncogene function may be biased by the genetic background into which a particular gene is introduced.

Clones designated FR or R-2 are derived from FR3T3 and Rat-2 cell lines, respectively. Clones bearing the names FVXM c-myc, SV_2NEO, V-RAS and RAS-NEO refer to the expression vectors FVXM c-myc (see text), pSV2NEO (Southern and Berg 1982) and HrasNVX(see text) respectively. c-myc levels were determined from densitometric tracings of autoradiograms such as that represented in Figure 4 and are expressed relative to the FR SV NEO pool. The quantity of GAPDH RNAs in each sample served as an internal standard. Sizes of soft agar colonies were measured after six weeks. Tumorigenicity assays were performed by innoculating subcutaneously $1X10^6$ cells into seven day old Fisher F344 rats. LAT. (W) refers to the latency period in weeks. (ND), not determined.

REFERENCES

Cairns J (1975) Mutation selection and the natural history of cancer. Nature 255: 197-200.

Connan G, Rassoulzadegan M, Cuzin F (1985) Focus formation in rat fibroblasts exposed to a tumour promoter after transfer of polyoma plt and myc oncogenes. Nature 314:277-279.

Fort Ph, Marty L, Piechaczyk M, Sabrouty S El, Dani Ch, Janteur Ph, Blanchard JM (1985) Various rat adult tissues express only one major mRNA species from the glyceraldehyde-3-phosphate dehydrogenase multigenic family. Nucleic Acids Res. 13:1431-1442.

Jainchill JS, Aaronson SA, Todaro GJ (1969) Murine sarcoma and leukemia viruses: assay using clonal lines of contact-inhibited mouse cells. J. Virol. 4:549-553.

Kaczmarek L, Hyland JK, Watt R, Rosenberg M and Baserga R (1985) Microinjected c-myc as a competence factor. Science 228:1313-1315.

Keath EJ, Caimi PG, Cole MD (1984) Fibroblast lines expressing activated c-myc oncogenes are tumorigenic in nude mice and syngeneic animals. Cell 39:339-348.

Kelekar A, Cole MD (1986) Tumorigenicity of fibroblast lines expressing the adenovirus Ela, cellular p53, or normal c-myc genes. Mol Cell Biol 6:7-14.

Klein G, Klein E (1985) Evolution of tumours and the impact of molecular oncology. Nature 315: 190-195.

Kriegler M, Perez CF, Hardy C and Botchan M (1984) Transformation mediated by SV40 T antigens: separation of overlapping SV40 early genes with a retroviral vector. Cell 38:483-491.

Land H, Parada LF, Weinberg RA (1983) Tumorigenic conversion of primary embryo fibroblasts requires at least two cooperating oncogenes. Nature 304:596-602.

Lee WF, Schwab M, Westway D, Varmus HE (1985) Augmented expression of normal c-myc is sufficient for cotransformation of rat embryo cells with a mutant ras gene. Mol Cell Biol 5:3345-3356.

Mougneau E, Lemieux L, Rassoulzadegan M, Cuzin F (1984) Biological activities of the v-myc and of rearranged c-myc oncogenes in rat fibroblast cells in culture. Proc Natl Acad Sci USA 81:5758-5762.

Rassoulzadegan M, Cowie A, Carr A, Glaichenhaus N, Kamen R, Cuzin F (1982) The roles of individual polyoma virus early proteins in oncogenic transformation. Nature 300: 713-718.

Seif R, Cuzin F (1977) Temperature-sensitive growth regulation in one type of transformed rat cells induced by the tsa mutant of polyoma virus. J. Virology 24:721-728.

Southern PJ, Berg P (1982) Transformation of mammalian cells to antibiotic resistance with a bacterial gene under the control of the SV40 early region promoter. J Mol Appl Genet 1:327-341.

Stanton LW, Watt R, Marcu KB (1983) Translocation, breakage, and truncated transcripts of c-myc oncogene in murine plasmacytomas. Nature 303:401-406.

Stern DF, Roberts AB, Roche NS, Sporn MB, Weinberg RA (1986) Differential responsiveness of myc and ras-transfected cells to growth factors: selective stimulation of c-myc transfected cells by epidermal growth factor. Mol Cell Biol 6:870-877.

Thomas PS (1980) Hybridization of denatured RNA and small DNA fragments transferred to nitrocellulose. Proc Natl Acad Sci USA 77:5201-5205.

Thompson CB, Challoner PB, Neiman PE and Groudine M (1985) Levels of c-myc oncogene are invariant throughout the cell cycle. Nature 314:363-366.

Topp WC (1981) Normal rat cell lines deficient in nuclear thymidine kinase. Virology 113:408-411.

Zeevi M, Nevins JR, Darnell JE Jr (1981) Nuclear RNA is spliced in the absence of $poly(A)^+$ addition. Cell 26:39-46.

Acknowledgements: The authors are very grateful to Dr. Michael Kriegler (Institute for Cancer Research, Fox Chase Cancer Center, Philadelphia, PA.) for making available to us the FVXM vector prior to publication and, to Dr. Francois Cuzin (Centre de Biochimie du CNRS, Universite de Nice, France) for providing us with FR3T3 late and early passage cell lines. We wish to thank Ms. Barbara Springhorn for care taken in preparing the manuscript and Chris Helmke, Mary Ann Huntington and Joyce Schirmer for graphic arts assistance. This research was supported by a fellowship to MZ from the Consejo Nacional de Investigaciones Cientificas y Tecnologicas, Caracas, Venezuela and by NIH grants awarded to KBM. KBM is a research career development awardee of the NIAID.

A Transfected c-*myc* Oncogene Inhibits Mouse Erythroleukemic Differentiation

E. Dmitrovsky, W.M. Kuehl, G.F. Hollis, I.R. Kirsch, T.P. Bender, and S. Segal

NCI-Navy Medical Oncology Branch, National Cancer Institute, National Institutes of Health, and Department of Medicine, Uniformed Services University of the Health Sciences, National Navy Medical Center, Bethesda, Maryland 20814

Cellular differentiation is a complex process for which the molecular mechanisms are poorly understood. One useful model for the study of differentiation is the Friend virus derived (Friend 1971) mouse erythroleukemia (MEL) cell lines. These transformed early erythroid precursors can be induced to terminally differentiate into mature erythroid cells by a variety of seemingly unrelated agents including dimethyl sulfoxide (DMSO) (Marks 1978). Following DMSO induction, the majority of cells become irreversibly committed to differentiation, undergoing several rounds of cell division before ceasing to replicate (Gusella 1976; Fibach 1977). These terminally differentiated cells express high levels of hemoglobin (Boyer 1972; Ostertag 1972). After DMSO induction of MEL cells there is a biphasic decline in steady state levels of c-myc (Lachman 1984; Kirsch 1985) and c-myb mRNAs (Kirsch 1985). We sought to determine if the down regulation of c-myc mRNA is a necessary step for DMSO induced differentiation. Our experiments indicate that expression of a transfected human c-myc gene inhibits the terminal differentiation of MEL cells.

To study whether the c-myc oncogene is involved in the terminal differentiation of MEL cells, we transfected into the 745 MEL cell line a plasmid containing the human c-myc oncogene. A modified (Davis 1986) calcium-phosphate transfection procedure (Graham 1973) was used. This plasmid called $PL^1hmcneo^r$ (kindly provided to us by Dr. Lee at the University of San Francisco) is a derivative of the pCV108 vector which contains pSV2neo inserted into pJB8 (Lau 1983). A genomic human c-myc fragment with the XhoI site in the first exon fused to the enhancer-promoter region of the Moloney murine leukemia virus LTR is inserted into pCV108.

After G418 selection, six stable transfectants were obtained from three independent transfection experiments and were designated T55-57 and T60-62. All expressed on Northern analysis the neomycin resistance gene while T55, T56, and T60-62 also expressed the introduced human c-myc gene when probed with the nick-translated 1.5 kb human c-myc ClaI/EcoRI 3'flanking and third exon fragment. When stringently washed, the human c-myc can be distinguished from the murine c-myc mRNA. The obtained transfectants were all single cell subcloned by limiting dilution in 96 well microtiter plates.

As the first step in our analysis, all six subclones were induced with DMSO. These inductions were performed in two ways. In the first method (designated stationary phase induction), exponentially growing cells were seeded at a density of $5x10^5$ cells/ml on day -1, and split to 10^5 cells/ml one day later (day 0) in medium supplemented with or without 1.5% DMSO (SIGMA). Cells were harvested at various time points by centrifugation at 1000 rpm x 5 minutes and washed twice with phosphate buffer

Current Topics in Microbiology and Immunology, Vol. 132

saline and then resuspended in guanidine thiocyanate for RNA and DNA isolation (Chirgwin 1979). The second method (designated logarithmic phase induction) differed from the first in that exponentially growing cells were maintained in continuous logarithmic growth. This was achieved by splitting clones daily at their respective doubling times and replacing the cultures with fresh medium supplemented with or without DMSO. The removed cells were harvested and stored for subsequent mRNA analysis.

Strikingly, we found that all clones which expressed the human c-myc gene failed after 7 days of stationary phase induction with DMSO to generate either a red pellet or benzidine positivity of single cells, which is an assay for hemoglobin synthesis (Fibach 1977). In contrast, clone 57 which expressed only the neomycin resistance gene and not the human c-myc gene induced by day 7 both a red pellet and 90% benzidine positive single cells. To maximize DMSO response, logarithmic phase inductions were performed on clones of all six transfectants. The accumulation of acid-benzidine reactive cells is depicted in Fig. 1. As shown, despite a 14 day induction period with DMSO, only clone 57 generated a majority of benzidine reactive cells while all the clones which expressed the human c-myc gene produced negligible levels of benzidine reactivity.

To better define the effect of exogenous human c-myc expression on the DMSO induction of MEL cells, two transfectants were selected for further analysis: T56 which expressed high levels of the human c-myc gene and T57 which did not. Southern blot analysis demonstrated that the human c-myc gene was integrated into the genome of clone 56 whereas clone 57 did not contain an intact human c-myc gene (data not shown). Four parameters were used to assess the response of clones 56 and 57 to DMSO induction. These included: cell pellet color, acid-benzidine staining of single cells, induced α-globin mRNA, and cell cloning efficiency. The results of these experiments clearly indicate a failure of clone 56 to differentiate normally in contrast either to clone 57 or the MEL parent. Clone 57, like the MEL parent, induced with DMSO by day 7 a red pellet with the majority of cells benzidine reactive. There was an approximate 20 fold increase of α-globin mRNA over basal levels. These cells also lost their clonability, suggesting they have undergone with differentiation terminal rounds of division. In contrast, clone 56 which has minimal induction of α-globin mRNA by day 10, continued to generate subclones despite a 14 day logarithmic phase induction with DMSO.

We conclude from these experiments that expression of the introduced human c-myc oncogene inhibits the DMSO induced differentiation of MEL cells. We are attempting to define the lowest level of exogenous c-myc mRNA expression that will alter the DMSO mediated differentiation. We are presently deterimining if HMBA (N,N'-hexamethylene-bisacetamide) induced differentiation will also be altered in these stable transfectants. Future studies will examine if other oncogenes can substitute for c-myc in this inhibitory effect.

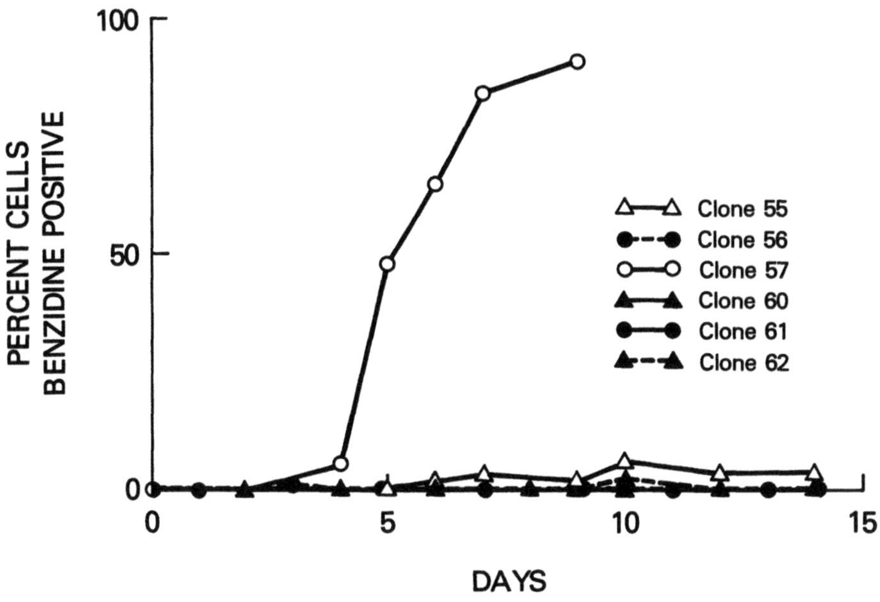

Fig. 1. Single cell benzidine assay for hemoglobin during a 14 day logarithmic phase induction with DMSO of clones 55, 56, and 60-62 which expressed the introduced human c-*myc* gene and clone 57 which did not.

REFERENCES

Boyer SH, Wuu KD, Noyes AN, Young R, Scher W, Friend C, Preisler HD, Bank A (1972) Hemoglobin biosynthesis in murine virus-induced leukemic cells in vitro: structure and amounts of globin chains produced. Blood 40:823-835

Chirgwin JM, Przybyla AE, MacDonald RJ, Rutter WJ (1979) Isolation of biologically active ribonucleic acid from sources enriched in ribonuclease. Biochem 18:5294-5299

Davis L, Dibner M, Battey J (1986) In: Methods in molecular biology, Elsevier Publishing Co. (in press)

Fibach E, Reuben RC, Rifkind RA, Marks PA (1977) Effect of hexamethylene bisacetamide on the commitment to differentiation of murine erythroleukemia cells. Cancer Res 37: 440-444

Friend C, Scher W, Holland JG, Sato T (1971) Hemoglobin synthesis in murine virus-induced leukemic cells *in vitro*: stimulation of erythroid differentiation by dimethyl sulfoxide. Proc Natl Acad Sci USA 68: 378-382

Graham FL, Van der Eb AJ (1973) A new technique for the assay of infectivity of human adenovirus 5 DNA. Virology 52:456-467

Gusella J, Geller R, Clarke B, Weeks V, Housman D (1976) Commitment to erythroid differentiation by Friend erythroleukemia cells: a stochastic analysis. Cell 9:221-229

Kirsch IR, Bertness V, Silver J, Hollis G (1985) Oncogene regulation

during erythroid differentiation. In: Leukemia: recent advances in biology and treatment, Alan R Liss, Inc. p 91
Lachamn HM, Skoultchi AI (1984) Expression of c-myc changes during erythroid differentiation of mouse erythroleukemia cells. Nature 310:592-594
Lau Y-F, Kan YW (1983) Versatile cosmid vectors for the isolation, expression, and rescue of gene sequences: studies with the human α-globin gene cluster. Proc Natl Acad Sci USA 80:5225-5229
Marks PA, Rifkind RA (1978) Erythroleukemic differentiation. Ann Rev Biochem 47: 419-448
Ostertag W, Melderis H, Steinheider G, Kluge N, Dube S (1972) Synthesis of mouse haemoglobin and globin mRNA in leukaemic cell cultures. Nature (London) New Biol 239:231-234

Addendum in proof

Recently similar findings were reported in Nature (Coppola, J.A. and Cole, M.D. Nature 320: 760-763, 1986).

Altered c-myc RNA Metabolism in Burkitt's Lymphomas and Mouse Plasmacytomas

M. Piechaczyk, A. Bonnieu, D. Eick(1), E. Remmers(2), J-Q. Yang(2), K. Marcu(2), Ph. Jeanteur and J-M Blanchard

Laboratoire de Génétique Moléculaire, UA CNRS 1191, U.S.T.L., 6 place E. Bataillon, 34060, Montpellier Cedex, France; (1) Institüt fur Virologie, Zentrum für Hygiene der Universität Freiburg, Hermann-Herder Strasse 11, 7800, Freiburg, FRG; (2) Dpt of biochemistry, SUNY at Stony Brook, Stony Brook, NY 11794, USA

SUMMARY:

Exon 1 deleted c-myc RNAs found in some mouse plasma cell tumors (Piechaczyk et al., 1985) and Burkitt's lymphomas (Eick et al., 1985) are more stable than their normal counterparts in control cells. In this paper we extend our original observations to other B cell tumors and we prove that the structural modification of c-myc RNA is responsible for its stabilization. However, we also show that exon 1 by itself does not account for the extreme instability of normal c-myc RNAs. Finally our results suggest that abnormal c-myc transcripts, while always stabilized in the cytoplasm, may sometimes be more actively degraded in the nucleus than normal ones in reference cell lines.

INTRODUCTION:

The c-myc gene is reputed to immortalize fibroblasts. It was shown to participate in tumor induction in transgenic mice and to impart tumorigenic potential to immortalized mouse and rat fibroblasts. Although no role has been assigned to its protein it has been proposed that c-myc may function in the process of cell proliferation (for review see Klein and Klein, 1985).

The c-myc gene is made up of three exons. The last two exons encode a protein of 439 amino acids. No translation initiation site is found in the first exon. Consequently c-myc RNAs, initiated at two promoters separated by about 150bp, bear unusually long 5' non coding sequences of about 600 and 450 nucleotides whose role remains obscure. We have shown that c-myc RNA is extremely unstable in normal and tumor cells and suggested that its degradation involves factors that would be differentially affected in various cell types (Dani et al., 1984). Indeed we have pointed out that c-myc gene expression is modulated at the post-transcriptional level in various situations. First, the destabilization of cytoplasmic mRNA dramatically contributes to c-myc down-regulation in the lymphoblastoid cell line Daudi when growth has been inhibited by interferon (Dani et al., 1984b) and during the terminal differentiation of Friend erythroleukemia cells (Mechti et al., submitted for publication). Second, the stabilization of nuclear or cytoplasmic transcripts accounts for its up-regulation in quiescent hamster fibroblasts stimulated by addition of purified growth factors (Blanchard et al., 1985).

Alteration of c-myc gene expression either by amplification, retroviral insertion or chromosome translocation is probably an important step in the development of a large variety of neoplasms (reviewed by Klein and Klein, 1985). In murine plasma cell tumors (MPCs) and Burkitt's lymphomas (BLs) c-myc is

---

(abbreviations: BL: Burkitt's lymphoma, MPC: mouse plasma cell tumor, kb: kilobases)

Current Topics in Microbiology and Immunology, Vol. 132

frequently rearranged via reciprocal chromosome translocations with immunoglobulin heavy or light chain loci (reviews: Klein et al., 1983; Leder et al., 1983; Perry, 1983; Klein and Klein, 1985). Often in MPCs and less frequently in BLs the breakpoint is situated within the c-myc gene either in exon 1 or intron 1. In this case high levels of truncated mRNAs are produced from normally silent promoters located in the gene's first intron and sometimes in the immunoglobulin locus while no transcripts of the normal allele can be detected. We have recently shown in two MPCs (Piechaczyk et al., 1985) and two BLs (Eick et al., 1985) that a significant stabilization of abnormal c-myc RNAs contibutes to their accumulation to high levels in these tumors. In this report we extend our original observations to new MPCs and BLs. Moreover we show that the increased half-lives of truncated molecules is a direct consequence of the structural alteration and does not result from a stabilizing cellular context. We also suggest that the first exon by itself does not account for the extreme instability of normal c-myc RNAs. Finally we point out that the cytoplasmic stabilization of c-myc RNAs may sometimes be surprisingly counterbalanced by an active nuclear turn-over.

MATERIALS AND METHODS:

RNA analysis and run-on experiments were performed as described (Dani et al., 1984a, 1984b; Piechaczyk et al., 1984, 1985; Blanchard et al., 1985). Descriptions of cells lines are referenced in the text. Manca cells were a gift of S-M Fu and S. Chen-Kiang. LY65 and IARC 316 were provided by G. Lenoir and MOPC 315 by F. Mushinski. Hind III/Sst I and Sst I/Hind III fragments from pMYC 54 cloned in pSP65 and pSP64 were kind gifts of S. Bauer.

RESULTS:

ABNORMAL c-MYC RNAs FOUND IN SOME MPCs AND BLs ARE MORE STABLE THAN THEIR NORMAL COUNTERPARTS IN CONTROL CELLS.

In two MPCs (Piechaczyk et al, 1985) and in two BLs (Eick et al., 1985) abnormal c-myc RNAs generated from truncated c-myc gene were shown to be significantly more stable than their normal counterparts in reference cells. Here we extend our survey to two other MPCs: X63 (Dunnick et al., 1983) and MOPC 315 (Keath et al., 1984a), and to two BLs: Manca (Hayday et al., 1984) and LY 65 (Taub et al., 1984). The mouse pre-B cell line 1881.5 and the ABPC 20 MPC (Piechaczyk et al.,1985) as well as the immortalized human B cell line IARC 309 (Eick et al., 1985) and the IARC 316 BL, in which c-myc gene gives rise to normally sized mRNAs, were used as controls. RNAs turn-overs were determined by actinomycin D chase (Dani et al., 1984). RNAs were analysed by Northern blotting with the mouse cDNA clone pMYC 54 (Stanton et al., 1983). Half-lives were estimated after densitometer scanning of RNA blot autoradiographs. Results are listed in table 1 and compared to our previous data. They show that abnormal c-myc RNAs generated from genes broken either in exon 1 or intron 1 are significantly more stable than their normal homologues.

THE STRUCTURAL ALTERATION ACCOUNTS FOR c-MYC RNA STABILIZATION

The increased stability of abnormal c-myc RNAs in MPCs and BLs in which the gene is broken is likely a consequence of the structural alteration of the molecule. However one cannot exclude the possibility of a stabilizing cytoplasmic context. To rule out this hypothesis we compared normal and truncated RNAs in the same cells. For this purpose the MPC 11 cell line, in which only the decapitated c-myc gene is expressed, was transfected with a 10.5 kb KpnI genomic fragment bearing the intact mouse gene. Turn-overs of various RNA species were determined in a transient assay after transformation by protoplast fusion. Normal RNAs were assayed by RNAse mapping essentially as described by Kruijer et al. (1984)by

	MAN		MOUSE	
		half-life (minutes)		half-life (minutes)
CONTROL CELL LINES (normal c-myc RNA)	IARC 309 (1) (N)	15	ABPC 20 (5) (N)	15
	IARC 316 (2) (N)	15	18-81.5 (5) (N)	25
	BURKITT's LYMPHOMA		MOUSE PLASMACYTOMA	
c-MYC GENE TRUNCATED IN EXON 1	BL 67 (1) (MR)		J558L (5) (HR)	70
	2.4 kb RNAs	50	MPC 11 (5) (HR)	70
	3.5 kb RNAs	180	X 63 (6) (HR)	60
c-MYC GENE TRUNCATED IN INTRON 1	BL 18 (1) (SR)	50	MOPC 315 (7) (HR)	50
	LY 65 (3) (SR)	50		
	MANCA (4) (MR)			
	2.4 kb RNAs	50		
	3 kb RNA	180		

Table 1: ABNORMAL c-myc RNA APPARENT HALF-LIVES IN BLs AND MPCs.

(1) IARC 309 is an immortalized B cell line isolated from the same patient as BL67; (2) IARC 316 is a BL presenting a duplication of exon 2 and 3 but giving rise to normal c-myc RNAs; (3)(4) LY65 and MANCA are described in Taub et al. (1984) and Hayday et al. (1984), respectively; (5) 18-81.5 (pre-B cell line), ABPC 20 (MPC presenting no c-myc abnormality), J558L and MPC 11 are referenced in Piechaczyk et al.(1985); (6)(7) X63 and MOPC 315 are described in Dunnick et al.(1983) and Keath et al. (1984a).

(N) normal c-myc RNAs of 2.2 and 2.4 kb; (MR) Manca and BL67 exhibit two major c-myc RNA species. The shorter ones are clearly initiated at cryptic promoters situated in the first intron. The longer ones are transcribed from the immunoglobulin locus in BL67. (SR) Single RNA species of 2.4 kb in BL18 and LY65; (HR) numerous cryptic promoters situated in the first intron and sometimes in the immunoglobulin locus give rise to an heterogeneous c-myc RNA population (1.6 to 3 kb).

The lag time necessary for actinomycin D to block the transcription (5-10mn) was not taken into account.

using the 0.4 kb HindIII/SstI fragment of exon 1 cloned in pSP65. Truncated RNAs were quantified by the same method with the 1.6 kb SstI/HindIII fragment of the mouse cDNA clone pMYC 54 cloned in pSP64 spanning the end of exon 1, exon 2 and part of exon 3. At first, no normal mRNA was detected when total RNA was analysed either by Northern blotting or S1 nuclease protection experiments. Latter it was assayed by using polyA$^+$ RNA from 200ug total cellular RNA, highly radioactive probes and long exposure of the analytical electrophoresis gel. The very low level of normal c-myc RNA (at least 20 to 50 fold less than truncated RNAs) is problably due to either the allelic exclusion occuring in MPC 11 (Fahrlander et al, 1985) or the loss of enhancer sequences rather than to low transfection yields since high levels of neomycin messenger RNA were transcribed from the co-transfected pSV$_2$neo plasmid (Southern and Berg, 1980). Figure 1 shows that normal c-myc RNA is nearly three times less stable than truncated RNA molecules naturally found in this MPC. This indicates that the structural alteration of the molecule is responsible for its stabilization.

EXON 1 IS NOT ABLE TO CONFER INSTABILITY UPON STABLE mRNA

The absence of exon 1 from the stabilized c-myc RNAs raises the possibility

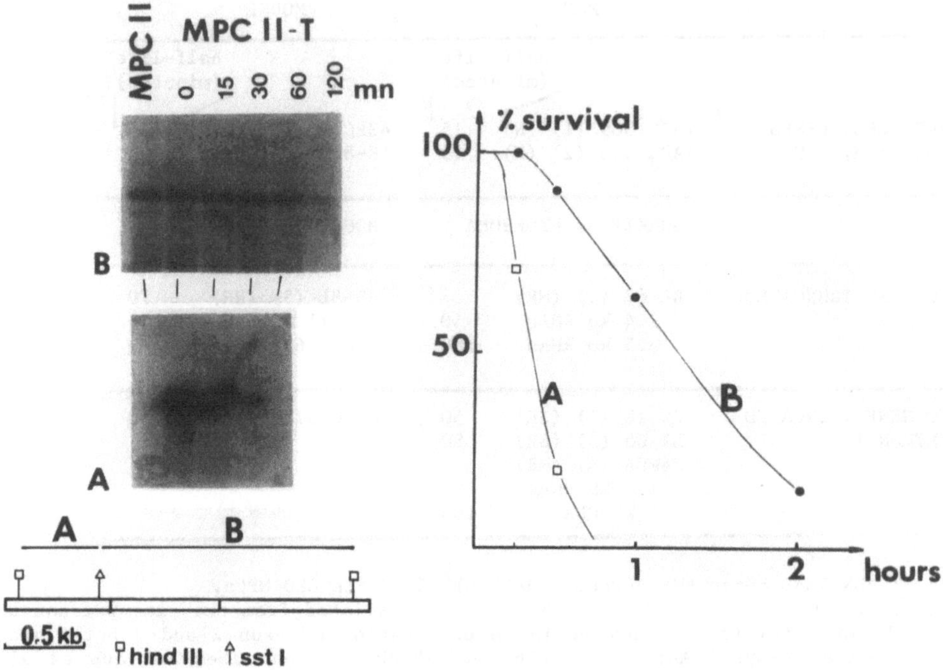

Figure 1: COMPARISON OF NORMAL AND ABNORMAL c-MYC RNAs IN THE MPC 11 MOUSE PLASMACYTOMA.

MPC 11 cells were transfected (MPC 11-T) by protoplast fusion mainly as described by (Rassoulzadegan et al., 1982) with the 10.5 kb Kpn I/Kpn I genomic fragment bearing the normal mouse c-myc gene cloned in pSV_2gpt (Muligan and Berg, 1981). Truncated RNAs were assayed by RNAse mapping by using the Sst I/Hind III fragment of the cDNA clone pMYC 54 (Stanton et al., 1984) spanning exon 2 and part of exon 3 cloned in the pSP64 vector (probe B). Normal RNAs were assayed with the first exon specific Hind III/Sst I fragment cloned in pSP65 (Probe A). Half-lives were determined by actinomycin D chase as described in Dani et al. (1984). RNAse mapping was essentially carried out according to Kruijer et al.(1984). 10ug total RNA samples were used for truncated RNA decay measurements while poly A^+ RNA from 200ug total RNA was used for normal c-myc RNA turn-over determination. Protected RNA fragments were fractionated by electrophoresis on an 8M urea-5% polyacrylamide gel. A and B correspond to 7 days and overnigth autoradiographs, respectively.

that target sequences for rapid and specific degradation are located within it. To test this hypothesis we planned to link exon 1 to a stable sequence and after cell transfection to assay for a possible destabilization of the chimaeric messenger. The 1.7 kb Bgl II/Bgl II mouse genomic fragment bearing all the first exon and 5' upstream sequences was linked to the bacterial chloramphenicol acetyltransferase gene from pSV_2CAT (Gorman et al., 1981) as described in figure 2 (E. Remmers, submitted for publication). Mouse NIH 3T3 fibroblasts were stably transformed by the calcium phosphate precipitation method with this construction and pSV_2CAT. mRNAs half-lives were determined after an actinomycin D transcriptional block by carrying out S1 nuclease protection experiment using a CAT mRNA specific probe. Figure 2 shows that CAT and myc-CAT mRNAs are stable over a period of 4 hours while c-myc RNA rapidly decays. This indicates that if exon 1 contributes to c-myc RNA instability it is unable by itself to confer any instability upon another messenger sequence.

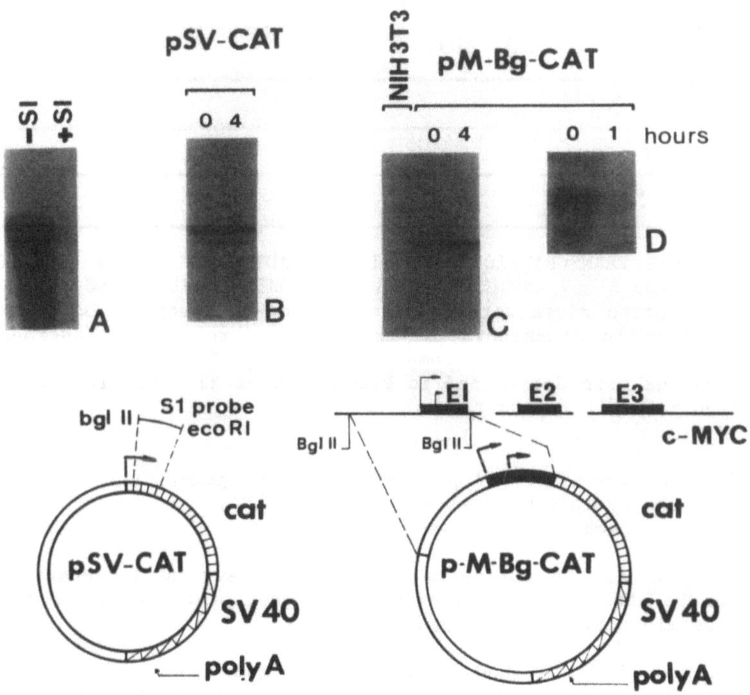

Figure 2: THE c-MYC GENE FIRST EXON IS NOT ABLE TO CONFER SOME INSTABILITY TO THE CHLORAMPHENICOL ACETYTRANSFERASE MESSENGER

Stable NIH 3T3 transformants were established by transfection by the calcium phosphate method with pSV_2CAT and p-M-Bg-CAT plasmids. p-M-Bg-CAT was constructed i) after deleting the SV 40 promoter-enhancer region and ii) inserting the 1.7 kb Bgl II/Bgl II fragment carrying the whole first exon of c-myc gene as well as upstream sequences so that CAT gene transcription is under the control of c-myc promoters (E. Remmers et al., submitted). Half-lives were determined by actinomycin D chase. For each time point 25 ug total RNA samples were assayed for CAT mRNA by S1 protection experiment using the 252 nucleotides Bgl II/Eco RI CAT specific fragment cloned in M13.

(A) CAT probe (+25ug tRNA) incubated in the presence or in the abscence of S1 nuclease,

(B) CAT mRNA stability analysis in transfected mouse NIH 3T3 cells,

(C) CAT mRNA assay in non transfected NIH 3T3 cells and myc-CAT mRNA stability analysis in transfected NIH 3T3 cells,

(D) to rule out a possible titration of c-myc specific RNAses by chimaeric messengers transcribed from p-M-Bg-CAT, the instability of normal c-myc RNA was controled by Northern blotting analysis.

TRUNCATED c-MYC TRANSCRIPTS ARE SOMETIMES ACTIVELY DEGRADED IN THE NUCLEUS

For a given gene, if we assume that RNA decay is exponential and if there is no differential nuclear regulation then we have the relationship:

$$\frac{N_A \times T_A}{n_A} = \frac{N_B \times T_B}{n_B}$$

in which: - A and B are two different cell lines,

	MAN		MOUSE	
	IARC 309	BL 67	18-81	J558L
mRNA steady-state levels	1	2.5	1	2.5
Half-lives	1	6	1	3.5
Transcription rates	1	3	1	1

Table 2: c-MYC GENE TRANSCRIPTIONS AND mRNA STEADY-STATE LEVELS AND STABILITIES IN HUMAN IARC 309 and BL 67 AND MOUSE 18-81.5 AND J558L CELL LINES.

c-myc transcription rates were compared by run-on assay on in vitro isolated nuclei as described in Piechaczyk et al. (1984). Probes are described in the text. Steady-state levels were compared both by Northern and dot blotting analysis. Half-lives were determined in Piechaczyk et al. and Eick et al. (1985). Values are given in arbitrary units.

- N is the number of RNA polymerases on the gene,
- T is the cytoplasmic half-live of the mRNA,
- n is the number of mRNA molecules.

The ratio N_A/N_B can be estimated by run-on assays on isolated nuclei. The ratio n_A/n_B can be estimated by comparing RNA steady state levels in the two cell lines. T is determined by actinomycin D chase.

We have compared N, T and n for c-myc gene in a BL (BL67) and an immortalized human B cell line (IARC 309) isolated from the same patient (Eick et al., 1985) as well as in the MPC J558L and the pre-B cell line 18-81.5 (Piechaczyk et al., 1985). The Pst I/Pst I fragment of the human cDNA clone pRYC 7.4 spanning part of the second exon and the entire third exon and the Xba I/Xho I mouse genomic fragment spanning exon 2, intron 2 and exon 3 cloned in M13 phages were used as homologous probes for run-on assays. Two major abnormal c-myc RNAs are synthesized in BL67. We have considered the half-life of the whole population since our run-on assay on isolated nuclei does not allow to discriminate the two units of transcription. Results are presented in table 2. The relationship presented above is obviously not observed in the case of BL 67 and IARC 309 suggesting that abnormal c-myc transcripts are more actively degraded in the nucleus of the former than normal ones in the reference cell line. At variance the increased stability of truncated c-myc RNAs found in J558L accounts for their higher steady-state levels as compared to normal RNAs synthesized in 18-81.5 (Piechaczyk et al., 1985).

DISCUSSION:

What are the determinants for rapid c-myc RNA degradation?

It is clear from our results (Piechaczyk et al.,1985; Eick et al., 1985; this paper) that its structural alteration entails c-myc RNA stabilization in MPCs and BLs in which the gene is decapitated. However it is not clear if the loss of exon 1 or, alternatively, the acquisition of new sequences is responsible for the increased half-life. Consequently no role can be assigned yet to exon 1 in normal c-myc RNA degradation. As a matter of fact we have found that chimaeric myc-CAT messengers carrying the first exon (this work) as well as naturally occuring RNAs made up of exon 1 and part of intron 1 (Eick et al., 1985) are stable molecules. This idea is reinforced by the finding of abnormally sized c-myc RNAs bearing all or nearly all exon 1 in the plasmacytomas TEPC 2027 and TEPC 1165, respectively which are also very stable (S. Bauer et al., this volume).

If truncated c-myc RNAs found in MPCs are stabilized ($t_{1/2}$=50-70 mn) we must remark that they are still unstable compared to the average half-life of 8-10 hours of mRNAs in dividing cells. This leads us to speculate that targets for specific degradation might reside in the 3' moiety of the molecule. However, when different abnormal RNAs are found in the same BL such as Manca (this work) or BL 67 (Eick et al., 1985) the longer species are more stable than the shorter ones. This indicates that additional sequences can decrease the turn-over of unstable RNAs. In other words they probably diminish the ability of target sequences to be recognized (or cut) by specific degradation enzymes probably by modifying the secondary or tertiary structure of the RNA.

In conclusion we would like to suggest that: i) important determinant(s) for rapid c-myc RNA degradation might be located in the 3' part of the molecule, ii) the structure of the molecule is probably an important parameter for its rapid decay, iii) if exon 1 contributes to extreme c-myc RNA instability it must act either in association with downstream sequences or by contributing to the nucleation of an optimal configuration of this messenger.

Abnormal c-myc RNAs transcripts may be actively degraded in the nucleus.

A previous study showed that their longer half-lives account for the higher steady-state levels of truncated c-myc RNAs in two plasmacytomas as compared to their normal homologues in control cells. The comparison of transcription rates of normal and rearranged c-myc genes in two human cell lines as well as the steady-state levels and turn-overs of their respective mRNAs suggests that abnormal c-myc transcripts are more actively degraded in the nucleus than their normal counterparts. In conclusion we would like to suggest that, in addition to possible enhanced transcription, various post-transcriptional mechanisms may play a significant role in the accumulation of truncated myc RNAs in murine plasma cell tumors and Burkitt's lymphomas. The more documented one is the cytoplasmic stabilization of RNA species (Piechaczyk et al., 1985; Eick et al., 1985; Rabbitts et al., 1985). However, we believe that this deregulation can sometimes be counterbalanced by an active degradation of abnormal c-myc transcripts in the nucleus. In agreement with this idea it was found in an independant study (S. Bauer et al., this volume) that the abnormally high levels of atypically large c-myc RNAs in the TEPC 1165 and TEPC 2027 plasmacytomas probably result from a balance between an enhanced transcription of c-myc locus and a perturbed nuclear and cytoplasmic metabolism of its RNA.

ACKNOWLEDGMENTS:

We are grateful to S. Bauer, Ph. Fort, F. Mushinski and Ch. Theillet for fruitful discussions and for critical reading of the manuscript. This work was supported by grants from the CNRS, INSERM, Ligue nationale contre le cancer, CRAM, and ARC.

REFERENCES:

Blanchard, J-M., Piechaczyk, M., Dani, Ch., Chambard, J-C., Franchi, A., Pouysegur, J. and Jeanteur, Ph. (1985) c-myc gene is transcribed at high rate in G_0 arrested fibroblasts and is post-transcriptionally regulated in response to growth factors. Nature 317: 443-445

Dani, Ch., Blanchard, J-M., Piechaczyk, M., El-Sabrouty, S. and Jeanteur, Ph. (1984) Extreme unstability of c-myc RNA in normal and tumor cells. Proc. Natl. Acad. Sci. USA 81: 7046-7050

Dani, Ch., Mechti, N., Piechaczyk, M., Lebleu, B., Jeanteur,Ph. and Blanchard J-M. (1985) Increased rate of degradation of c-myc RNA in Interferon-treated Daudi cells. Proc. Natl. Acad. Sci. USA 82: 4896-4899

Dunnick, W., Schell, B.E. and Dery, C. (1983) DNA sequences near the site of reciprocal recombination between a c-myc oncogene and an immunoglobulin switch region. Proc. Natl. Acad. Sci. USA 80: 7269-7273

Eick, D., Piechaczyk, M., Henglein, B., Blanchard, J-M., Traub, B., Koffler, E., Wiest, S. Lenoir, G. and Bornkamm, G. (1985) Abberant c-myc RNAs have long half-lives in Burkitt's lymphomas. EMBO J. 4:3717-3725

Fahrlander, P., Piechaczyk, M. and Marcu, K.B. (1985) Chromatine structure of the mouse c-myc gene. EMBO J. 4: 3195-3202

Gorman, C.M., Moffat, L.F. and Howard, B.H. (1981) Molec. Cell Biol. 2: 1044-1051

Hayday, A.C., Gilies, S.D., Saito, H., Wood, C. and Tonegawa, S. (1984) Activation of a translocated c-myc gene by an enhancer in the immunoglobulin heavy chain locus. Nature 307: 334-340

Keath, E.J., Keletar, A. and Cole, M.D. (1984) Transcriptional activation of the translocated c-myc oncogene in mouse plasmacytomas: similar RNA levels in tumor and proliferating cells. Cell 37: 581-528

Klein, G. and Klein, E. (1985) Evolution of tumors and the impact of molecular biology. Nature 315: 190-195

Kruijer, W., Cooper, J.A., Hunter, T. and Verma. I. (1984) PDGF induces rapid but transient expression of the c-fos gene and protein. Nature 310 711-716

Leder, P., Battey, J., Lenoir, G., Moulding, C., Murphy, W., Potter, H., Stewart, T. and Taub, R. (1983) Translocations among antibody genes in human cancer. Science (Wash.) 222: 765-771

Mulligan, R.C. and Berg, P. (1981) Selection for animal cells that express the Escherichia coli gene coding for xanthine-guanine phosphorybosyltransferase Proc. Natl. Acad. Sci. USA 78:2072-2076

Perry, R.P. (1983) Consequences of c-myc invasion of immunoglobulin loci: facts and speculations. Cell 33: 647-650

Piechaczyk, M., Blanchard, J-M., Marti, L., Dani, Ch., Panabieres, F., El Sabrouty, S. and Jeanteur, Ph. (1984) Post-transcriptional regulation of GAPDH gene in rat tissues. Nucl. Acids, Res. 12: 6951-6963

Piechaczyk, M., Yang, J-Q., Blanchard, J-M., Jeanteur, Ph. and Marcu, K. (1985) Post-transcriptional mechanisms are responsible for the accumulation of abnormal c-myc RNAs in mouse plasmacytomas. Cell 42: 589-597

Rabbitts, P.H., Forster, A., Stinsen, M.A. and Rabbitts, T.H. (1985) Exon 1 deletion stabilizes c-myc RNA. EMBO J. 13B: 3727-3733

Southern, P.J. and Berg, P. (1982) Mammalian cell transformation with SV40 hybrid plasmid vectors J. Mol. Appl. Gen. 1 327-332

Stanton, L.W., Watt, R. and Marcu, K.B. (1983) Translocation, breakage and truncated transcripts of c-myc oncogene in murine plasmacytomas. Nature 303: 401-406

Stanton, L.W., Farhlander, P.D. and Marcu, K.B. (1984a) Nucleotide sequence comparison of normal and translocated murine c-myc gene. Nature 310: 423-425

Taub, R., Moulding, C., Battey, J., Murphy, W., Vasicek, T., Lenoir, G. and Leder, P. (1984) Activation and somatic mutation of the translocated c-myc gene in Burkitt lymphoma cell. Cell 36: 339-348

Watt, R., Stanton,L.W., Marcu, K.B., Gallo, R.C., Croce, C.M. and Rovera,G. (1983) The structure and nucleotide sequence of the 5' end of the human c-myc gene. Nature 303: 725-728

Mutations which Stabilize *myc* Transcripts and Enhance *myc* Transcription in Two Mouse Plasmacytomas

S.R. Bauer[1], M. Piechaczyk[2], K.B. Marcu[3], R.P. Nordan[1], M. Potter[1], and J.F. Mushinski[1]

[1]Laboratory of Genetics, National Cancer Institute, National Institutes of Health, Bethesda, MD 20892 USA; [2]Laboratoire de Biologie Moleculaire, USTL, 34 060 Montpellier, Cedex, France; [3]Biochemistry Department, S.U.N.Y. at Stony Brook, Stony Brook, NY 11794 USA

INTRODUCTION

We previously reported preliminary findings concerning two mouse plasmacytomas, TEPC 1165 and TEPC 2027 which make abundant myc transcripts of 3.9 and 4.0 kb, respectively. A Northern blot of poly(A)$^+$ RNAs from TEPC 1165 and TEPC 2027 probed with various portions of the myc gene showed that the first intervening sequence (IVS-I) ends up in mature myc mRNAs of both tumors (Mushinski 1985). All three myc gene exons are present as well.

More extensive Northern blot analysis of myc RNAs in TEPC 1165 and TEPC 2027 revealed additional smaller myc RNA bands of 3.0 kb (TEPC 1165) and 2.4 kb (TEPC 2027). The TEPC 1165 3.0 kb myc RNA also contained myc exons I-III and 5' portions of IVS-I. However, the 3' portions of IVS-I were not present in the 3.0 kb myc RNA. The TEPC 2027 2.4 kb myc RNA contained all three myc exons but no IVS-I sequences and thus resembled the normal 2.4 kb myc RNA (Bauer et al. 1986).

S1 nuclease protection studies and restriction mapping of the cloned rearranged TEPC 1165 myc gene revealed a 200 bp deletion at the 3' end of exon 1 which could have removed the exon 1 splice donor site (Yang et al. 1985). The deletion could then lead to longer transcripts containing IVS-I. Subsequently, the rearranged EcoRI myc gene fragment from TEPC 2027 was cloned and mapped (see Results). We thought that a study of myc mRNA expression and gene structure in these two tumors might reveal information concerning regulation of myc gene expression in tumors and normal cells, since these tumors do not have interruptions in the myc coding sequence.

RESULTS

Restriction mapping of the rearranged myc gene from TEPC 2027 (Bauer et al. 1986) revealed that the 3 myc exons were in germline configuration. No deletions of the exon I-IVS-I junction were detected. However, the presence of IVS-I in the 4.0 kb myc RNA suggested that TEPC 2027 might have a splicing defect, so the exon I-IVS-I junction site was subcloned and sequenced in the M13 sequencing system (Messing and Vieria 1982). The same was done for TEPC 1165 to confirm the location of the deletion.

Current Topics in Microbiology and Immunology, Vol. 132

TEPC 1165 has suffered a continuous deletion of 194 bp which extends 69 bp into exon I and 125 bp into IVS-I. This removed the splice donor sequence and prevented IVS-I from being removed from the mature myc mRNA. No such deletion was discovered in TEPC 2027. However, the core sequence of the exon I splice donor site has undergone transversion mutation from GT to GA. Mutations within the core splice donor sequence have previously been shown to abolish splicing in human β-globin transcripts (Cech 1983). Thus, both tumors have IVS-I sequences in their myc RNA due to problems at the splice donor region of exon I. The lack of deletion in TEPC 2027 explains why its myc mRNA appears longer than that of TEPC 1165.

We next endeavored to understand the causes for the great abundance of myc mRNA in TEPC 1165 and TEPC 2027. An earlier study (Piechaczyk et al. 1985) had shown that in certain plasmacytomas truncated myc gene transcripts, which contained IVS-I sequences, had half-lives of 50-70 minutes, considerably prolonged from the short span of 20 minutes characteristic of most normal cells. Similar experiments were performed on TEPC 1165 and TEPC 2027 to determine if the abundant steady state levels of myc mRNA might be partially a result of transcript stabilization. Northern blots of RNAs were isolated from tissue culture lines of TEPC 1165, TEPC 2027 and 18-81 after increasing lengths of exposure to Actinomycin D. 18-81 is a pre-B cell line with an intact myc gene. The plasmacytoma lines were adapted to tissue culture in the presence of plasmacytoma growth factor (Nordan 1986). The Northern blots were probed with a full length myc cDNA, pMc-myc54 (Stanton et al. 1984). Intensity of myc RNA hybridization was measured by scanning densitometry. The results are summarized in Table 1. At time zero the amount of plasmacytoma myc RNA was increased 4-fold (TEPC 2027) and 11-fold (TEPC 1165) compared to the AMuLV transformed pre-B cell line 18-81. In contrast to this result, 18-81 and other plasmacytomas were shown to contain very similar amounts of myc RNA at steady state (Yang et al. 1985).

The 2.4 kb transcripts in 18-81 and TEPC 2027 had half-lives of 20 minutes which agrees with reported values for normal myc RNA half-life (Piechaczyk et al. 1985). The 4.0 kb myc RNA of TEPC 2027 had a half-life of 2 1/2 hours which is at least twice as long as the longest half-life reported in other plasmacytomas. TEPC 1165 transcripts were even more stable. The 3.0 kb message half-life was 5 hours, while the 3.9 kb mRNA half-life was almost 8 hours. It is clear that half-life elongation is at least one important contribution to the great abundance of myc mRNA in TEPC 1165 and TEPC 2027.

Enchanced transcriptional activation of the myc gene is another potential mechanism that could play a role in achieving the unusual abundance of myc mRNA in TEPC 1165 and TEPC 2027. Nuclear run-on assays were performed on nuclei from TEPC 1165 and TEPC 2027 to examine the rate of myc transcription in these tumors. Scanning densitometry data, taken from nuclear run-on autoradiograms (Fig. 1), were normalized to the invariant standard GAPDH (Piechaczyk et al. 1984) and showed that the rate of transcription of the myc gene was increased 4 fold in TEPC 1165 and 3 fold in TEPC 2027.

Results of half-life and nuclear run-on data are summarized in Table 1.

Table 1. Comparison of *myc* mRNA steady state levels, half-lives and transcription rates

	mRNA size (kb)	18-81	TEPC 1165	TEPC 2027
Steady state levels[a] (Relative)	4.0			2.5
	3.9		3.8	
	3.0		7.5	
	c-*myc* - 2.4	1		1.5
	Total *myc* mRNA	1	11.3	4.0
Half-lives [b] (Hours) [Relative to c-*myc* 2.4 kb RNA half-life]	4.0			2.5 [8]
	3.9		7.8 [24]	
	3.0		5.0 [15]	
	c-*myc* - 2.4	0.33 [1]		0.33 [1]
Transcription rates[c] (Relative)		1	4.3	3.5

[a]Relative steady state levels were estimated from densitometry scans of two independent Northern blots and normalized to 18-81 2.4 kb mRNA

[b]Half-life estimates based on densitometry of four independent Northern blots (two for TEPC 2027) and compared to 18-81 and TEPC 2027 2.4 kb mRNA

[c]Transcription rates based on densitometry of three independent nuclear run-on assays (two for TEPC 2027) normalized to GAPDH (known to be regulated post-transcriptionally, Piechaczyk et al. 1984)

DISCUSSION

DNA sequence analysis, nuclear run-on assays and mRNA half-life measurements showed that the unusual transcript sizes of TEPC 1165 and TEPC 2027 *myc* RNA resulted from the presence of IVS-I sequences due to structural alterations of the exon I splice donor sequence which inhibited splicing. The presence of these IVS-I sequences was responsible, in part, for the great abundance of these *myc* mRNAs since these and other transcripts containing IVS-I sequences appear to have prolonged half-lives. There may be multiple regions which affect *myc* transcript stability. For instance the 3.9 *myc* mRNA of TEPC 1165 is much more stable than the 4.0 kb mRNA of TEPC 2027. The

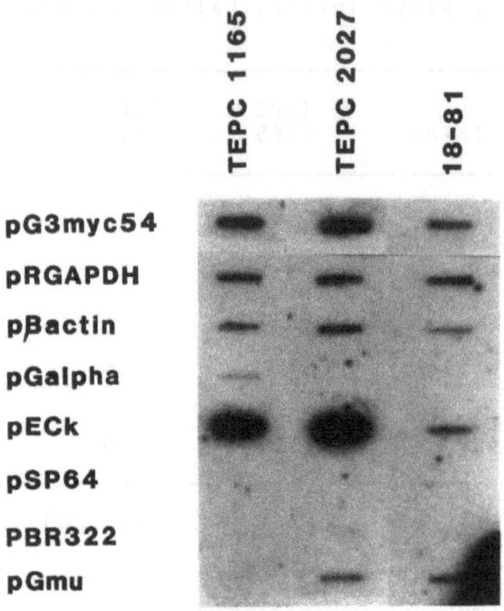

Fig. 1. Nuclear run-on assay for transcription rates. Nascent ^{32}P-labeled nuclear transcripts from TEPC 1165, TEPC 2027 and 18-81 were hybridized to nitrocellulose strips bearing a series of spots of 5 μg linearized plasmid DNAs. pG3myc54 was constructed by inserting the 1.7 kb HindIII myc fragment of pMc-myc54 (Stanton et al. 1983) into pGEM-3 (Promega Biotec). pGmu is a 670 bp Bam HI-PstI fragment from pμ3741 (Marcu et al. 1980) subcloned in pGEM-4 (Promega Biotec). pGalpha is a 560 bp EcoRI fragment from p107 alpha R5 (Early et al. 1979) cloned in pGEM-4. pRGAPDH (Piechaczyk et al. 1984), pECK (Coleclough et al. 1981) and pβactin (pAL41, Alonso et al. 1986) are described elsewhere. pSP64 and pBR322 were intact plasmids (Promega Biotec) used as negative controls.

only structural difference between the 3.9 kb transcript and the 4.0 kb transcript is the 200 bp deletion which includes sequences from exon I and IVS-I. Perhaps a destabilizing sequence resides within the deleted region. Also, the TEPC 1165 3.0 kb myc RNA is less stable than the 3.9 kb RNA (half-lives of 5.0 hr and 7.8 hr, respectively), while both TEPC 1165 myc RNAs are more stable than the 4.0 kb TEPC 2027 myc RNA (half-life of 2.5 hr). The TEPC 1165 3.0 kb myc RNA possibly arises from cryptic splicing within IVS-I sequences found in the 3.9 kb myc RNA. Cryptic splicing has been previously observed in mouse plasmacytomas where myc RNAs originate in IVS-I of myc genes truncated by DNA rearrangement (Marcu 1985). Removal of some IVS-I sequences by cryptic splicing may also remove stabilizing sequences, thus shortening the half-life of the 3.0 kb TEPC 1165 myc RNA relative to the 3.9 kb myc RNA.

In TEPC 2027 a normal 2.4 kb and a large 4.0 kb myc RNA have different half-lives. The normal 2.4 kb RNA has a half-life of 20 minutes while the large 4.0 kb RNA has a half-life of 2.5 hours. From this result it seems unlikely that the presence of exon I in myc RNAs is the cause of myc RNA instability but, rather, that inclusion of IVS-I sequences stabilizes myc RNA. This suggests that plasmacytomas with rcpt(12;15) translocations accumulate myc RNA because of prolonged half-lives that result from inclusion of IVS-I in truncated myc RNAs rather than the loss of exon I sequences.

In addition to the changed half-lives of the myc mRNAs, increased transcription of the myc gene also contributes to the great abundance of myc mRNA in these two tumors. We do not have many clues as yet to explain what factors are involved in this increased transcription rate. However, the myc gene rearrangements 5' of the myc gene exons in both TEPC 1165 and TEPC 2027 may have removed or disrupted a recently identified dehancer sequence located 428-1188 bp 5' of myc exon I (Remmers et al. 1986). Also, the mutations at the end of exon I in both tumors may reside within areas of the myc gene putatively identified as regions which bind soluble negative transcriptional regulatory factors.

Although we do not yet understand all the factors involved in these cells, these two plasmacytomas have provided significant clues regarding mechanisms that control the levels of steady state myc mRNA in normal cells and how they can be dysregulated in plasmacytomas. Both these tumors had undergone rcpt(12;15) chromosomal translocations. This karyological abnormality, typical of mouse plasmacytomas, is thought to be instrumental in causing a modestly elevated, constitutive steady state level of myc mRNA. The deletion and transversion detected in TEPC 1165 and TEPC 2027, respectively, are additional (probably subsequent) mutations that affect the myc gene and its transcription. This is an important documentation of one form of a second mutation that may be required to turn a cell with rcpt(12;15) into a malignantly transformed cell.

REFERENCES

Alonso S, Minty A, Bourlet Y, Buckingham M (1986) Comparison of three actin-coding sequences in the mouse; evolutionary relationships between actin genes of warm-blooded vertebrates. J Molec Evol 23:11-22

Bauer SR, Piechaczyk M, Marcu KB, Nordan RP, Potter M, Mushinski JF (1986) Mutations present in two mouse plasmacytomas increase abundance of myc mRNA by increasing both transcription and mRNA stability. (manuscript in preparation)

Cech T (1983) RNA splicing: three themes with variations. Cell 34: 713-716

Coleclough C, Perry RP, Karjalainen K, Weigert M (1981) Aberrant rearrangements contribute significantly to the allelic exclusion of immunoglobulin-gene expression. Nature 290:372

Early PW, Davis MM, Kaback DB, Davidson N, Hood L (1979) Immunoglobulin heavy chain gene organization in mice: analysis of a myeloma genomic clone containing variable and alpha constant regions. Proc Natl Acad Sci USA 76:857-861

Marcu KB, Banerji J, Penncanage NA, Lang R, Arnheim N (1980) 5' flanking region of immunoglobulin heavy chain constant region genes displays length heterogeneity in germ-lines of inbred mouse strains. Cell 22:187

Marcu KB (1985) In: Melchers F, Potter M (eds) Mechanisms of B cell neoplasia 1985. Editiones Roche, Basle Switzerland, p 225

Messing J, Vieira J (1982) A new pair of M13 vectors for selecting either DNA strand of double-digest restriction fragments. Gene 19:269-276

Mushinski JF (1985) In: Melchers F, Potter M (eds) Mechanisms of B cell neoplasia 1985. Editiones Roche, Basle Switzerland, p 237

Nordan RP, Potter M (1986) A growth factor required by plasmacytoma cells *in vitro*. In: Melchers F, Potter M (eds) Mechanisms of B cell *neoplasia* 1986.

Piechaczyk M, Blanchard JM, Marty L, Dani C, Panabieres F, El Sabouty S, Fort P, Jeanteur P (1984) Post-transcriptional regulation of glyceraldehyde-3-phosphate dehydrogenase gene expression in rat tissues. Nucl Acids Res 12:6951-6963

Piechaczyk M, Yang JQ, Blanchard JM, Jeanteur P, Marcu KB (1985) Post-transcriptional mechanisms are responsible for accumulation of truncated c-myc RNAs in murine plasma cell tumors. Cell 42: 589-597

Remmers EF, Yang J-Q, Marcu KB (1986) A negative transcriptional control element located upstream of the murine c-*myc* gene. EMBO J 5 (in press)

Stanton LW, Watt R, Marcu KB (1983) Translocation, breakage and truncated transcripts of the c-myc oncogene in murine plasmacytomas. Nature 303:401-406

Yang JQ, Bauer SR, Mushinski JF, Marcu KB (1985) Chromosome translocations clustered 5' of the murine c-*myc* gene qualitatively affect promoter usage: implications for the site of normal c-myc regulation. EMBO 4:1441-1447

Studies on c-*myc* Regulation in Normal and Transformed Cells

K. B. Marcu, P. D. Fahrlander, M. A. Julius, A. Nepveu, E. F. Remmers and J. Q. Yang

Biochemistry Dept., SUNY at Stony Brook, Stony Brook, NY, 11794

INTRODUCTION

Structural alterations involving the c-myc locus and concomitant dysregulation of this proto-oncogene's normal pattern of expression are common features of a variety of tumors and transformed cells. The structural changes which have been identified thus far are chromosome translocation, retroviral insertion and DNA amplification (Klein and Klein, 1985; Cory, 1986).

The c-myc proto-oncogene is expressed from two promoters (P_1 and P_2) in a wide variety of cell types (Stewart et al, 1985; Yang et al., 1985). Normal c-myc RNAs (Dani et al, 1984) and the 62-64 KD c-myc polypeptide (Hann and Eisenman, 1984) are highly unstable in vivo. The c-myc protein has been localized within the nucleus and has been proposed to contribute to a cell's competence to enter and progress through the cell cycle (Thompson et al, 1985). Transcriptional and post-transcriptional mechanisms are responsible for alterations in c-myc expression. The addition of serum or defined growth factors to growth-arrested fibroblasts results in transient increases in c-myc RNA levels as a consequence both of increased transcription and enhanced messenger stability (Greenberg and Ziff, 1984; Blanchard et al, 1985), although the relative contributions of these two factors to c-myc induction remain controversial. The contribution(s) of the c-myc gene product (which seems to be qualitatively normal in most tumors exhibiting abnormal c-myc expression) to the proliferation of normal cells or to the development of a transformed phenotype are subjects of intense investigation. In murine plasma cell tumors (PCTs) and Burkitt lymphomas (BL) in humans, c-myc is generally rearranged via reciprocal chromosome translocation with the immunoglobulin heavy or light chain loci (reviewed in Klein and Klein, 1985; Cory, 1986). C-myc genes regulated by immunoglobulin gene enhancers were recently shown to generate B lymphoid malignancies at high frequencies in transgenic mice (Adams et al, 1985). In this report, we have summarized some of our recent studies on the regulation of c-myc expression in normal and transformed cells.

CHROMATIN STRUCTURE OF MURINE C-MYC LOCI

We have recently completed a detailed analysis of the chromatin structures of c-myc genes in different contexts in normal and transformed murine cells. In analogy to earlier work on the human myc locus (Siebenlist et al., 1984), a regular pattern of DNase I hypersensitive sites (DH) were observed upstream and within the gene in cell lines with actively transcribed, intact c-myc loci (Fahrlander et al., 1985b). The DH sites in the c-myc genes of a pre B lymphoma (18-81), a PCT with a 6;15 variant translocation (ABPC4) and in an A-MuLV (P160 strain) transformed NIH3T3 line (54c12) are shown in Figure 1. Four major DH sites are present in all three lines while a fifth site at the 5' end of intron 1 is uniquely present in 54c12. The c-myc locus in 54c12 is 40 fold amplified (Nepveu et al., 1985 and see section below). A summary of these results along with data on myc loci in other cell types is presented in Table I. We observed that c-myc genes broken by a 12;15 chromosome translocation retain only DH site V which may be associated with the cryptic intron transcripts commonly detected in this class of PCTs. DH site V is equally predominant in intact and broken myc genes and the broken c-myc loci do not appear to have other novel DH sites. It is particularly noteworthy that the normal untranslocated myc alleles in PCTs were found to be devoid of all five DH sites (Table I and Fahrlander et al., 1985b). The absence of DH sites in these normal myc alleles is directly correlated with their transcriptional inactivity (Fahrlander et al., 1985b). This observation is in contrast with the results obtained in Burkitt lymphomas (BLs) wherein the unexpressed normal alleles uniquely retain DH site I which is located 2 Kb 5' of c-myc (Siebenlist et al., 1984, Fahrlander et al., 1985b). The DNA sequence near DH site I of mouse c-myc was determined and compared with the analogous region of the human myc gene (Figure 2, Fahrlander et al., 1985b). The overall homology of these sequences was 58% while five lengthy stretches were >90% homologous. These regions of extensive homology are essentially the same distance from the P_1 start sites of the mouse and human myc loci and may define conserved regulatory sequences.

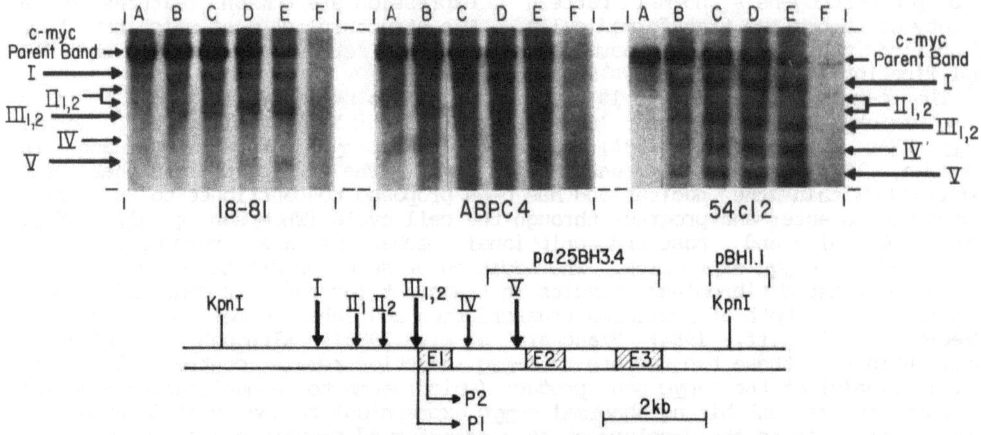

Fig. 1 DNase I hypersensitivity within and upstream of unrearranged c-myc. DNA from DNase I-treated nuclei was digested with KpnI and analyzed by Southern blotting; filters were probed with p 25BH3.4 (Stanton et al, 1983). 18-81 is an A-MuLV derived pre-B lymphoma, ABPC4 is a plasma cell tumor with an rcpt(6;15), 54C12 is an A-MuLV transformed fibroblast line with an amplified myc locus (Nepveu et al, 1985). Sub-bands generated by cleavage at different DNase I hypersenstive sites are indicated. Levels of DNase I were as follows (units/$2x10^7$ nuclei): 0, 1.0, 2.0, 4.0, 8.0 and 16.0 for lanes A-F respectively (Fahrlander et al., 1985b). The three exons and two promoters of c-myc are indicated.

TABLE I DH sites within the c-myc loci of different murine cell lines

Cell line[a]	Description[b]	Hypersensitive Site I	II	III	IV	V
NIH3T3	fibroblast	+	+	+	-	+
54cl2	A-MuLV fibroblast	+	+	+	+	+
18-81	A-MuLV pre-B	+	+	+	-	+
EA3-17	pre-B	+	+	+	-	+
FDC-P1	myeloid	+	+	+	-	+
MPC-11	PCT,rcpt(12;15)	-	-	-	-	+[c]
J558L	PCT,rcpt(12;15)	-	-	-	-	+[c]
C6T TEPC1156	PCT,rcpt(12;15)	+	+	+	-	+
CAK TEPC1198	PCT,inv(6;15)	+	+	+	-	+
ABPC4	PCT,rcpt(6;15)	+	+	+	-	+
ABPC20	PCT,rcpt(6;15)	+	+	+	-	+

a Origins of cell lines can be found in Fahrlander et al., (1985b).
b A-MuLV, Abelson murine leukemia virus; PCT, plasma cell tumor; rcpt, reciprocol chromosome translocation; inv, pericentric inversion.
c DH site V was only found on the translocated allele.

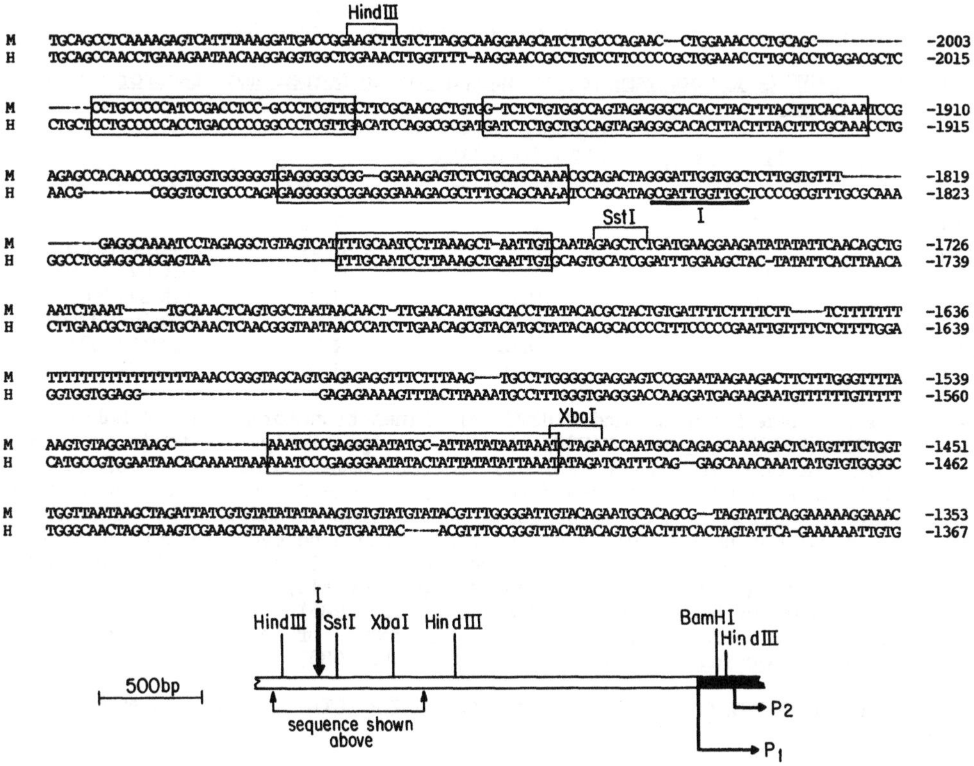

Fig. 2 Comparison of mouse (M) and human (H) myc DNA sequences near DH site I. Homologies were maximized by computer analysis. Regions of >20 nucleotides that are >90% homologous are boxed. Sequences are numbered with respect to the P_1 initiation site (+1). The position of DH site I in the human (Siebenlist et al, 1984) and mouse (Fahrlander et al 1985b) sequences is indicated.

The chromatin structure associated with DH site I may be necessary for transcription of a myc gene whose 5' flanking region is in germ line configuration, but is not, of itself, sufficient to result in transcriptional activity (Fahrlander et al., 1985b).

AMPLIFICATION AND ABNORMAL EXPRESSION OF C-MYC LOCI IN A-MuLV TRANSFORMED FIBROBLASTS

We have observed c-myc amplifications in three independent lines of NIH3T3 cells transformed by three different strains of A-MuLV (Nepveu et al., 1985). The c-myc RNAs in these cell lines are not elevated more than 2 fold over NIH 3T3 controls and they possess atypical promoter ratios with very low usage of the P_1 start site (see Table II). As shown in Figure 1, the majority if not all copies of the c-myc locus in 54cl2 reside in open chromatin. However, preliminary results of *in vitro* transcription studies with isolated nuclei indicate that the transcription of the sense strand of the myc coding exons is down-regulated (Nepveu and Marcu, unpublished results). Experiments performed with protein synthesis inhibitors suggest that c-myc expression is repressed at the transcriptional and post-transcriptional levels by labile factors in these cells (Nepveu and Marcu, unpublished results). It would follow that myc DNA amplifications in these cell lines did not result in commensurate increases in c-myc RNAs suggesting that other factors responsible for normal c-myc control must also be disrupted to result in deregulated myc expression.

TABLE II: c-MYC Gene Copy Number and Expression in Normal and Transformed NIH3T3 Lines

Cell line[a]	c-myc gene copy number[b]	Amounts of c-myc mRNAs (relative to NIH3T3 cells)[c]	P_1/P_2[c]	Retroviral Strains[a]
NIH3T3	1	1	0.33	
54cl2	19	2	0.07	A-MuLV(P160)
ANN-I	13	1.6	0.12	A-MuLV(P120)
N-25	8	N.D.	N.D.	A-MuLV(P90)
Ab92td	1	N.D.	N.D.	A-MuLV(P92td)
HA-821	1	N.D.	N.D.	MuSV(HA-821)
Hras(mx)6	1	N.D.	N.D.	HrasNVX

a 54cl2, ANN-1 and N25 and NIH3T3 cell lines transformed with A-MuLV(P160), A-MuLV(P120) and A-MuLV(P90) strains, respectively. 92td is an NIH3T3 cell infected with A-MuLV(P92td), a transformation-defective mutant. HA-821 is an NIH3T3 line transformed with the HA-821 strain of Harvey murine sarcoma virus. Hras(mx)6 is an NIH3T3 line transformed by HrasNVX, a moloney murine retroviral vector containing a neomycin selection gene and the Harvey murine sarcoma virus oncogene. References for the origins of cell lines and viruses are given in Nepveu et al., (1985).

b Expressed per haploid genome (Nepveu et al. 1985)

c Data was obtained from densitometric scans of autoradiographs of S_1 nuclease mapping experiments (Nepveu et al. 1985)

ANTI-SENSE IMMUNOGLOBULIN GENE PROMOTERS CONTRIBUTE TO TRANSLOCATED C-MYC EXPRESSION

The role of the immunoglobulin loci in activating the expression of translocated c-myc genes remains an enigma. That immunoglobulin switch regions are selected as targets for c-myc translocation is puzzling since the c-myc locus and the repeated sequence motifs of Ig gene switch regions are not significantly homologous (Stanton, Watt and Marcu, 1983; Stanton et al., 1984b). Furthermore, in most cases the known enhancer element of the C_H locus is present on the reciprocal product of the 12;15 translocation in PCTs. We therefore undertook a study to assess whether Ig heavy chain constant region (C_H) genes and their associated switch regions directly confer transcriptional competence to a rearranged myc gene. In order to address this question, we prepared a cDNA library according to Okayama and Berg to localize the promoters responsible for the expression of the disperse sizes of aberrant myc RNAs in the MPC-11 PCT which harbors a 12;15 translocation within the c-myc first exon (Stanton et al., 1984). Fifteen independent myc cDNA clones were isolated from such a cDNA library (Julius et al., unpublished results). As expected from earlier studies, a number of myc cDNAs were derived from transcripts that initiated from cryptic promoters within the c-myc first intron (Stanton et al., 1983; Keath et al., 1984). However, the largest cDNA clones, which presumably correspond to rearranged myc RNAs 2.4-2.8 Kb in length, had an unexpected structure as shown for one representative clone, pOBc-myc-12, in Figure 3. pOBc-myc-12 contains 400 bp of γ2a switch region sequence demonstrating that some of the myc transcripts in MPC-11 initiated to the 5' side of the broken first exon. The joining of the first and second exons is mediated by the normal myc splice donor and acceptor sites within the first intron. S_1 nuclease protection experiments and DNA sequence analysis demonstrated that the 5' end of pOB-c-myc 12 is colinear with the genomic DNA, that it is most likely full length and initiates from a promoter on the anti-sense strand of the γ2a switch region (Julius et al, unpublished results). Furthermore, these data also indicated that about 20% of MPC-11 c-myc RNAs at steady state derive from promoters that reside in the Sγ2a region.

These findings suggest that translocated c-myc transcription is under the control of promoters that are in association with C_H genes and in an opposite orientation with respect to them. We are also aware of an analogous case in a Burkitt lymphoma in which the transcription of an Sμ-c-myc translocation is contributed by a promoter that lies upstream of Sμ (Eick et al., 1985). Therefore, C_H switch regions seem to be transcriptionally competent in the absence of the known Igh enhancer element. Several reports in the literature have shown that the Igh enhancer is not required for the *in situ* maintenance of expression of a rearranged H-chain gene (Wabl and Burrow, 1984; Zaller and Eckhardt, 1985). We suspect that the Sγ2a region and possibly other regions within the C_H locus are transcriptionally competent prior to a c-myc translocation. It is important to note that a novel class of truncated constant region transcripts has recently been described in a mouse B-cell lymphoma that has the proclivity to undergo switch region recombination (Stavnezer and Sirlen, 1986). These novel transcripts are encoded specifically by C_H genes to which these μ^+ cells switch preferentially (Stavnezer and Sirlin, 1986). It has been suggested that regions accessible to RNA polymerase may also be more accessible to switch region mediated recombination (Stavnezer and Sirlin, 1986) and in this regard possibly to c-myc translocation as well.

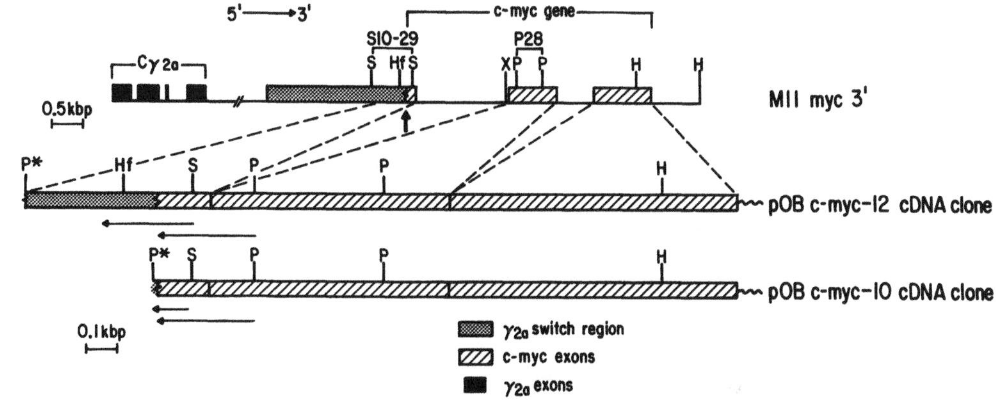

Fig. 3 Structural comparison of a genomic clone of the translocated myc gene derived from the MPC-11 tumor (M11 myc 3') and two myc cDNA clones derived from MPC-11 poly A^+ RNA. Restriction sites are: H, Hind III; Hf, Hinf I, P, PstI, P^*, PstI site introduced by cloning; S, SstI and X, XbaI. M11 myc 3' is described in Stanton et al, (1984a). cDNA clones were isolated from a library prepared from MPC-11 poly A^+ RNA according to Okayama and Berg (1983) (Julius et al., unpublished results).

A NEGATIVE TRANSCRIPTIONAL CONTROL ELEMENT IS LOCATED UPSTREAM OF THE MURINE C-MYC GENE

In this study, we have investigated the properties of cis-acting regulatory sequences within the vicinity of the murine c-myc locus by analyzing the expression of myc-CAT hybrid gene vectors transfected into a human lymphoblastoid cell line (BJAB) (Zech et al., 1976) and a monkey fibroblast line (COS) (Gluzman, 1981). Hybrid gene constructs were made by fusing portions of the murine c-myc gene to the bacterial chloramphenicol acetyl transferase (CAT) gene in a CAT vector, pCAT(ΔEP), which lacks enhancer and promoter elements (Gorman et al., 1982) (see pM(Bg)CAT and pM(Sm-Bg)CAT in Figure 4A) (Remmers et al., 1986). As shown for BJAB cells in Figure 5A and Table III, pM(Sm-Bg)CAT is about 3x more active than pM(Bg)CAT. Both of these vectors contain the entire c-myc first exon. However, the larger myc-CAT vector, pM(Bg)CAT contains 1.7 Kb of 5' flanking sequences while pM(Sm-Bg)CAT has only about 0.4 Kb of upstream sequences. This result suggests that a negative element may reside in the 760 bp BglII-SmaI segment at the 5' end of pM(Bg)CAT. S_1 nuclease analysis of RNAs isolated from HeLa cells stably transfected with either of these myc-CAT vectors demonstrated that the majority of the myc-CAT transcripts initiate from the normal myc second promoter, P_2 (Yang et al., in preparation).

We next assessed the ability of the putative negative element in the 760 bp BglII-SmaI fragment to repress the expression of a heterologous promoter. We inserted this 760 bp 5' flanking myc segment in either orientation 3' of the poly A addition site of an SV40 promoter and enhancer driven CAT gene, pSV2CAT (Gorman et al., 1982) (see pSV2CAT (Bg-Sm 3') and pSV2CAT(Sm-Bg 3') in Figure 4B). As controls for these vectors, we inserted other portions of the 1.7 Kb myc BglII segment into the same site 3' of the CAT gene in pSV2CAT (see pSV2CAT (Sm-Bm 3') and pSV2CAT(Bg-Hd 3') in Figure 4B). Results of experiments presented in Figure 5B and Table III show that only the 760 bp BglII-SmaI fragment dramatically inhibits the activity of the pSV2CAT vector. To directly demonstrate that attachment of the BglII-SmaI fragment 3' of pSV2CAT resulted in the reduction of CAT RNAs initiated at the SV40 early promoters, we assayed for CAT transcripts in COS cells transiently transfected with pSV2CAT(Bg-Sm 3') by S_1 nuclease protection (see Figure 6). COS cells were used to increase the sensitivity of RNA detection since vectors with SV40 replication origins are amplified in these cells (Gluzman, 1981). We also included an SV40-rabbit β globin expression vector, pSV2 βG, as an internal transfection control. As shown in Figure 6 in comparison to pSV2CAT and pSV2CAT(ΔE) (an enhancer deleted vector), no SV40 driven CAT transcripts are apparent in COS cells transfected with pSV2CAT(Bg-Sm 3').

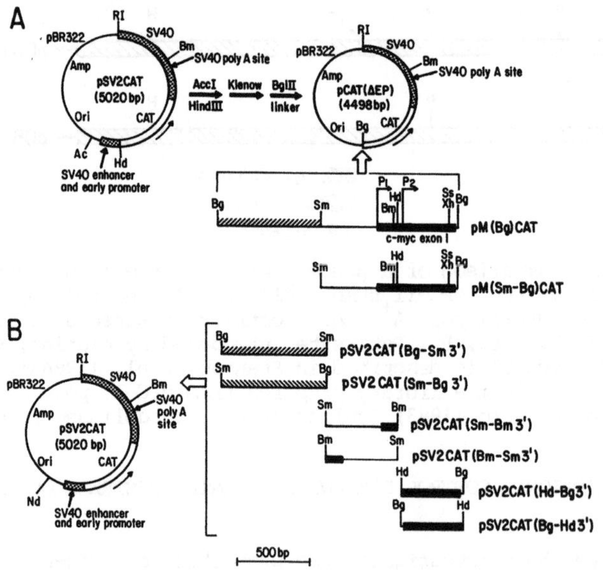

Fig. 4 Myc-CAT Vectors
(A) A 1.7 Kb BglII fragment containing the c-myc first exon and 5' flanking DNA was inserted in pCAT(ΔEP) as indicated for pM(Bg)CAT. pM(Sm-Bg)CAT was prepared by deletion of myc sequences 5' of the SmaI site.
(B) The indicated c-myc fragments were inserted in the BamHI site of pSV2CAT. Restriction enzyme sites are labeled as follows: Ac, Acc I; Bm, BamHI; Bg, Bgl II; Hd, Hind III; Nd, Nde I; RI, EcoRI; Ss, Sst I; Xh, Xho I.

We conclude from these independent experiments that the 760 bp Bg-Sm myc segment contains a negative control element which functions at the transcriptional level since it is located outside of the c-myc transcription unit. Enhancer elements have the opposite effect on gene expression (Banerji et al., 1981; Moreau et al., 1981). We propose the term "dehancer" for this 5' c-myc segment since it mediates many of the corresponding opposite effects. The myc "dehancer's" properties include: (1) acting at a distance of 400 bp 5' of c-myc and 1.7 Kb 3' of the SV40 promoter in pSV2CAT, (2) inhibiting expression in either orientation and (3) inhibiting the expression of a heterologous promoter. We speculate that this "dehancer" element may contribute to normal c-myc control by modulating the usage of the gene's promoters or by contributing to the down-regulation of c-myc expression in differentiated, non-proliferating cells. It is also conceivable that this negative region may protect c-myc from the influence of other nearby transcription units. The removal of the "dehancer" and/or its insertion into the chromatin domain of an immunoglobulin locus by chromosome translocation could contribute to the abnormal myc expression observed in a variety of B-cell tumors. Future experiments will investigate the physiological significance of this "dehancer" segment for c-myc gene expression in normal and transformed cells.

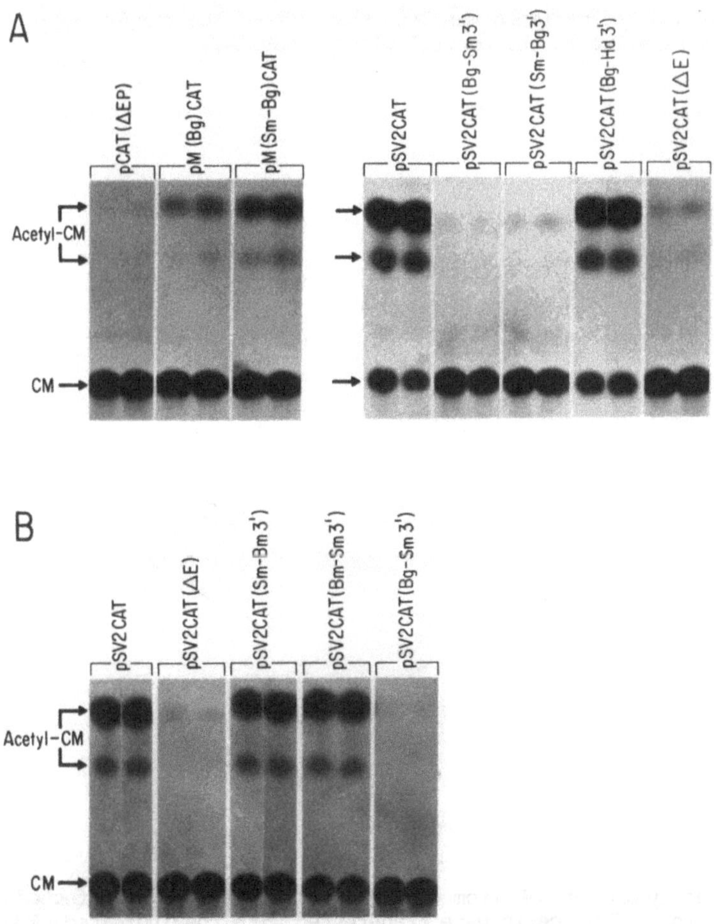

Fig. 5 CAT activity in BJAB cell lysates. A and B: BJAB cells transfected with the CAT vectors described in Figure 1 A and B were lysed and assayed for CAT enzymatic activity (Gorman et al., 1982). The two adjacent lanes represent independent transfections of each plasmid DNA.

TABLE III Relative Expression of myc-CAT vectors

Transfected plasmid DNAs	Relative CAT Activity of BJAB Cell Lysates*
pSV2CAT	100
pCAT(ΔEP)	0.9
pSV2CAT(ΔE)	2.8
pM(Bg)CAT	8.0
pM(Sm-Bg)CAT	23.5
pSV2CAT(Bg-Sm 3')	2.2
pSV2CAT(Sm-Bg 3')	3.3
pSV2CAT(Sm-Bm 3')	103
pSV2CAT(Bm-Sm 3')	116
pSV2CAT(Hd-Bg 3')	109
pSV2CAT(Bg-Hd 3')	110

* Cells were transfected by the DEAE dextran technique (Lopata et al, 1984, Mosthof et al., 1985). Lysates were prepared, assayed and counted as described (Lopata et al., 1984). Data presented are averaged from three independent transfections and the variance was less than 20% of the sample mean. All values are expressed relative to the control plasmid pSV2CAT.

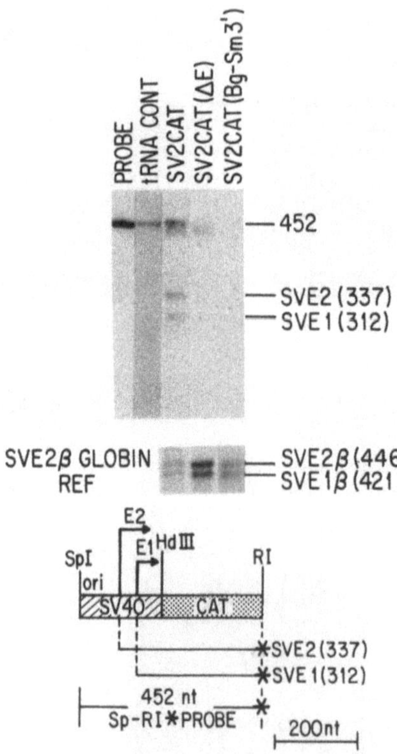

Fig. 6 S_1 analysis of RNA from COS cells transiently transfected with CAT vectors. COS cells were transfected with the indicated CAT vectors and an SV_2 β globin vector as a reference control. pSV2CAT(ΔE) lacks the SV40 72 bp repeat region in pSV2CAT but retains the SV40 ori and early promoters. The S_1 nuclease protected bands correspond to CAT or βglobin RNAs which initiated at the two SV40 early start sites in their respective vectors. Variations in $SVE_2\beta$ and $SVE_1\beta$ band intensities in independent samples are due to differences in gene transfer efficiencies which become more pronounced in preparative transfections.

REFERENCES

Adams JM, Harris AW, Pinkert CA, Corcoran LM, Alexander WS, Cory S, Palmiter RD and Brinster RL (1985) The c-myc oncogene driven by immunoglobulin enhancers induces lymphoid malignancy in transgenic mice. Nature 318:533-538

Banerjee M, Wiener F, Spira J, Babonits M, Nilsson MG, Sumegi J and Klein G (1985) Mapping of the c-myc, pvt-1 and immunoglobulin kappa genes in relation to the mouse plasmacytoma-associated variant (6;15) translocation breakpoint. EMBO J 4:3183-3188

Banerji J, Rusconi S and Schaffner W (1981) Expression of a β-globin gene is enhanced by remote SV40 sequences. Cell 27:299-308

Blanchard J-M, Piechaczyk M, Dani Ch, Chambard J-C, Franchi A, Pouysegur J. and Jeanteur Ph. (1985) c-myc gene is transcribed at high rate in G_o arrested fibroblasts and is post-transcriptionally regulated in response to growth factors. Nature 317:443-445

Corcoran LM, Cory S and Adams JM (1985) Transposition of the immunoglobulin heavy chain enhancer to the myc oncogene in a murine plasmacytoma. Cell 40:71-79

Cory S, Graham M, Webb E, Corcoran L and Adams JM (1985) Variant (6;15) translocations in murine plasmacytomas involve a chromosome 15 locus at least 72 kb from the c-myc oncogene. EMBO J 4:675-681

Cory S (1986) Activation of cellular oncogenes in hematopoietic cells by chromosome translocation. Adv Cancer Res (in press)

Eick D, Piechaczyk M, Henglein B, Blanchard J-M, Traub B, Kofler E, Wiest S, Lenoir GM and BornKamm GW (1985) Aberrant c-myc RNAs of Burkitt's lymphoma cells have longer half-lives. EMBO J 4:3717-3725

Dani Ch, Blanchard J-M, Piechaczyk M, El Sabouty S and Jeanteur Ph (1984) Extreme instability of myc mRNA in normal and transformed human cells. Proc Natl Acad Sci USA 81:7046-7050

Fahrlander PD, Sumegi J, Yang JQ, Wiener F, Marcu KB and Klein G (1985a) Activation of the c-myc oncogene by the immunoglobulin heavy chain gene enhancer after multiple switch region mediated chromosome rearrangements in a murine plasmacytoma. Proc Natl Acad Sci USA 82:3746-3750

Fahrlander PD, Piechaczyk M and Marcu KB (1985) Chromatin structure of the murine c-myc locus: implications for the regulation of normal and chromosomally translocated genes. EMBO J 4:3195-3202

Gluzman Y (1981) SV40 transformed simian cells support the replication of early SV40 mutants. Cell 23:175-182

Gorman CM, Moffat LF and Howard BH (1982) Recombinant genomes which express chloramphenicol acetyltransferase in mammalian cells. Mol Cell Biol 2:1044-1051

Greenberg ME and Ziff EB (1984) Stimulation of mouse 3T3 cells induces transcription of the c-fos oncogene. Nature 311:438-442

Hann SR and Eisenmann RN (1984) Proteins encoded by the human c-myc oncogene: differential expression in neoplastic cells. Mol Cell Biol 4:2486-2497

Keath EJ, Kelekar A and Cole MD (1984) Transcriptional activation of the translocated c-myc oncogene in mouse plasmacytomas: similar RNA levels in tumor and proliferating normal cells. Cell 37:521-528

Klein G and Klein E (1985) Evolution of tumors and the impact of molecular oncology. Nature 315:190-195

Lopata MA, Cleveland DW and Sollner-Webb B (1984) High level transient expression of a chloramphenicol acetyl-transferase gene by DEAE dextran mediated DNA transfection coupled with a dimethyl sulfoxide or glycerol shock treatment. Nuc Acids Res 12:5707-5717

Moreau P, Hen R, Wasylyk B, Everett R, Gaub MP and Chambon P (1981) The SV40 72 bp repeat has a striking effect on gene expression both in SV40 and other chimeric recombinants. Nucl Acids Res 9:6047-6068

Mosthof L, Pawlita M and Gruss P (1985) A viral enhancer element specifically active in human haematopoietic cells. Nature 315:597-600

Nishikura K, Ar-Rushdi A, Erikson J, Watt R, Rovera G and Croce CM (1983) Differential expression of the normal and of the translocated human c-myc oncogenes in B cells. Proc Natl Acad Sci USA 80: 4822-4826
Okayama H and Berg P (1983) A cDNA cloning vector that permits expression of cDNA inserts in mammalian cells. Mol Cell Biol 3:280-289
Nepveu A, Fahrlander PD, Yang J-Q and Marcu KB (1985) Amplification and altered expression of the c-myc oncogene in A-MULV transformed fibroblasts. Nature 317:440-443
Piechaczyk M, Yang JQ, Blanchard J-M, Jeanteur P and Marcu KB (1985) Post-transcriptional mechanisms are responsible for accumulation of truncated c-myc RNAs in murine plasma cell tumors. Cell 42:589-597
Remmers EF, Yang J-Q and Marcu KB (1986) A negative transcriptional control element located upstream of the murine c-myc gene. EMBO J 5 (in press)
Siebenlist U, Hennighausen L, Battey J and Leder P (1984) Chromatin structure and protein binding in the putative regulatory region of the c-myc gene in Burkitt lymphoma. Cell 37: 381-391
Stanton LW, Watt R and Marcu KB (1983) Translocation, breakage and truncated transcripts of the c-myc oncogene in murine plasmacytomas. Nature 303:401-406
Stanton LW, Yang J-Q, Eckhardt LA, Harris LJ, Birshtein BK and Marcu KB (1984a) Products of a reciprocal chromosome translocation involving the c-myc gene in a murine plasmacytoma. Proc Natl Acad Sci USA 81:829-833
Stanton LW, Fahrlander PD, Tesser P and Marcu KB (1984b) Nucleotide sequence comparison of normal and translocated murine c-myc genes. Nature 310:423-425
Stavnezer-Nordgren J and Sirlin S (1986) Specificity of immunoglobulin heavy chain switch correlates with activity of germline heavy chain genes prior to switching. EMBO J 5:95-102
Stewart TA, Bellve AR and Leder P (1984) Transcription and promoter usage of the myc gene in normal somatic and spermatogenic cells. Science 226:707-710
Taub R, Moulding C, Battey J, Murphy W, Vasicek T, Lenoir GM and Leder P (1984) Activation and somatic mutation of the translocated c-myc gene in Burkitt lymphoma cells. Cell 36:339-348
Thompson CB, Challoner PB, Nieman PE and Groudine M (1985) Levels of c-myc oncogene mRNA are invariant throughout the cell cycle. Nature 314:363-366
Wabl MR and Burrows PD (1984) Expression of immunoglobulin heavy chain at a high level in the absence of a proposed immunoglobulin enhancer in cis. Proc Natl Acad Sci USA 81:2452-2455
Yang J-Q, Bauer SR, Mushinski JF and Marcu KB (1985) Chromosome translocations clustered 5' of the murine c-myc gene qualitatively affect promoter usage: implications for the site of normal c-myc regulation. EMBO J 4:1441-1447
Zaller DM and Eckhardt LA (1985) Deletion of a B-cell specific enhancer affects transfected but not endogenous immunoglobulin heavy-chain gene expression. Proc Natl Acad Sci USA 82:5088-5092
Zech L, Haglund U, Nilsson K and Klein G (1976) Characteristic chromosomal abnormalities in biopsies and lymphoid-cell lines from patients with Burkitt and non-Burkitt lymphomas. Int J Cancer 17:47-56

Acknowledgements: This research was supported by NIH grants awarded to KBM. KBM is a research career development awardee of the National Institutes of Health and AN is the recipient of an FRSQ (Quebec) fellowship.

Characterization and Nuclear Localization of the v- and c-*myc* Proteins

N. Sullivan**, C. Green*, M. Pasdar*** and R. Watt*

*Smith Kline and French Laboratories, Swedeland PA 19479
**Cold Spring Harbor Laboratory, Cold Spring Harbor NY 11724
***Fox Chase Cancer Center, 7701 Burholme Avenue, Philadelphia PA 19111

INTRODUCTION

Both the human c-myc protooncogene and its avian retroviral counterpart, v-myc, have been associated with the malignant phenotype (Bishop 1983). In particular, alterations of the human c-myc gene, whether by translocation or amplification, have been associated with a wide range of human neoplasms (Yokota et al. 1986; Leder et al. 1983). Both proteins are known to be located in the cell nucleus and have been shown to bind to DNA in in vitro assays (Eisenman et al. 1985; Persson and Leder 1984; Watt et al. 1985). However the functions of the v- and c-myc proteins are still unknown.

To further characterize the c-myc protein and its nuclear localization, we have expressed and purified the full length human c-myc protein in bacteria. This protein has been used to produce both polyclonal and monoclonal antibodies, which specifically recognize the recombinant protein. These antibodies have allowed us to examine the subnuclear localization of the v- and c-myc proteins and the effect of selected treatments upon the nuclear translocation of the c-myc protein following microinjection. In addition, using a novel microinjection assay, we demonstrate that the recombinant c-myc protein can cooperate with the product of the Ha-ras gene to cause transient morphological transformation of primary rat embryo fibroblasts.

MATERIALS AND METHODS

Construction of Full Length c-myc Expression Vector

The full length c-myc protein expression vector was constructed by modifying a previously described vector, pOTS-myc (Fig. 1A) (Watt et al. 1985). Briefly, oligonucleotide-directed mutagenesis (Zoller and Smith 1982) was used to introduce a T to A transversion in the ninth codon of the myc coding region. This creates a new HindIII restriction site, without alteration of the amino acid sequence. Restriction with NdeI and HindIII, followed by addition of synthetic oligonucleotides, reconstructs the correct 5' end of the coding sequence. The resultant expression vector, c*-myc, encodes the full length c-myc protein with no additional amino acids at the amino terminus (Fig. 1A).

Protein Purification

The full length c-myc protein described above was expressed in the thermoinducible E. coli strain, AR68, transformed with the c*-myc plasmid construction and purified as previously described (Watt et al. 1985).

Current Topics in Microbiology and Immunology, Vol. 132

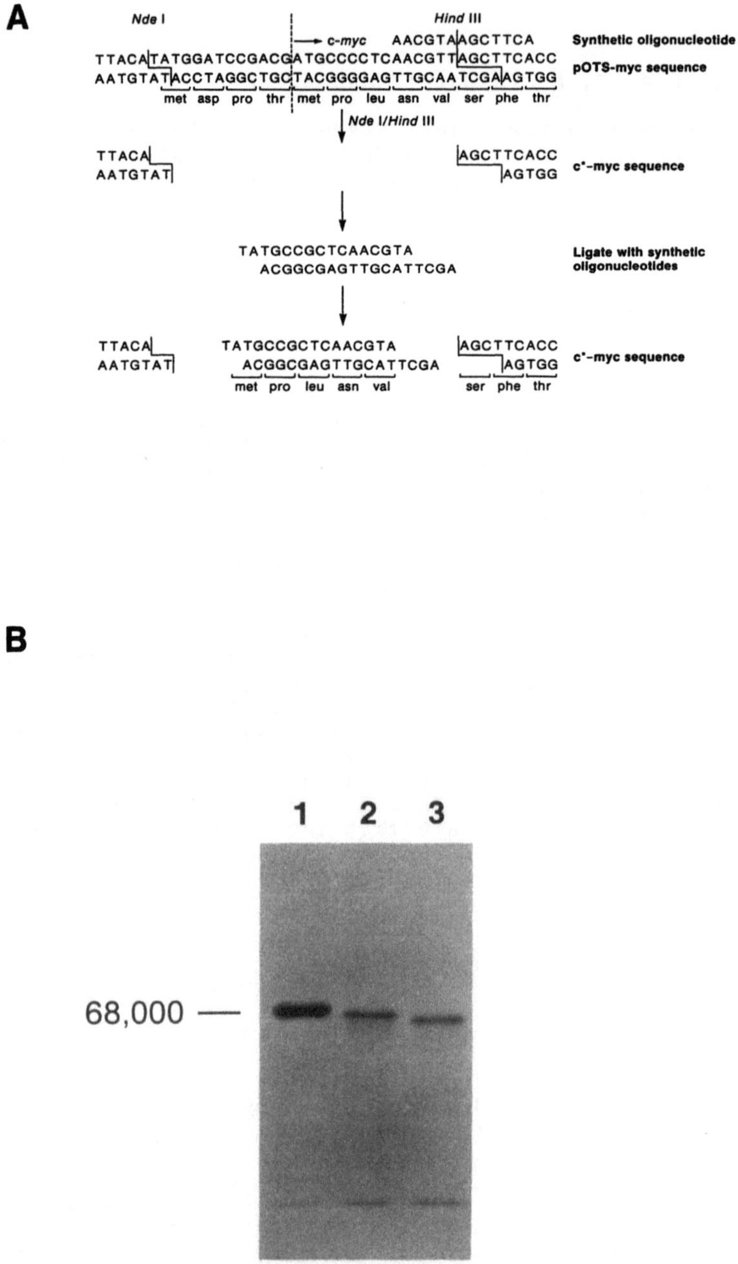

Fig. 1 Construction of c*-myc expression vector and protein purification. (A) Strategy for reconstructing the 5' end of the c-myc coding sequence (B) Purified proteins from the pOTS-myc and c*-myc expression vectors, analysed by SDS-PAGE. Lane 1, BSA marker; lane 2, pOTS-myc protein; lane 3, full length c-myc protein.

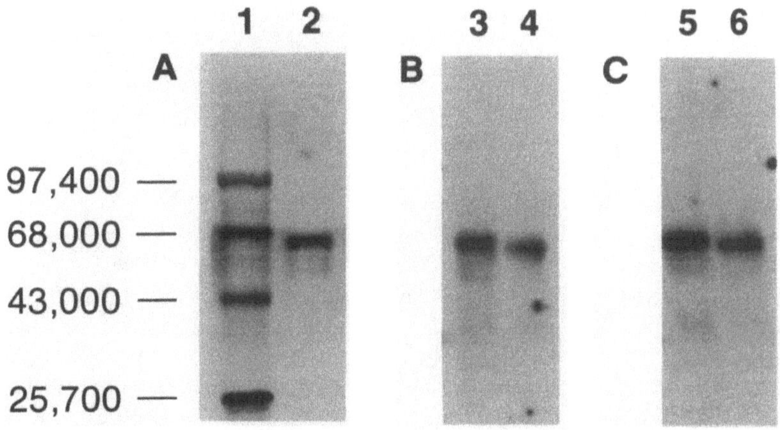

Fig. 2 Immunoblot of recombinant myc proteins with polyclonal and monoclonal antibodies. Samples were analysed by SDS-PAGE, transferred to nitrocellulose, incubated with anti-myc antibodies, followed by ^{125}I-labeled protein A. Panel A, rabbit polyclonal antiserum; panel B, mouse monoclonal antibody, B3; panel C, mouse monoclonal antibody, F5. Lane 1, labeled molecular weight markers; lanes 2, 3 and 5, purified pOTS-myc protein; lanes 4 and 6, purified full length c-myc protein.

Production of Monoclonal Antibodies

Hybridomas secreting monoclonal antibodies were produced by fusion of a mouse plasmacytoma cell line, SP2/0, with spleen cells from a 10 week old female BALB/c mouse immunized with recombinant human c-myc protein. The mouse was initially injected subcutaneously with 100ug of protein in Freund's complete adjuvant, followed by three boosts of 35ug of protein each at two week intervals. The serum was tested in an enzyme-linked immuno-absorbant assay (ELISA) (Voller et al. 1978). A final intraperitoneal injection of 35ug of protein in phosphate buffered saline was given three days before fusion. Hybridomas were cloned using the limiting dilution procedure. Of those hybridomas which reacted strongly in the ELISA, two (B3 and F5) were tested further by immunoblottting against the c-myc protein.

Affinity Purification of Antibodies

Monoclonal antibodies were purified from cell supernatants by diluting 1:1 with 0.1M phosphate buffer (pH8.0) and loading onto a 5ml column of protein A sepharose (Pharmacia), preequilibrated in the same buffer. After extensive washing, the antibody was eluted with 0.15M NaCl: 0.58% glacial acetic acid, followed by dialysis against PBS and concentration by ultrafiltration.

Immunofluorescence and Microinjection

Cells grown on coverslips were fixed in either methanol (30 secs., -20°C) or paraformaldehyde (2%, 20mins.) followed by treatment with

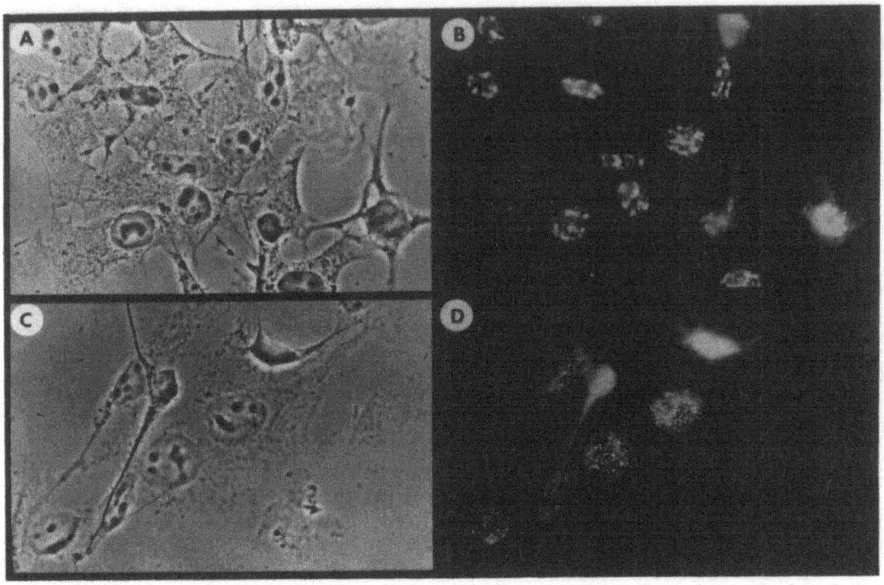

Fig. 3 Localization of the v-myc protein in Q8 cells. Panels A and C, phase-contrast micrographs; panel B, immunofluorescence with rabbit polyclonal serum; panel D, immunofluorescence with mouse monoclonal antibody, B3.

0.2% Triton X-100 in PBS. After washing in PBS, the first antibody, diluted in PBS (1:200 for the polyclonal antiserum, 1:50 for the monoclonal antibodies), was added for 20 min. at 37°C, followed by either rhodamine conjugated goat anti-rabbit IgG or rhodamine conjugated goat anti-mouse IgG for the polyclonal and monoclonal antibodies respectively. For fluorescence, cells were mounted in gelvatol (Monsanto) and viewed using a Zeiss fluorescence microscope. Microinjection was performed as previously described (Sullivan et al 1985).

RESULTS AND DISCUSSION

Construction of the Full Length c-myc Expression Vector and Protein Purification

We have previously described the construction of a myc expression vector, pOTS-myc, which encodes a fusion protein consisting of the full length c-myc protein with an additional 4 amino acids at the amino-terminus (Watt et al. 1985). As described in Fig. 1A and the Materials and Methods section, a modified vector, c*-myc, has been constructed, which expresses the full length c-myc protein unfused to any other sequence. This vector was transformed into the E. coli strain, AR68, from which the recombinant c-myc protein was purified after thermoinduction (Watt et al. 1985). The purified protein has an apparent molecular weight of 64,000 daltons as determined by SDS-PAGE electrophoresis (Fig. 1B) and has a slightly lower apparent molecular weight than the protein encoded by the original pOTS-myc vector, due to the removal of the four amino-terminal amino acids (Fig. 1B). This protein was used for the production of both polyclonal and monoclonal

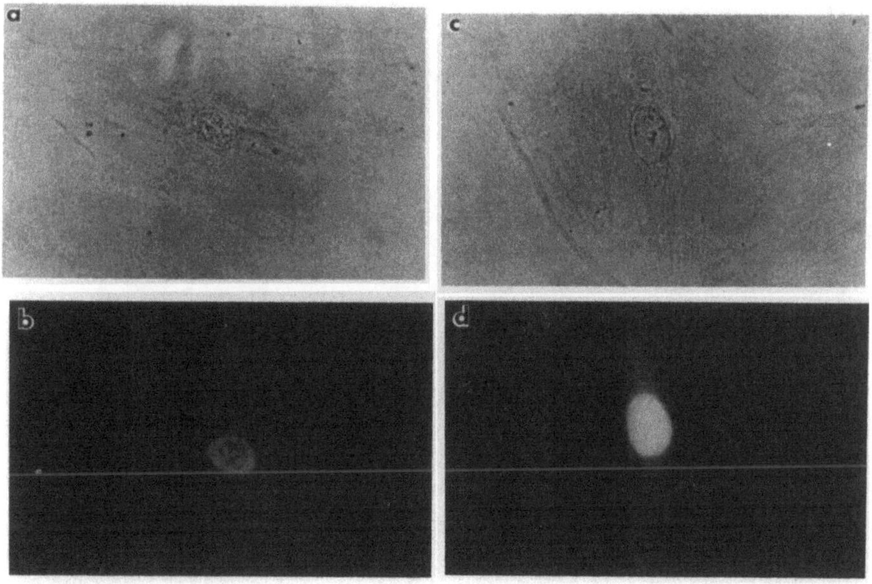

Fig. 4 Localization of microinjected recombinant human c-myc protein in REF52 cells, with (panels C and D) or without (panels A and B) treatment with actinomycin D. Panels A and C, phase-contrast micrographs; panels B and D, immunofluorescence with rabbit polyclonal antiserum.

antibodies, which are specific for the recombinant human c-myc protein (Fig. 2).

Detection of myc Protein by Immunofluorescence

The subnuclear localization of the 110kDa gag-myc fusion protein ($p110^{gag-myc}$ or v-myc) was examined in quail embryo fibroblasts retrovirally transformed with the avian myelocytomatosis virus, MC29, (the Q8 cell line) using both the polyclonal and monoclonal antibodies directed against the recombinant c-myc protein. It has previously been demonstrated that the polyclonal antiserum can selectively immunoprecipitate the v-myc protein from Q8 cells (Watt et al. 1985). As shown in Fig. 3B, the polyclonal antiserum shows v-myc to be localized to the nucleus and exhibits a non-nucleolar punctate staining pattern. Immunofluorescence using the monoclonal antibody, B3, shows a similar, but somewhat more punctate, pattern of staining (Fig. 3D).

To compare the localization of the recombinant human c-myc protein with the v-myc protein, the c-myc protein was microinjected into the cytoplasm of the established rat embryo fibroblast cell line, REF52 (10^{-14}l of a 1mg/ml solution of purified protein). When stained with the polyclonal antiserum against c-myc and a rhodamine conjugated goat anti-rabbit second antibody, the c-myc injected cells exhibited nuclear fluorescence with a similar punctate subnuclear localization to that seen with v-myc (Fig. 4B). Thus the v-myc and recombinant c-myc proteins similarly localize to discrete regions of the cell nucleus. Furthermore, after microinjection, the c-myc protein translocated to the nucleus within 5 minutes after injection and

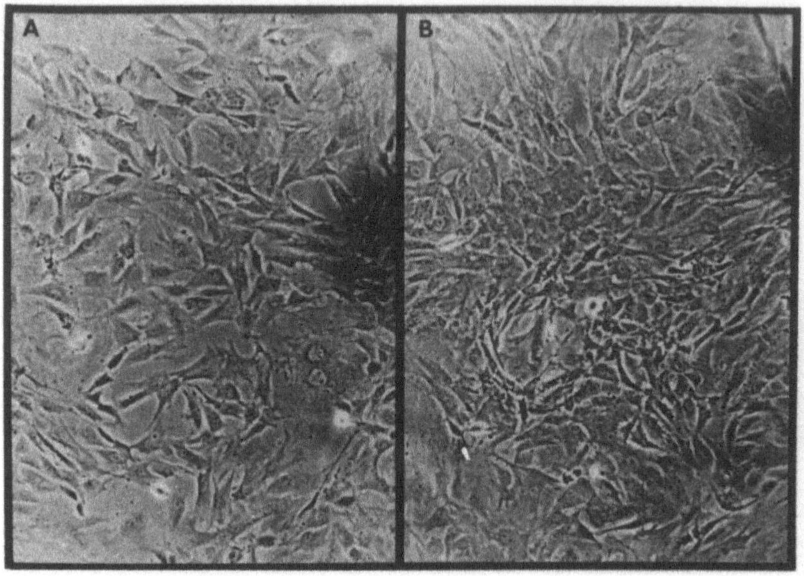

Fig. 5 Co-microinjection of recombinant human c-*myc* and Ha-*ras* proteins into primary rat embryo fibroblasts. Panel A, cells microinjected with Ha-*ras* protein alone; panel B, cells co-microinjected with c-*myc* and Ha-*ras* proteins.

remained detectable by immunofluorescence for 6-8 hours. To examine further the factors involved in the nuclear translocation of the microinjected protein, an attempt was made to block this translocation by treatment with a number of agents. Prior to microinjection, the REF52 cells were treated for three hours with cycloheximide (50ug/ml), actinomycin D (10ug/ml), monensin (100uM), or combinations of ATP depleting agents eg. a) 2-deoxyglucose (20mM) plus antimycin A (1uM), b) 2-deoxyglucose plus sodium azide (10uM), c) potassium cyanide (1uM) or d) dinitrophenol (1uM). None of these treatments appeared to affect the translocation of c-*myc* to the nucleus. Furthermore, heat shock treatment (2 hours at 42°C) either pre- or post-injection failed to prevent the protein from localizing to the nucleus. The only difference observed was in the case of treatment with actinomycin D, in which the microinjected c-*myc* protein exhibits a more homogeneous immunofluorescence pattern in the nucleus, lacking the discrete regions of punctate staining (Fig. 4D). This suggests that the *myc* protein may be associated with nuclear RNA, either as part of a transcription complex or some other RNA containing structure.

Cooperation of Microinjected c-*myc* and Ha-*ras* Proteins

The biological activity of the recombinant c-*myc* protein has been examined by testing its ability to complement the activity of the Ha-*ras* protein. Previous studies have shown that microinjection of the oncogenic (but not the proto-oncogenic form) of the Ha-*ras* protein into serum starved primary rat embryo fibroblasts (1°REFs) results in the initiation of DNA synthesis as determined by ^{3}H-thymidine incorporation, in a manner dependent on the amount of injected *ras* protein (Sullivan et al. 1985). Furthermore, microinjection of the oncogenic *ras* protein (10^{-14}l of a 0.5mg/ml solution) into these cells fails to induce morphological changes in the monolayer (Fig. 5A). However, when co-injected with the recombinant human c-*myc* protein (at 0.5mg/ml), the action of the *ras* protein was potentiated such that a focus appeared in the monolayer after 24 hours (Fig. 5B). This focus lasted for approximately one cell cycle after which the cells flattened out and resumed essentially normal morphology. Thus the recombinant c-*myc* protein can potentiate the action of *ras* in a manner analogous to that observed after cotransfection of the *myc* and *ras* genes into primary fibroblasts (Land et al. 1983).

ACKNOWLEDGEMENTS

We thank James D. Watson and Philip S. Schein for their support of this work, Ganesh Sathe for synthesizing the synthetic oligonucleotides and Ray Sweet for providing the Ha-*ras* protein.

REFERENCES

Bishop JM (1983) Cellular oncogenes and retroviruses. Annu. Rev. Biochem. 52: 301-354

Eisenman RN, Tachibana CY, Abrams HD, Hann SR (1985) v-*myc* and c-*myc* encoded proteins are associated with the nuclear matrix. Mol. Cell. Biol. 5: 114-126

Land HL, Parada LF, Weinberg RA (1983) Tumorigenic conversion of primary embryo fibroblasts requires at least two cooperating oncogenes. Nature 304: 596-602

Leder P, Battey J, Lenoir G, Moulding C, Murphy W, Potter H, Stewart T, Taub R (1983) Translocations among antibody genes in human cancer. Science 222:766-771

Persson H, Leder P (1984) Nuclear localization and DNA binding properties expressed by human c-*myc* oncogene. Science 225: 718-721

Sullivan N, Welsh W, Watt R, Bar-Sagi D, Ferguson B, Chao T, Kamata T, Sweet R, Gross M, Rosenberg M, Feramisco J (1985) Microinjection of oncogene proteins causes DNA synthesis and proliferation in nonestablished cells. In: Feramisco J (ed) Cancer Cells, vol. 3. Cold Spring Harbor Laboratory, p 243

Sullivan NF, Watt RA, Spector DL (1986) Association of the *myc*-oncogene protein with small nuclear ribonucleoprotein particles (snRNPs) Nature submitted

Voller A, Bartlett A, Bidwell DE (1978) Enzyme immunoassay with special reference to ELISA techniques. J. Clin. Path. 31: 507-520

Watt RA, Shatzman AR, Rosenberg M (1985) Expression and characterization of the human c-*myc* DNA binding protein. Mol. Cell. Biol. 5: 448-456

Yokota J, Tsunetsugu-Yokota Y, Battifora H, Le Fevre C, Cline MJ (1986) Alterations of *myc*, *myb* and *ras*Ha proto-oncogenes in cancers are frequent and show clinical correlation. Science 231: 261-265

Zoller MJ, Smith M (1982) Oligonucleotide-directed mutagenesis using M13-derived vectors: and efficient and general procedure for the production of point mutations in any fragment of DNA. Nuc. Acids Res. 10: 6487-6500

Characterisation of Human *myc* Proteins

Gerard. I. Evan, David. C. Hancock, Trevor. D. Littlewood, Nicolas. S. Gee.
Ludwig Institute for Cancer Research, MRC Centre, Hills Road, Cambridge CB2 2QH, England.

INTRODUCTION

The c-myc oncogene, the cellular homologue of the v-myc transforming gene of the avian myelocytomatosis viruses, is a highly conserved cellular gene found in species throughout the vertebrate phylum. C-myc can contribute to transformation of cultured primary fibroblasts when transfected together with the EJ ras gene (Land et al, 1983). Moreover, alterations in the structure or regulation of the c-myc gene are associated with a number of human tumours and transformed cell lines. In particular, genomic amplification of c-myc has been observed in cell lines derived from several tumour types such as small cell lung carcinomas (Little et al, 1983), promyelocytic leukaemia (Collins and Groudine, 1982) and colonic apudoma cell (Alitalo et al, 1983a) whilst chromosomal translocations involving both the c-myc and the immunoglobulin gene locus are ubiquitous in Burkitt's lymphoma (reviewed in Rabbitts, 1985).

The c-myc gene is just one of a family of mammalian genes each of which shares sequence homology. To date, this family comprises c-myc, N-myc (Schwab, 1985) and L-myc (Nau et al, 1985). The homology between these myc gene is most marked at two discontinuous regions located within exon 2 of c-myc, the so-called myc boxes (Schwab, 1985). The known myc genes also share similar structural organisation in the genome. However, whereas expression of c-myc appears to be common in many diverse cell types, both transformed and untransformed, expression of N-myc and L-myc is much more restricted. N-myc is expressed in teratocarcinoma stem cells (Jakobvits et al, 1985) and is amplified in certain types of neuroectoderm derived tumour, notably neuroblastoma (Schwab, 1985). L-myc is expressed and amplified in a significant number of small cell lung carcinoma cell lines. All the myc genes are expressed in early embryogenesis (Zimmerman et al, 1986) and they may play important roles in development.

PREPARATION OF ANTIBODIES SPECIFIC FOR THE HUMAN c-myc PROTEIN

To prepare antibodies against the human c-myc protein we synthesised a number of synthetic peptides containing sequences encoded by the c-myc open reading frame. The peptides were covalently conjugated to keyhole limpet haemocyanin and the conjugates used to immunise NZW rabbits. Two of these peptides (A and B corresponding to amino acid residues 171-188 and 408-439 of the inferred human c-myc protein sequence respectively) elicited antibodies which reacted with a 62/64 kDa phosphoprotein in cell lines expressing c-myc (Ramsay et al, 1984). Analysis clearly demonstrated that this 62/64 kDa protein was the human c-myc

Current Topics in Microbiology and Immunology, Vol. 132

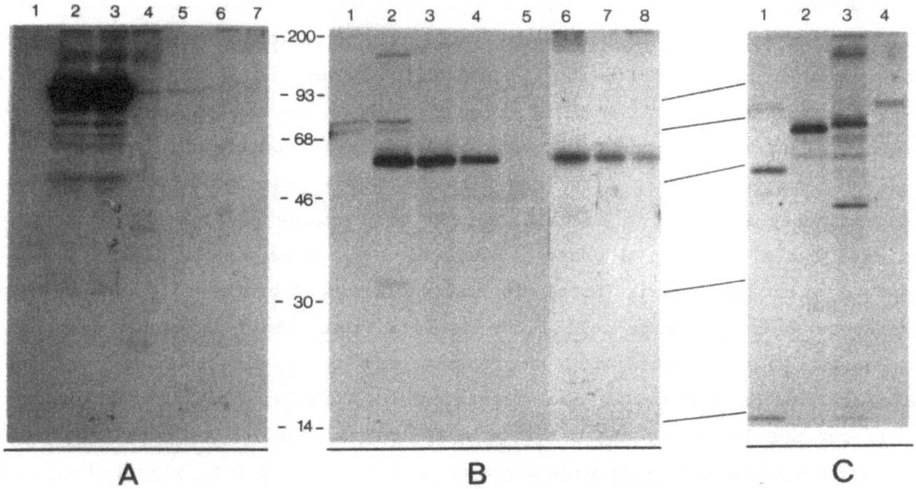

Figure 1 Immunoprecipitation of *myc* proteins from human, mouse and quail cells. Human Colo 320 HSR cells (B, and C tracks 1 and 2), mouse Rec2A fibroblasts (C tracks 3 and 4) and MC29 virus transformed quail fibroblasts were all labelled with ^{3}[H]-lysine for 1 h as described (Evan *et al*, 1985). Detergent extracts derived from each labelled cell type were then immunoprecipitated with various antibodies as follows: (A) Tracks 1, pre-immune rabbit serum; 2, rabbit anti-peptide B antibody; 3, rabbit anti v-*myc* protein antibody (Alitalo *et al*, 1983b); 4, MAb CT9-B7 anti-peptide B; 5, MAb CT14-G4 anti-peptide B; 6, MAb Myc1-8F9 anti-peptide A; 7, MAb Myc1-6E10 anti-peptide A. (B) Tracks 1, pre-immune rabbit serum; 2, rabbit anti-peptide B serum; 3, MAb CT9-B7; 4, MAb CT14-G4; 5, MAb Myc1-9E10 anti-peptide B; 6, MAb Myc1-8F9; 7, MAb Myc1-3C7 anti-peptide A; 8, MAb Myc1-6E10. (C) Tracks 1, anti HLA MAb W6/32.1; 2 and 3, MAb Myc1-8F9; 4, MAb W6/32.1. Molecular weights were determined using appropriate markers.

gene product, p62$^{c\text{-}myc}$. The same two synthetic peptides were then used to immunise BALB/c mice from which were isolated a number of hybridomas secreting monoclonal antibodies (MAbs). These MAbs also react with the c-*myc* protein as assayed by both immunoprecipitation and immunoblotting (figure 1). We decided to use these p62$^{c\text{-}myc}$-specific monoclonal antibodies to examine the characteristics and properties of the human c-*myc* protein.

CHARACTERISTICS OF THE HUMAN c-myc PROTEIN

Expression of the c-*myc* gene is regulated in a number of unusual and characteristic ways. C-myc mRNA is not expressed in quiescent untransformed cells but it is rapidly induced upon mitogenic stimulation (Kelly et al, 1983). This rapid induction following a mitogenic signal is a feature shared with several other genes, of which a notable example is the proto-oncogene c-fos. Together these mitogen-induced genes comprise the "competence" (Cochran et al, 1984) or "immediate early" (Lau and Nathans, 1985) gene family, members of which are presumably involved in enabling a cell to progress through the first part of the cell cycle and into S phase. Elevated c-myc mRNA levels (i.e. elevated as compared with the levels found in untransformed fibroblasts) are a frequent occurrence in many tumour cell lines derived from widely differing tissues. In some cases such elevated mRNA expression may be a direct result of genomic amplification of the c-myc gene (reviewed in Alitalo, 1985) or of chromosomal translocations involving the c-myc gene (Rabbitts, 1985). We were interested to know whether elevated c-myc mRNA expression invariably led to elevated expression of the c-myc protein. Accordingly, we compared the steady state $p62^{c-myc}$ and c-myc mRNA levels in a variety of cell lines by immunoblotting and northern blotting analyses respectively. The results are shown in figure 2. Clearly, the steady state levels of both c-myc mRNA and protein vary considerably in different cells and there appears to be an excellent correlation between the two. Of the cell lines tested, the lowest levels of c-myc expression are consistently observed in untransformed primary fibroblastic lines (lanes 1-3). In contrast to this, transformed cell lines with amplified copies of the c-myc gene (Colo 320 HSR, HL60 and N417) show much higher levels of both c-myc mRNA and protein. Of particular interest, however, is the finding that the transformed cell lines HeLa and CCRF CEM also have substantially elevated levels of c-myc expression although neither of these cells possesses a c-myc amplification. Our further analyses have shown that elevated c-myc expression is a common feature of many diverse transformed cell lines lacking detectable c-myc amplification. Thus, genomic amplification is not the only means by which a cell can accumulate elevated c-myc protein levels.

A further characteristic of the c-myc gene is its rapid repression when a susceptible transformed cell is induced to differentiate by one of a number of polar compounds (Westin et al, 1982; Lachman et al, 1984). The promyelocytic leukaemia cell line HL60 (Collins and Groudine, 1982) can be induced to differentiate along the granulocytic lineage with the concomitant repression of the c-myc gene by the addition of dimethyl sulphoxide (DMSO) to the growth medium (Westin et al, 1982). Our analysis showed that the disappearance of $p62^{c-myc}$ was very rapid and virtually complete by three hours post induction (figure 2; tracks 6 and 7). A more detailed analysis of the kinetics of disappearance of $p62^{c-myc}$ is shown in figure 3. In this experiment we have also investigated the fate of the c-myc gene product $p75^{c-myb}$ using anti-peptide antibodies. $P75^{c-myb}$ is

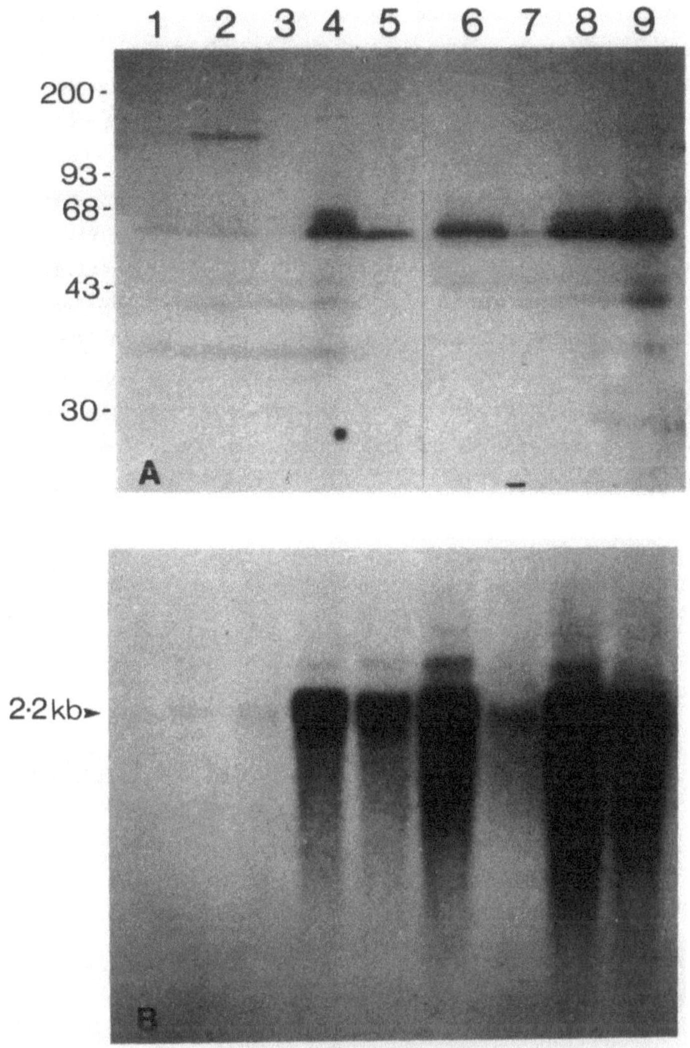

<u>Figure 2</u> Comparison of c-<u>myc</u> protein and mRNA levels in various cell lines. (A) Samples of 10^6 cell equivalents of each cell type were fractionated on a 10% SDS polyacrylamide gel and electroblotted onto nitrocellulose paper. The blot was probed with the human c-<u>myc</u> protein-specific MAb Myc1-9E10 followed by labelled anti-mouse Ig antibody. (B) Samples of 10µg total RNA from each cell type were fractionated on an agarose gel and probed with a c-<u>myc</u> probe.

another nuclear proto-oncogene product whose expression is common in cells of haemopoietic lineages. Figure 3 shows that levels of p62$^{c\text{-}\underline{myc}}$ begin to fall almost immediately following addition of DMSO to the medium, arguing that the protein is being rapidly degraded. Levels of p75$^{c\text{-}\underline{myb}}$ also fall but rather more slowly. At first sight these data appear consistent with the attractive model that high levels of c-myc protein prevent the HL60 cell from embarking on its differentiation programme, thereby giving rise to a self-perpetuating "transformed" clone. However, further analysis (unpublished data) has shown that the cells do not become irreversibly committed to differentiation unless they have been in contact with DMSO for at least 10 hours. If the DMSO is removed before this time, the HL60 cells do not differentiate even though both c-myc and c-myb proteins have virtually vanished from the cells after only 5 or 6 hours. Instead, c-myc and c-myb protein levels rapidly rise to their previous levels and the cells start dividing again.

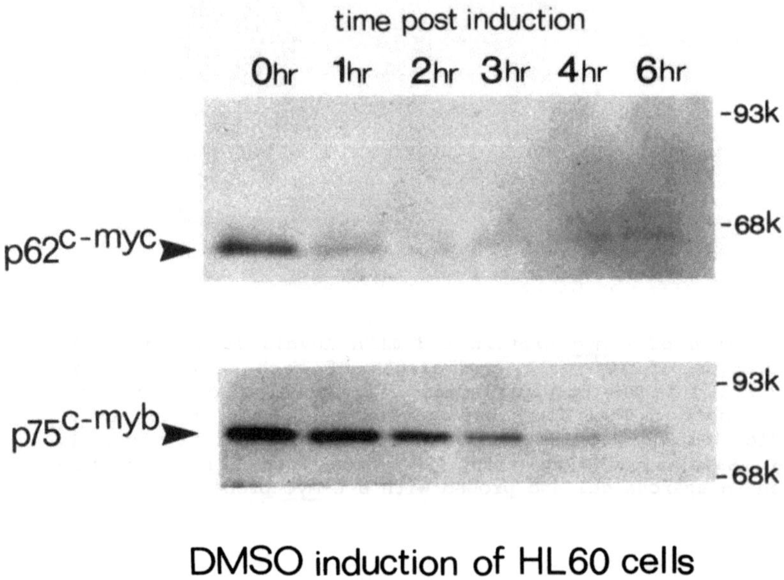

Figure 3 Expression of c-myc and c-myb proteins in HL60 promyelocytic leukaemia cells following induction with DMSO. Log phase HL60 cells were induced by addition of DMSO to the growth medium to a final concentration of 1.2%. Various times after addition of DMSO, 2 million cells were removed and fractionated on an SDS polyacrylamide gel. Duplicate fractions were probed with antibodies to the c-myc protein (MAb Myc1-9E10) or to the c-myb protein (rabbit polyclonal antibody).

SUBCELLULAR LOCALISATION OF THE HUMAN c-myc PROTEIN

Analysis of the avian v-*myc* proteins has shown that they all localise to the nucleus of cells (Abrams *et al*, 1982; Donner *et al*, 1982; Alitalo *et al*, 1983b). During metaphase, however, v-*myc* proteins become dispersed throughout the cell and show no association with condensed chromosomes (Winqvist *et al*, 1984). Presumably, therefore, it is within the interphase nucleus that v-*myc* proteins exert their transforming effect. We were therefore interested to know whether the human c-*myc* protein was also localised to the nucleus. We prepared nuclei by a variety of different methods from the two cell lines Colo 320 HSR and HeLa, both of which express c-*myc*. When cells were fractionated under conditions of low ionic strength, nearly all the $p62^{c\text{-}myc}$ in the cell is found associated with the nuclei, a result in agreement with those of others (Persson and Leder, 1984; Ramsay *et al*, 1984; Hann and Eisenman, 1984). The small fraction of $p62^{c\text{-}myc}$ not associated with the nuclei (about 5% of the total) is presumably nascent $p62^{c\text{-}myc}$ en route to the nucleus. However, when we fractionated cells in isotonic salt buffers (144 mM NaCl or KCl), we observed quantitative extraction of $p62^{c\text{-}myc}$ from the nuclei. This suggests the possibility that $p62^{c\text{-}myc}$ may be bound to its nuclear target(s) by an interaction which is largely ionic in nature and which may be quite weak and easily reversible under the ionic conditions prevailing within the cell nucleus.

We next sought to fractionate further cell nuclei so as to determine the subnuclear compartment containing the c-*myc* protein. The ultrastructure of the interphase nucleus is largely speculative. However, in the presence of non-ionic detergents and high salt buffers, nuclease-treated nuclei can be depleted of the majority of chromatin components to leave a residual "nuclear matrix". This nuclear matrix retains some of the morphological features of the intact nucleus. It comprises the nuclear lamina, three related proteins forming a proteinaceous shell around the nucleus, plus a number of other poorly defined proteins probably associated with the lamina via metalloprotein interactions (Lebkowski and Laemmli, 1982). Unfortunately, the composition of the nuclear matrix can vary considerably, depending upon the method used to prepare it and the cell type used as its source. This makes the precise definition of the nuclear matrix difficult.

A number of nuclear functions are reportedly associated with the nuclear matrix, including transcription, DNA replication and RNA processing. Because of this we felt it important to establish whether or not the c-*myc* protein was localised to the nuclear matrix or the soluble chromatin fraction. Such information might suggest a function for the c-*myc* protein. We prepared nuclear matrices by a number of different established methods, although all followed the basic pattern of exhaustive nuclease treatment followed by extraction with high salt (2M NaCl)

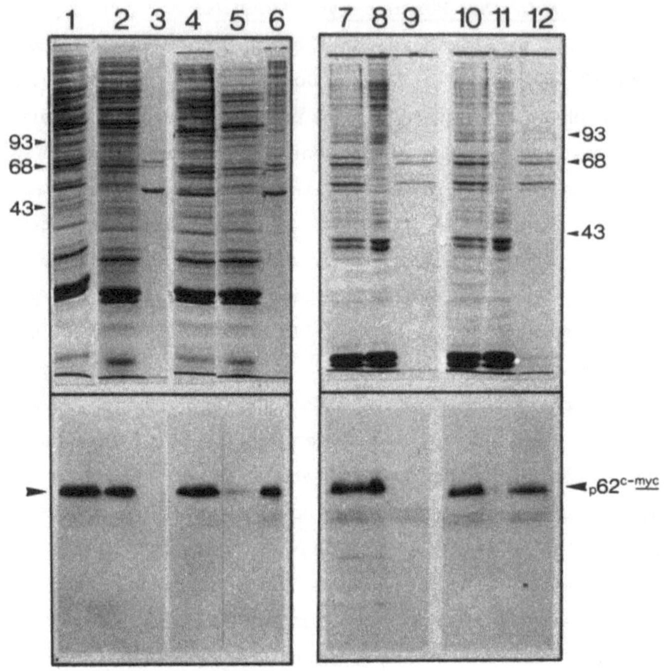

Figure 4 Fractionation of Colo 320 HSR and HeLa cell nuclei. Nuclei were purified as described (Lebkowski and Laemmli, 1982) from Colo 320 HSR cells (tracks 1-6) and Hela cells (tracks 7-12) and treated with DNase I at either 4°C (tracks 1-3 and 7-9) or 37°C (tracks 4-6 and 10-12). Nuclei were then extracted with 2M NaCl buffer pH 9.6 to give a soluble "chromatin" (tracks 2, 5, 8, 11) and an insoluble "matrix" (tracks 3, 6, 9, 12) fraction. Whole nuclei were run in tracks 1, 4, 7 and 10. Fractions were run on a 10% SDS polyacrylamide gel and probed for total protein (top) or c-*myc* protein (bottom).

buffers to yield a soluble (chromatin) and an insoluble fraction (matrix). Our preliminary results suggested that p62$^{c\text{-}myc}$ was present in the insoluble nuclear matrix fraction, in agreement with Eisenman *et al*, (1985). However, this was difficult to reconcile with our earlier observation that p62$^{c\text{-}myc}$ was completely extracted from nuclei by salt concentrations as low as 144 mM. Moreover, when we used somewhat different methods to prepare nuclear matrices, p62$^{c\text{-}myc}$ was completely soluble in the high salt buffer and there appeared to be no co-purification of p62$^{c\text{-}myc}$ with the nuclear matrix. A detailed analysis demonstrated that the key variable affecting the behaviour of p62$^{c\text{-}myc}$ in different nuclear matrix preparation was the temperature at which the nuclease digestion was carried out. In some procedures this was at 37°C and in others at 4°C. P62$^{c\text{-}myc}$ becomes insoluble in high salt buffers whenever isolated nuclei are exposed to temperatures of 37°C (figure 4). In an effort to understand better the nature of this temperature-dependent insolubilisation of $p62^{c\text{-}myc}$, we investigated the precise temperature requirements for insolubilisation. We found the nuclease treatment to be irrelevant to the process and that insolubilisation occurred in isolated nuclei only if heated above a critical temperature of 35°C. Below this temperature $p62^{c\text{-}myc}$ never becomes insoluble even after extended periods. Above 35°C, $p62^{c\text{-}myc}$ becomes rapidly resistant to high salt extraction and thereafter co-fractionates with the operationally defined "nuclear matrix" (Evan and Hancock, 1985).

It is clear from figure 4 that $p62^{c\text{-}myc}$ is not the only protein which becomes insoluble in nuclei at 37°C. Of the order of 20-30 other proteins, corresponding to about 20% of the total nuclear protein by weight, are similarly affected. Included within this group of nuclear proteins are, in appropriate cells, SV40 large T antigen, p53, adenovirus Ela protein and the product of the human N-*myc* gene (see below). We feel it unlikely that each of the proteins in the complex is intrinsically insoluble above the critical temperature of 35°C. Instead, we suggest that the complex may form around one, or a few, thermally sensitive components localised in a specific nuclear compartment. The complex may thus involve components lying in close physical proximity within the nucleus.

Clearly, the insolubilisation of nuclear proteins which we observe in isolated nuclei at 37°C does not occur in intact cells at this temperature because no such complexes are found in nuclei prepared from cells cultured at 37°C. However, similar complexes are found in the nuclei of cells subjected to transient heat shock at 41°C (Evan and Hancock, 1985). Thus, formation of insoluble nuclear complexes appears to be a major consequence of transient hyperthermia in mammalian cells, a process which can be mimicked in isolated nuclei but at a slightly lower temperature (i.e. *in vitro* heat shock).

From the above studies, we believe there to be little evidence that the c-*myc* protein is associated with the classically defined nuclear matrix. Instead our evidence suggests that $p62^{c\text{-}myc}$ binds to the nucleus via an ionic interaction that may be quite weak under the ionic conditions prevailing within the nucleus of an intact cell. Thus the interaction between $p62^{c\text{-}myc}$ and its site(s) of action in the nucleus may be of low affinity and easily reversible.

SOME CONCLUSIONS CONCERNING THE HUMAN c-*myc* PROTEIN

Certain conclusions can be made concerning the properties of the human c-*myc* protein:

1) The c-*myc* protein is a 62 kDa phosphoprotein, $p62^{c\text{-}myc}$. At least two distinct polypeptide species can be discerned on SDS polyacrylamide gels although the relationship between these different species is obscure.

2) The c-*myc* protein has a very short biological half life (c. 20 minutes).

3) $p62^{c\text{-}myc}$ is expressed at elevated levels in many transformed cell types.

The level of c-myc genomic amplification does not exactly correlate with the steady state levels of p62$^{c\text{-}myc}$ in each cell type, although all tested cells containing amplified c-myc genes do express elevated levels of c-myc mRNA and protein.

4) p62$^{c\text{-}myc}$ localises in the cell nucleus and is bound there by a very salt-labile interaction.

5) p62$^{c\text{-}myc}$ is absent from quiescent cells and induced rapidly following mitogenic stimulation.

6) p62$^{c\text{-}myc}$ is also rapidly repressed in susceptible transformed cells which are induced to differentiate. However, this rapid repression may be more a factor of growth arrest than of committment to differentiation.

Any model for p62$^{c\text{-}myc}$ action must take into account the rapid turnover of p62$^{c\text{-}myc}$, its nuclear location and its induction following mitogenic stimulation. A model satisfying these criteria proposes the c-myc protein as a cell-cycle "enabling" signal whose presence is required, either continually or else during a sensitive temporal window, to allow a cell to progress through its cycle. Disappearance of p62$^{c\text{-}myc}$ would thus signal a cell to enter quiescence at the end of that replication round. Such a scenario requires that p62$^{c\text{-}myc}$ have a short biological half life and be reversibly bound by an appropriate "receptor" within the nucleus. Thus repression of p62$^{c\text{-}myc}$ synthesis would rapidly lead to clearing of the intracellular pool of p62$^{c\text{-}myc}$ and an empty "receptor." Of course, this model makes no predictions as to what p62$^{c\text{-}myc}$ binds in the nucleus, or what its function is when it does so. Rather, the model relegates p62$^{c\text{-}myc}$ to the role of an intracellular messenger. Clearly, testing such a model biochemically is likely to be very difficult.

THE HUMAN N-myc PROTEIN

One strategy, albeit indirect, for elucidating the function of the c-myc protein is to examine the properties of proteins encoded by other members of the mammalian myc family, N-myc and L-myc. From such studies, it might be possible to distinguish important general properties of myc proteins from any idiosynchratic attributes possessed by the c-myc protein. Like c-myc, both N-myc and L-myc are present as amplified genes in various types of neoplasm. Such amplification appears to be restricted to tumours of certain lineages: these include neuroblastoma, retinoblastoma and small cell lung carcinoma in the case of N-myc, whilst L-myc amplification has so far been observed only in small cell lung carcinoma. N-myc is also expressed in teratocarcinoma stem cells and in mid-gestation mouse embryos (Jakobvits *et al*, 1985). However, it is as yet unclear precisely in which normal somatic lineages N-myc is expressed or whether N-myc fulfills analagous or different functions to the c-myc gene. In particular, it is not known whether N-myc functions as a mitogen-induced "competence" gene in the manner suggested for c-*myc*.

To investigate the N-*myc* protein we raised antibodies against several peptide sequences encoded by the human N-*myc* gene. Two of these peptides (peptides A and B, corresponding to residues 367-381 and 336-348 of the inferred N-*myc* protein sequence respectively) contain sequences specific to the N-*myc* protein sequence whilst a third (peptide C) contains a sequence conserved in all mammalian *myc* genes, c-*myc*, N-*myc* and L-*myc*, examined to date. All three peptides elicited antibodies which recognise a 66/68 kDa phosphoprotein in neuroblastoma cell lines expressing N-*myc*. Antibodies to peptide C also recognise the 62 kDa c-*myc* and 64 kDa L-*myc* proteins in appropriate cells (manuscript in preparation) whereas antibodies to peptides A and B are specific for the N-*myc* protein, $p66^{N\text{-}myc}$.

We used these N-*myc* specific antibodies to examine the half life of the 66 kDa N-*myc* protein in the human neuroblastoma cell line Kelly which contains a 200 fold genomic N-*myc* amplification and to compare it to that of the c-*myc* protein in Colo 320 HSR cells (figure 5a). Clearly, the half lives of both the N-*myc* and c-*myc* proteins are of the same order, both being about 20 minutes. We next analysed the subcellular distribution of $p66^{N\text{-}myc}$ in Kelly cells (figure 5b). Like $p62^{c\text{-}myc}$, almost all $p66^{N\text{-}myc}$ co-fractionates with the nuclear fraction at low ionic strengths. However, whereas $p62^{c\text{-}myc}$ is quantitatively extracted from nuclei by elevated salt concentrations, only about 50% of $p66^{N\text{-}myc}$ is extracted under similar conditions. The remaining $p66^{N\text{-}myc}$ is resistant to extraction even in 2M NaCl buffer. *In vitro* heat shock of nuclei (i.e. incubating isolated nuclei at 37°C) insolubilises all nuclear $p62^{c\text{-}myc}$ as expected. *In vitro* heat shock also insolubilises the previously extractable fraction of $p66^{N\text{-}myc}$. Thus, in Kelly cells a portion of the N-*myc* protein behaves exactly like its c-*myc* counterpart, but a significant fraction of $p66^{N\text{-}myc}$ behaves like a classical nuclear matrix protein.

CONCLUSION

It is clear that we have only just begun to compare the biological properties of the various *myc* proteins. Nonetheless, our preliminary do studies suggest that the N-*myc* protein has very similar biological properties to the c-*myc* protein in terms of its subcellular localisation, its phosphorylation, its heterogeneous appearance on SDS polyacrylamide gels and its unusually short biological half life. It remains to be seen what the significance is, if any, of its different behaviour from $p62^{c\text{-}myc}$ in terms of its extractability from cell nuclei. Fractionation of nuclei into meaningful nuclear compartments is fraught with a lack of detailed knowledge concerning nuclear architecture as well as with many technical artefacts. Hopefully, the roles of *myc* proteins in the control of cell cycle, differentiation and neoplasia will become clearer as our knowledge of this interesting family of proteins increases.

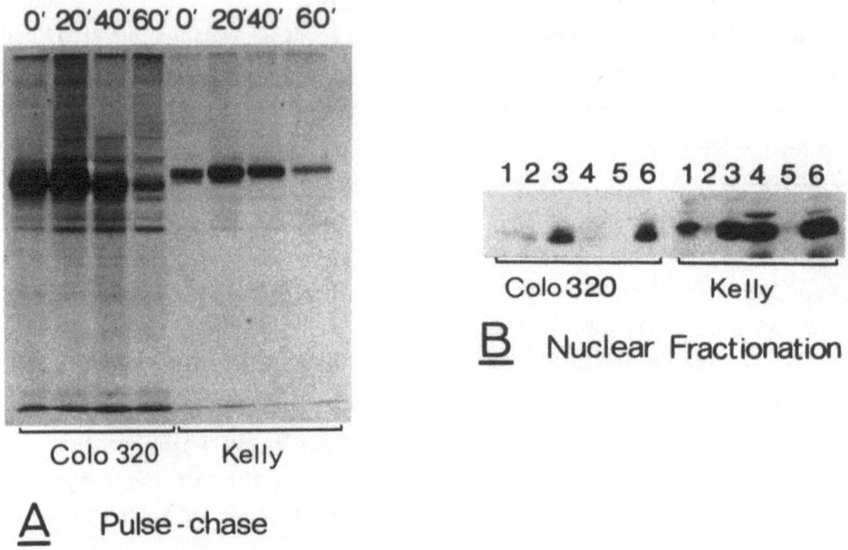

Figure 5 ANALYSIS OF THE HUMAN N-*myc* PROTEIN. (A) Pulse chase labelling of c-*myc* and N-*myc* proteins in Colo 320 HSR and Kelly cells respectively. Cells were pulsed with ^{35}[S]-methionine for 10 minutes and chased in medium containing 10x normal cold methionine. At various times (0, 20, 40, 60 minutes) equal aliquots of the cells were lysed and immunoprecipitated with either anti-c-*myc* or anti-N-*myc* antibodies, as appropriate. Immunoprecipitated fractions were analysed by SDS polyacrylamide gel electrophoresis. (B) Subcellular fractionation of human c-*myc* and N-*myc* proteins. Colo 320 HSR or Kelly cells were lysed in low ionic strength buffer containing 0.1% digitonin (Evan and Hancock, 1985) to give a soluble (track 1) and a nuclear fraction. Nuclei were washed and exhaustively treated with nuclease. The nuclear were then pelleted and any materail released by the nuclease kept (track 2) Half the nuclei were then kept at 4°C (tracks 3 and 4), the other half were incubated at 37°C for 10 minutes (i.e. *in vitro* heat shock - tracks 5 and 6). Nuclei were maintained throughout in RSB buffer containing digitonin as described (Evan and Hancock, 1985). Nuclei were then extracted with 2M NaCl buffer pH 9.6 to yield a soluble chromatin (tracks 3 and 5) and an insoluble matrix (tracks 4 and 6) fraction. Fractions were resolved on an SDS gel, electroblotted and probed with antibodies to the c-*myc* (Colo 320 HSR) or N-*myc* (Kelly) protein.

REFERENCES

Abrams HD, Rohrshneider LR, Eisenman RN (1982) Nuclear location of the putative transforming protein of the avian myelocytomatosis virus. Cell 29: 427-439.

Alitalo K, Schwab M, Lin CC, Varmus HE, Bishop JM (1983a) Homogeneously staining chromosomal regions contain amplified copies of an abundantly expressed cellular oncogene (c-myc) in malignant neuroendocrine cells from a colonic carcinoma. Proc. Nat. Acad. Sci. (USA) 80: 1707-1711.

Alitalo K, Ramsay G, Bishop JM, Ohlsson S, Colby WW, Levinson AD (1983b) Identification of nuclear proteins encoded by viral and cellular myc genes. Nature (London) 306: 274-277.

Alitalo K (1985) Amplification of cellular oncogenes in cancer cells. Trends in Biochem. Sci. 10: 194-197.

Cochran BH, Zuller J, Verma IM, Stiles CD (1984) Expression of the c-fos gene and of a fos-related gene is stimulated by platelet-derived growth factor. Science 226: 1080-1082.

Collins SJ, Groudine MT (1982) Amplification of endogenous myc-related sequences in a human myeloid cell line. Nature (London) 298: 679-681.

Donner P, Greiser-Wilke I, Moelling K (1982) Nuclear localisation and DNA binding of the transforming gene product of avian myelocytomatosis virus. Nature (London) 296: 262-266.

Eisenman RN, Tachibana CY, Abrams HD, Hann SR (1985) V-myc and c-myc proteins are associated with the nuclear matrix. Mol. Cell. Biol. 4: 114-126.

Evan GI, Hancock DC (1985) Studies on the interaction of the human c-myc protein with cell nuclei: $p62^{c\text{-}myc}$ as a member of a discrete subset of nuclear proteins. Cell 43: 253-261.

Evan GI, Lewis GK, Ramsay G, Bishop JM (1985) Isolation of monoclonal antibodies specific for human c-myc proto-oncogene product. Mol. Cell. Biol. 5: 3610-3616.

Hann SR, Eisenman RN (1984) Proteins encoded by the human c-myc oncogene: differential expression in neoplastic cells. Mol. Cell. Biol. 4: 2486-2498.

Jakobvits A, Schwab M, Bishop JM, Martin GR (1985) Expression of N-myc in teratocarcinoma stem cells and mouse embryos. Nature (London) 318: 188-191.

Kelly K, Cochran B, Stiles C, Leder P (1983) Cell-specific regulation of the c-myc gene by lymphocyte mitogens and platelet-derived growth factor. Cell 35: 603-610.

Lachman HM, Skoultchi AI (1984) Expression of c-myc changes during differentiation of mouse erythroleukaemia cells. Nature (London) 310: 592-594.

Land H, Parada L, Weinberg RA (1983) Tumourigenic conversion of primary embryo fibroblasts requires at least two cooperating oncogenes. Nature (London) 304: 596-602.

Lau LF, Nathans D (1985) Identification of a set of genes expressed during the G0/G1 transition of cultured mouse cells. EMBO J. 4: 3145-3151.

Lebkowski JS, Laemmli UK (1982) Non-histone proteins and long range organisation of HeLa interphase DNA. J. Mol. Biol. 156: 325-344.

Little CD, Nau MM, Carney DN, Gazdar AF, Minna JD (1983) Amplification and expression of the c-myc oncogene in human lung cancer cell lines. Nature (London) 306: 194-196.

Nau MM, Brooks BJ, Battey J, Sausville E, Gazdar AF, Kirsch IR, McBride OW, Bertness V, Hollis GF, Minna JD (1985) L-myc, a new myc-related gene amplified and expressed in human small cell lung cancer. Nature (London) 318: 69-73.

Persson H, Leder P (1984) Nuclear localisation and DNA binding properties of a protein expressed by human c-myc oncogene. Science 225: 718-720.

Rabbitts TH (1985) The c-myc proto-oncogene's involvement in chromosomal abnormality. Trends in Genetics 1: 327-331.

Ramsay G, Evan GI, Bishop JM (1984) The protein encoded by the human proto-oncogene c-myc. Proc. Nat. Acad. Sci. (USA) 81: 7742-7746.

Schwab M, Alitalo K, Klempnauer K-H, Varmus HE, Bishop JM (1983) Amplified DNA with limited homology to myc cellular oncogene is shared by human neuroblastoma cell lines and a neuroblastoma tumour. Nature (London) 305: 245-248.

Schwab M (1985) Amplification of N-myc in human neuroblastomas. Trends in Genetics 1: 271-275.

Westin EH, Wong-Staal F, Gelmann EP, Favera RD, Papas TS, Lautenberger JA, Eva A, Reddy EP, Aaronson SA, Gallo RC (1982) Expression of cellular homologues of retroviral onc genes in human haematopoietic cells. Proc. Nat. Acad. Sci. (USA) 79: 2490-2492.

Winqvist R, Saksela K, Alitalo K (1984) The myc proteins are not associated with chromatin in mitotic cells. EMBO J. 3: 2947-2950.

Zimmerman KA, Yancopoulos GD, Collum RG, Smith RK, Kohl NE, Denis KA, Nau MM, Witte ON, Toran-Allerand D, Gee CE, Minna JD, Alt FW (1986) Differential expression of myc family genes during murine development. Nature (London) 319: 780-783.

MIX
Papier aus verantwortungsvollen Quellen
Paper from responsible sources
FSC® C105338

If you have any concerns about our products,
you can contact us on
ProductSafety@springernature.com

In case Publisher is established outside the EU,
the EU authorized representative is:
Springer Nature Customer Service Center GmbH
Europaplatz 3, 69115 Heidelberg, Germany

Printed by Libri Plureos GmbH
in Hamburg, Germany